Resilience in Aging

Barbara Resnick · Lisa P. Gwyther
Karen A. Roberto
Editors

Resilience in Aging

Concepts, Research, and Outcomes

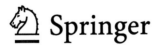 Springer

Editors
Barbara Resnick
University of Maryland School of Nursing
Baltimore, MD
USA
barbresnick@gmail.com

Lisa P. Gwyther
Duke University
Center for the Study of Aging and Human
Durham, NC
USA
lpg@geri.duke.edu

Karen A. Roberto
Center for Gerontology
Virginia Polytechnic Institute and
State University
Blacksburg, VA
USA
kroberto@vt.edu

ISBN 978-1-4419-0231-3   e-ISBN 978-1-4419-0232-0
DOI 10.1007/978-1-4419-0232-0
Springer New York Dordrecht Heidelberg London

Library of Congress Control Number: 2010938435

Printed on acid-free paper

Springer is part of Springer Science+Business Media (www.springer.com)

We dedicate this book to the GSA 2008 annual meeting researchers who took resilience seriously, to those who have been studying resilience, and to the wonderful older adults who have led the way and taught us all what it truly means to be resilient.

Foreword

Gerontology has advanced far beyond the problem-focused approach prevalent in the past decades. Now, scholars are increasingly interested in uncovering the strengths of older individuals and the benefits they contribute to society. From the medical sciences that stress health practices to prevent or slow the onset of disability to the behavioral sciences that demonstrate the value of positive thinking and close relationships, evidence of a balanced approach to understanding aging is widespread. *Resilience in Aging: Concepts, Research, and Outcomes*, situated in this multifaceted context of contemporary aging scholarship, presents a comprehensive set of theory and research on resilience in old age. Chapters on health, illness, and physiological aspects of aging; personality, motivation, and other psychological dimensions; culture and ethnicity; work and civic engagement; spirituality and the environment; and care settings and community interventions all offer important insights about many ways that older adults can achieve and display resilience, the benefits of being resilient for aging well, and steps community service providers can take to foster resilience in the older population. This volume is a key resource for gerontologists, researchers and students of aging, and professionals who work with and on behalf of older adults.

Blacksburg, VA   Rosemary Blieszner, PhD

Preface

Like every book, this book has a story behind the making. First and foremost kudos for every moment you enjoy reading this book should go to Janice Stern, our Springer editor. Janice initially pursued me with the idea of a book about resilience in older adults, similar to a book that Springer had published about children. The Handbook of Resilience in Children. She contacted me around the time I was living and breathing resilience as I was recovering from microfracture surgery on my knee and was unhappily non-weight bearing on my left lower extremity for 2 months. That and my own research in the area of motivation of older adults inspired me to seize this opportunity. Simultaneously, the Gerontological Society of America (GSA) was planning the 61st annual scientific meeting with the theme set at "Resilience in an Aging Society: Risks and Opportunities." As the Health Section Chair for the GSA that year (2008), I was part of the conference planning committee and had the opportunity to learn about the many sessions highlighting and addressing resilience in older adults. Fascinated with the wide array of presentations focused on different areas of resilience, I gathered the names of individuals to contact post presentation to invite them to turn their presentations into chapters for us to have and to hold. In addition, I asked the 2008 GSA President, Lisa Gwyther, and the 2008 Behavioral Science Section Chair, Karen Roberto, to join me as coeditors of the book. Together we divided and conquered and share with you more than you could ever want to know about resilience in older adults, and what we believe is the true key to successful aging.

Contents

Editor Biographies

Barbara Resnick, PhD, CRNP, FAAN, FAANP, is a professor in the Department of Organizational Systems and Adult Health at the University of Maryland School of Nursing, holds the Sonya Ziporkin Gershowitz Chair in Gerontology at the School of Nursing, and does clinical work at Roland Park Place, a Lifecare community. Dr. Resnick holds a BSN from the University of Connecticut, an MSN from the University of Pennsylvania, and a PhD from the University of Maryland. Research interests and expertise focus on: health promotion and disease prevention; outcomes following rehabilitation, functional performance, motivation related to function and exercise, testing outcomes of restorative care nursing programs and other innovative long-term care projects, and dissemination and implementation of innovative approaches to health care across a variety of clinical settings. Dr. Resnick has over 150 published articles, numerous chapters in nursing and medical textbooks, and books on restorative care and assisted living nursing. She has also presented on these topics nationally and internationally. Dr. Resnick's professional activities include membership in numerous nursing and interdisciplinary organizations, and she has served as a board member in many of these organizations and serves on many editorial boards, is the editor of a journal, Geriatric Nursing, and serves on boards of organizations focused on care of the older adult. Dr. Resnick has been recognized through receipt of numerous awards, such as the University of Connecticut Researcher of the Year Award, 2001, University of Pennsylvania 2003 Award for Clinical Excellence, the 2003 Founders Week Researcher award at the University of Maryland, 2004 Distinguished Scholar Award from University of Connecticut, 2004 Springer Geriatric Nursing Research Award, the Doris Schwartz award in 2008, and the 2009 Nurse Leader in Gerontology award among others. Dr. Resnick's clinical practice involves providing primary medical management to older adults in a variety of settings, and she bases her work on over 35 years of experience in providing care to older adults.

Lisa P. Gwyther, MSW, LCSW, is a social worker with more than 38 years of experience in aging, Alzheimer's disease and family caregiver research and services. She is an associate professor in the Department of Psychiatry and Behavioral Sciences at the Duke University School of Medicine, a senior fellow of the Duke Center for the Study of Aging, founder and director of the Duke Aging Center Family Support

Program, and education director of the Bryan Alzheimer's Disease Research Center at Duke. She was the 2008 president of the Gerontological Society of America. Her annual meeting theme, "Resilience in an Aging Society: Risks and Opportunities," was the genesis for this book. Ms. Gwyther was the first John Heinz Senate Fellow in Aging and Health in 1993. She served as a member of the health staff of former Senate Majority Leader, George J. Mitchell. In May 2003, she was inducted into the National Academies of Practice as a Distinguished Practitioner in Social Work. Ms. Gwyther has published over 114 peer-reviewed journal articles, book chapters and books, the latest of which, The Alzheimer's Action Plan: A Family Guide (2009), won two consumer health awards and a coveted star rating from the Library Journal.

Karen A. Roberto, PhD, is professor and director of the Center for Gerontology and the Institute for Society, Culture and Environment at Virginia Polytechnic Institute and State University, Blacksburg, VA. Her research examines the intersection of health and social support in later life. Her primary interests include older women's adaptation to chronic health conditions, family relationships and caregiving, and elder abuse and mistreatment. She is the author of over 140 scholarly articles and book chapters and the editor or author of 8 books, including Pathways of Human Development: Explorations of Change (with J. Mancini, 2009). Dr. Roberto is past-chair of the Behavioral and Social Sciences section of the Gerontological Society of America. She is a fellow of the Association for Gerontology in Higher Education, the Gerontological Society of America, the National Council on Family Relations, and the World Demographic Association. Dr. Roberto is a recipient of the Gordon Streib Academic Gerontologist Award from the Southern Gerontological Society and the Virginia Tech University Alumni Award for Excellence in Research.

Contributors

Rebecca S. Allen, PhD
The University of Alabama, Tuscaloosa, AL, USA

Arlene Astell, PhD, BSc (Hons.)
University of St. Andrews, St. Andrews, Fife, Scotland

Anne Davis Basting, PhD
University of Wisconsin Milwaukee, Milwaukee, WI, USA

Elyssa Besen, BA, PhD(c)
Boston College, Boston, MA, USA

Bryan Blissmer, PhD
University of Rhode Island, Kingston, RI, USA

Philip Bohle, PhD
University of Sydney, Sydney, NSW, Australia

Hayden B. Bosworth, PhD
Duke University Medical Center, Durham, NC, USA

Michelle Braun, PhD
Harvard Medical School and VA Boston Healthcare, Boston, MA, USA

Patricia M. Burbank, RN, DNSc
University of Rhode Island, Kingston, RI, USA

Linda Clare, PhD, CPsychol
Bangor University, Bangor, UK

Phillip G. Clark, ScD
University of Rhode Island, Kingston, RI, USA

Donna Cohen, PhD
University of South Florida, Tampa, FL, USA

Carol Ann Faigin, PhD
Togus VA Medical Center, 1VA Center, Augusta, Maine 04330, USA

Ruth Finkelstein, ScD
The New York Academy of Medicine, New York, NY, USA

Stevie N. Fowler, BS
The University of Alabama, Tuscaloosa, AL, USA

Paula Gardner, PhD
The New York Academy of Medicine, New York, NY, USA

Geoffrey Greene, RD, PhD
University of Rhode Island, Kingston, RI, USA

Jennifer C. Greenfield, MSW, PhD(c)
Washington University, St. Louis, St. Louis, MO, USA

Philip P. Haley, MA
The University of Alabama, Tuscaloosa, AL, USA

Jan P.H. Hamers, PhD
Maastricht University, Maastricht, The Netherlands

Grant M. Harris, BA
The University of Alabama, Tuscaloosa, AL, USA

Gregory Hicks, PhD
The University of Delaware, Newark, DE, USA

Angela K. Hochhalter, PhD
Scott & White Healthcare, Temple, TX and
Texas A&M Health Science Center, College Station, TX, USA

George L. Jackson, PhD, MHA
Duke University Medical Center, Durham, NC, USA

Jacquelyn B. James, PhD
Boston College, Boston, MA, USA

Rosalie A. Kane, PhD
University of Minnesota, Minneapolis, MN, USA

Elizabeth Kelson, MA, PhD(c)
University of British Columbia, Vancouver, BC, Canada

M. Denise King, PhD
University of Missouri, St. Louis, MO, USA

B.L. King-Kallimanis, MS, PhD(c)
University of Amsterdam, Amsterdam, The Netherlands

Glynda J. Kinsella, PhD
La Trobe University, Melbourne, VIC, Australia

Faith Lees, MS
University of Rhode Island, Kingston, RI, USA

Rebecca Logsdon, PhD
University of Washington, Seattle, WA, USA

Diane Martins, PhD, RN
University of Rhode Island, Kingston, RI, USA

Susan H. McFadden, PhD
University of Wisconsin Oshkosh, Oshkosh, WI, USA

Christopher McLoughlin, MSc
Monash University, Churchill, VIC, Australia

Ram R. Miller, MD
University of Maryland School of Medicine, Baltimore, MD, USA

Michelle E. Mlinac, PsyD
Boston Healthcare System, Harvard Medical School, Boston, MA, USA

Nancy Morrow-Howell, MSW, PhD
Washington University, St. Louis, MO, USA

Julie Netherland, MSW
The New York Academy of Medicine, New York, NY, USA

Greg O'Neill, PhD
National Academy on an Aging Society, Washington, DC, USA

Marcia G. Ory, PhD, MPH
Texas A&M Health Science Center, College Station, TX, USA

Norma Owens, PharmD, FCCP
University of Rhode Island, Kingston, RI, USA

Kenneth I. Pargament, PhD
Bowling Green State University, Bowling Green, OH, USA

Mary Hamil Parker, PhD
Institute for Palliative & Hospice Training, Inc, Oak Park, VA, USA

Alison Phinney, PhD, RN
University of British Columbia, Vancouver, BC, Canada

Joseph G. Pickard, PhD, LCSW
University of Missouri, St. Louis, MO, USA

Marcie Pitt-Catsouphes, PhD
Boston College, Boston, MA, USA

Roopwinder Pruthi, MA
The University of Alabama, Tuscaloosa, AL, USA

Barbara Purves, PhD
University of British Columbia, Vancouver, BC, Canada

Deborah Riebe, PhD
University of Rhode Island, Kingston, RI, USA

Francesca Rosenberg, BA
Museum of Modern Art, New York, NY, USA

Erlene Rosowsky, PsyD
Harvard Medical School and Massachusetts School of Professional Psychology,
Boston, MA, USA

Erik van Rossum, PhD
Maastricht University, Maastricht, The Netherlands

Robert E. Roush, EdD, MPH
Bastor College of Medicine, Houston, TX, USA

Marie Y. Savundranayagam, PhD
University of Wisconsin-Milwaukee, Milwaukee, WI, USA

Tom H. Sheeran, PhD, ME
Weill Cornell Medical College, White Plains, NY, USA

Ke Shen, PhD(c)
Peking University, Beijing, China

Matthew Lee Smith, PhD, MPH, CHES, CPP
Texas A&M Health Science Center, College Station, TX, USA

Philip Taylor, PhD
Monash University, Churchill, VIC, Australia

Ranak B. Trivedi, PhD
University of Washington, Seattle, WA, USA

Hilde Verbeek, MSc, PhD(c)
CAPHRI School for Public Health and Primary Care,
Maastricht University, Maastricht, The Netherlands

Carol J. Whitlatch, PhD
Benjamin Rose Institute, Cleveland, OH, USA

Jerald Winakur, MD, FACP, CMD
University of Texas Health Science Center at San Antonio, San Antonio, TX, USA

Darlene Yee-Melichar, EdD, CHES
San Francisco State University, San Francisco, CA, USA

Steven H. Zarit, PhD
Pennsylvania State University, University Park, PA, USA

Yi Zeng, PhD
Duke University, Durham, NC, USA
Peking University, Beijing, China
Max Planck Institute, Rostock, Germany

Chapter 1
Resilience: Definitions, Ambiguities, and Applications

Rebecca S. Allen, Philip P. Haley, Grant M. Harris, Stevie N. Fowler, and Roopwinder Pruthi

Resilience has been defined as a dynamic process of maintaining positive adaptation and effective coping strategies in the face of adversity (Luthar et al. 2000). Although most scholars and members of the general public have an intuitive understanding of resilience, ambiguities in definition, measurement, and application contribute to scientific criticism regarding the usefulness of resilience as a theoretical construct (Kaplan 1999; Tolan 1996). Previous reviews have addressed ambiguities and limitations of the research literature with a focus on children and adolescents facing adversity (Luthar et al. 2000). These authors call for greater research attention on resilience at different points in human development. This chapter focuses on the definition, ambiguity, and application of the construct of resilience across the adult lifespan as it relates to successful aging (see Chap. 2). Other chapters throughout this book focus on various domains of resilience including genetic, physical, and personality (see Chaps. 3 and 6), emotional (see Chap. 5), creative (see Chap. 7), and spiritual (see Chap. 11). Our goal in this initial chapter is to describe and define resilience as it relates to older adults and to operationalize this construct across various domains. In so doing, we expand the critical review provided by Luthar et al. (2000) to adult development and aging. Additionally, we address three controversies evident in our review of the literature on the construct of resilience within adult development and aging.

Definitions and Controversies Regarding Resilience and Aging

Resilience and Resiliency

One of the primary criticisms regarding literature on resilience is a lack of clarity in the definition, specifically confusion between resilience as a dynamic process and resiliency, or ego-resiliency, as an individual characteristic or trait (Luthar et al. 2000).

R.S. Allen (✉)
The University of Alabama, Tuscaloosa, AL, USA
e-mail: rsallen@ua.edu

B. Resnick et al. (eds.), *Resilience in Aging: Concepts, Research, and Outcomes*,
DOI 10.1007/978-1-4419-0232-0_1, © Springer Science+Business Media, LLC 2011

The most common definition of resilience is a dynamic *process* of adaptation to adversity (Luthar et al. 2000). Langer (2004) pointed out that everyday discussions among older adults often focus on deficits, such as their risk for encountering challenges associated with aging including chronic illness, caregiving, encountering ageist stereotypes and potential loss of roles, and the death of loved ones. Middle aged and older adults, however, have life experiences that result in significant strengths and capabilities allowing for successful coping with the multiple adversities they may encounter.

In contrast, Wagnild and Young (1993) define "resilience" as an individual difference, characteristic, or ability to successfully cope with change or misfortune. In their definition, resilient individuals are self-confident and know their own strengths and limitations. Although they regain *equilibrium* after a period of adversity or change, they do not necessarily regain their previous level of performance or functioning. Wagnild and Young have developed a psychometrically sound resilience scale that is available online at (http://www.resiliencescale.com/). The scale was developed through interviews with resilient individuals. Five themes of resilience emerge through factor analysis of this scale: equanimity, perseverance, self-reliance, existential aloneness, and spirituality/meaningfulness. Equanimity involves maintaining a balanced perspective on life. Perseverance means continuing to strive and cope in spite of adversity. Self-reliance encompasses belief in one's abilities. Existential aloneness involves reveling in one's own uniqueness and the belief in the continuity of the self across time. In Wagnild and Young's (1993) measure, spirituality and meaning play an important role in resilience through enabling the individual to draw conclusions as to why events occur and embrace the need for change, flexibility, and growth.

In this chapter, we operationalize "resilience" as encompassing the *developmental process* of being mindful of and prioritizing those behaviors, thoughts, and feelings that facilitate contentment within a specific developmental, physical, emotional, and spiritual context. We follow Luthar et al. (2000) approach of using more specific terms to describe the interplay of personal characteristics with the process of resilience, described below in the discussion of the second controversy within the resilience literature. However, we follow Richardson's (2002) approach and expand the definition of resilience to coping processes in the face of everyday life struggles as well as significant adverse events.

Terminology and Individual Difference Characteristics/Third Variable Problems

A second controversy in the resilience literature involves the role of covariates or moderator variables in understanding the impact of resilience on the person's adaptive capacity. Luthar et al. (2000) emphasize clarity in distinguishing the main effect of resilience on competence levels within specific risk conditions. The resilience process itself simply shows a main effect on competence or skill, but the interplay of the resilience process and individual difference characteristics produces interactions. In other words, those who engage in resilience processes perform at greater levels of competence than those who do not engage in these processes, regardless of the level of risk associated with the protective or vulnerable characteristic. Luthar et al. (2000) strongly encourage the use of more specific terminology to distinguish the discussion of moderator variables that may interact with resilience to produce different patterns with varying levels of competence or skill.

For example, *protective-stabilizing* attributes interact with resilience to decrease the decline in competence that comes with increased risk. An example of a protective-stabilizing attribute might be openness to learning new caregiving skills, as among dementia caregivers. Individuals in this at-risk group have been shown to use intervention strategies to maintain their well-being in the face of the deteriorating cognitive status of their care recipient (Belle et al. 2006; Pinquart and Sorensen 2003). Resilience is demonstrated when caregivers using intervention strategies do not display decreased caregiving competence across time in comparison with caregivers without the benefit of skills training interventions who are in the usual care or minimal support condition.

In the case of *protective-enhancing* attributes, the competence of individuals who engage in resilient practices is actually enhanced at levels of high risk. An example from the dementia caregiving literature might be cognitive appraisals that identify positive aspects of caregiving and the impact this process has on caregivers' response to intervention (Hilgeman et al. 2007). The influence of *protective* but-*reactive* attributes shows that, at high risk levels, the individual's competence is diminished but still greater than the competence of individuals who do not engage in resilient processes. An example of this might be the responsiveness of recently diagnosed terminally ill individuals or those undergoing palliative care to psychosocial interventions designed to improve emotional and spiritual outcomes in the face of declining physical function (Allen et al. 2008; Chochinov et al. 2005).

Thus, resilience, as opposed to resiliency, is seen as a dynamic process and not a static trait (Luthar et al. 2000). Therefore, it is important to examine the process by which a burdensome and adverse situation may lead to positive adaptations, emotions, and outcomes within particular domains. Ai and Park (2005) maintain that the positive psychology trend entering mainstream scientific inquiry, with its focus on positive outcomes including protection, growth, and resilience, provides a counterbalance to the traditional, predominantly negative outcome focus. Within this framework, a more complete understanding of the human experience of adversity emerges. Consideration of the concept of adversity leads us to the third major controversy in the resilience literature.

Must Adversity Be Present or Are Daily Life Disruptions Enough to Produce and Detect the Resilience Process?

Inasmuch as resilience is the surmounting of adversity, there must be adversity present for the process of resilience to take place (Doll and Lyon 1998). However, the meaning of a particular adverse event to the individual experiencing it can differ markedly from that held by the resilience researcher (Bartlett 1994; Gordon and

Song 1994; Luthar et al. 2000). The types of adversities faced in older adulthood are different than in other age groups. These adversities include everyday occurrences such as chronic illness and loss of role or of important relationships due to the death of loved ones in addition to more catastrophically adverse events such as dementia or the diagnosis of a terminal illness.

Richardson (2002) broadens the definition of resilience to encompass developmental adaptation in the face of disruptive events encountered in everyday life. Two postulates underlie Richardson's resilience meta-theory: (1) the source for actuating resilience comes from one's ecosystem, and (2) resilience is a capacity every person possesses. Richardson defines resilience as the motivational force within everyone that drives them to pursue wisdom, self-actualization, and altruism and to be in harmony with a spiritual source of strength within a period of biopsychospiritual homeostasis. This process of adaptation affords positive physical, mental, and spiritual outcomes.

Richardson further describes a process of reintegration to life disruptions that can be growth producing. Multiple positive and disruptive life events may be occurring simultaneously. This produces increasing opportunities for Richardson's "dynamic reintegration," illustrative of the process of resilience. However, individuals may choose for various reasons to turn down opportunities for growth and to avoid actively responding to life disruptions. Richardson states, "Without resilient reintegration in the face of disruptions, life prompts will continue to disrupt because people have not acquired resilient qualities" (p. 312).

Due to the specific life circumstances characteristic of adult development and aging, it makes sense to the current authors to expand the construct of resilience to adaptation processes associated with normative developmental change. Lamond et al. (2009) would agree with this expanded definition, as they posited a greater role for the resilience process in successful aging due to older adults' propensity to view their lives and health as satisfactory despite age-related disease and disability. Not all aging individuals, however, adapt to the aging process gracefully. Only some individuals embrace generative opportunities and actively engage in the challenges of older adulthood.

Having discussed three major controversies within the resilience literature, the rest of this chapter will attempt to provide operational definitions of the resilience process for domains of functioning covered within other chapters of this book. Specifically, we will address operational definitions of resilience in physiological (see Chaps. 3 and 6), emotional (see Chap. 5), and spiritual (see Chap. 11) domains.

Domains Within Which Resilience Operates

Physiological Resilience

Physiological resilience has been defined as "the capacity to maintain adequate function and structure at molecular and cellular levels by adapting or changing to specific challenges" (Franco et al. 2009). In physiology, the concept of *allostasis* refers to the maintenance of stability through change (Sterling and Eyer 1988; McEwen 2003). Physiological systems that involve glucocorticoids (e.g. cortisol; Sapolsky et al. 2000), adrenaline, and cytokines can produce physiological changes which are adaptive in the short run but maladaptive in the long run if these processes are not turned off. *Allostatic load* is the condition in which tissues can become damaged by chronic hormonal activation (McEwen 1998). Thus, preserving physical homeostasis to insure that the individual remains healthy and outside the realm of disease becomes more challenging across the older adult lifespan as physiological, environmental, social, emotional, and spiritual threats and individual responses to these threats accumulate. Therefore, within the physiological realm, the definition of the resilience process must include a developmental component of attempting to maintain adaptive functioning commensurate with one's definition of quality of life despite increasing functional limitation and chronic illness.

Societal factors such as socioeconomic privilege contribute to health disparities in physiological resilience (Pampel and Rogers 2004). Over the life course, members of high socioeconomic status groups develop greater resistance to disease because they enjoy better medical care, nutrition, and comfortable and safe living conditions in their neighborhoods. By contrast, members of lower socioeconomic groups face more assaults on health over the life course that can decrease the body's ability to fight off disease or to recover from it once ill. These disadvantaged environmental conditions lead to greater incidence of conditions such as high blood pressure, high cholesterol, and a weakened immune system. Conditions such as these are due to cumulative assaults on the body, secondary to chronically stressful conditions and inadequate health care.

Adequate definition and measurement of the process of resilience across the adult lifespan is key to identifying factors and individual attributes that promote successful aging in the physiological realm. The catechol-*O*-methyl transferase gene appears to be part of an interface that moderates physiological and emotional stress responses (Drolet et al. 2001; Craig 2002; Ribeiro et al. 2005), potentially suggesting a vulnerability to stress-related disorders such as Major Depressive Disorder (Jabbi et al. 2007). The physiological process of sleep has also taken on increasing importance as a mechanism by which some of the detrimental effects of physical and emotional stress can be undone. Restorative anabolic forces such as sleep counteract the forces that drain physiological reserves that shore up the individual against physiological assault. Age-related changes and potential deficits in sleep quantity or quality have consequences for learning, physiological functioning, health, and well-being (Lichstein et al. 2004).

There is ample support for the notion of developmental differences in the definition of resilience within the physiological realm. Notably, negative physical and mental health practices do not visibly induce morbidities at a young age. Hawkley et al. (2005) note that the marshaling of physiological resources and associated restorative processes can, across time, facilitate adaptive physiological responding to future physiological threats. In fact, episodic physical stressors may confer benefits in the absence of chronic physiological stressors (Boyce et al. 1995). For example, children in supportive environments may become "inoculated" against subsequent stressors due to supportive parenting history and environmental circumstance along with successful resolution to confrontations with physiological stressors and challenges (Boyce et al. 1995; Bugental 2005; Dienstbier 1989).

Adequate protection against external stressors, or individual differences in positive preventive health practices and adaptive coping, facilitate physiological resilience. Maintaining a physically and mentally active lifestyle, following a healthy diet, not smoking, avoiding excessive use of alcohol, establishing healthy sleep patterns, and using adaptive coping strategies for psychological distress contribute largely to individual differences in physiological resilience (Hawkley et al. 2005; Cacioppo et al. 2003). We turn now to a discussion of these factors.

Social Support and Resilience and Their Impact on Physical Processes

Loneliness contributes to and accelerates age-related decreases in physiological resilience through its influence on health behaviors, stress exposure, psychological stress responses and associated physiological responses, and restorative processes that replenish physiological reserves and fortify against future stress. Hawkley et al. (2007) have shown that loneliness interacts with age such that systolic blood pressure was higher by 0.85mmHg per standard deviation of loneliness for each additional year of age, suggesting that loneliness accelerates typical age-related reductions in physiological resilience. Moreover, feelings of helplessness and threat were greater among lonely individuals than among nonlonely individuals.

Other physiological risk factors present themselves more frequently among lonely individuals, accelerating the rate of decline in physiological reserves. Impairments in hypothalamic-pituitary-adrenocortical regulation across the adult years could play a particularly important role in the development of glucocorticoid insensitivity, a compromising of the normal feedback mechanism in which increasing levels of cortisol turn off the release of yet more cortisol, and impairments in the regulation of inflammatory processes. Apart from the direct influence of these physiological risks there are emotional stressors and burdens that befall individuals across the adult lifespan. These burdens and stressors do not occur solely among older adults but are particularly prevalent in this group (e.g. caregiving, chronic illness, loss due to death). The effects of these risks on older adults are sizeable and lead us to a discussion of the importance of the stress process and emotion regulation, or the process of emotional resilience.

Emotional Resilience

In Richardson's (2002) meta-theory of the resilience process, resilience is a motivating force and intuitive process by which individuals rely on an innate moral framework that facilitates energy and the experience of control and freedom. When someone is living outside their moral code, negative affect saps energy and the experience of control and freedom. To get a deeper understanding of emotional resilience, the stress and coping process must be examined.

The Stress and Coping Process

As Pearlin and Skaff (1996) note, successful adaptation to late life involves experiencing mastery within domains over which one can exert control and yielding mastery within domains where control is more difficult. Lazarus and Folkman's (1984) transactional model of the stress process and Folkman's (1997) revised model are useful frameworks that attempt to explain how an adverse event or ongoing situation may lead to various psychological outcomes. The original model stated that if a situation is appraised as burdensome a problem- or emotion-focused coping strategy would be used to deal with the negative appraisal. The coping strategy chosen leads to either a favorable resolution, no resolution (e.g. the problem persists without change), or an unfavorable resolution. Favorable resolutions lead to positive emotions and no resolution or unfavorable resolutions lead to emotional distress. If an unfavorable resolution is met with the resultant experience of distress, then the coping process is repeated. A state of chronic stress arises if the process repeatedly ends with unfavorable emotional outcomes.

Lazarus and Folkman's (1984) original model did not account for the impact of positive emotions in the stress and coping process. The revision of the model was prompted by the observation that caregivers of loved ones with AIDS were experiencing positive emotions independent of the distress associated with end-of-life caregiving (Folkman 1997). Thus, positive emotions may result from what seemingly is a situation with no resolution (e.g. the death of a loved one cannot be prevented). Folkman's revised model proposes that people facing an unfavorable resolution or no resolution to a problem may engage in meaning-based coping.

The Revised Stress and Coping Model

In Folkman's (1997) stress process model, "meaning-based coping" mediates the impact of negative event outcomes (e.g. unfavorable resolution or no resolution to a problem) on resulting emotions. Meaning-based coping includes positive reappraisal, revised goals, positive events or activities, and religious/spiritual beliefs. It serves as a resilient process of reducing the impact of negative life events such as illness and disability and leads to the experience of positive emotions.

Folkman (2008) reviewed the empirical research support for meaning-based coping as distinct from other forms of coping. She found that the evidence supports meaning-based coping as a distinct coping strategy because it is primarily associated with the creation of positive emotions rather than the direct regulation of distress. Thus, Folkman's model suggests that meaning-based coping sustains the coping process as a consequence of the creation of positive emotional outcomes. The attainment of positive emotions can be seen as a buffer/mediator between the stresses of an adverse event and the experience of negative emotions. Folkman (2009) reviewed the evolution of stress and coping theory and emphasized the challenges inherent in the scientific study of a dynamic, multilevel, recursive system anchored in the appraisal process of the individual in context. Clearly, ongoing longitudinal studies are needed to fully explore the nature of emotional resilience as it relates to stress and coping across the adult lifespan.

Spiritual/Religious Resilience

The spiritual/religious resilience process represents one aspect of meaning-based coping that leads to positive outcomes in adverse situations. One of the means of coping with and adapting to adversity is reliance on religion and spirituality. A substantial proportion of people in stressful situations use religion to cope with their hardships (Pargament 1997; Roff et al. 2004). Among older adults and individuals self-identifying as members of minority groups, religion is cited more frequently than any other form of coping (Koenig 1998). Spirituality and religion play an important role for older adults in adapting positively to negative situations, resulting in the process of spiritual/religious resilience.

Spiritual/religious resilience is a process in which a person uses spiritual and/or religious beliefs and behaviors as a means of coping in the face of adversity. The end-state of the process is a positive or peaceful emotional outcome. This domain of resilience stands in contrast to physiological resilience in which the goal is more "protective but reactive" (e.g. diminishment of negative outcomes) rather than "protective enhancing" (e.g. the attribute produces growth in interaction with the resilience process). As in Folkman's (2008) review, the production of positive emotional states is a positive event outcome in itself that also facilitates the ongoing coping process and may result in the decrease of negative event outcomes. To enact spiritual/religious resilience, one must use a spiritual or religious coping strategy and this coping strategy must lead to a positive emotional outcome. It is not sufficient to define spiritual/religious resilience as being comprised solely of the use of coping or as the experience of positive emotional outcomes during a negative situation. Spiritual/religious resilience can be described as the use of a spiritual/religious coping strategy, the resultant experience of positive emotional outcomes, and the consequential abatement of negative emotions.

Religion has been highlighted as one of the primary means of coping for caregivers (Caregiving in the U.S. 2004). Research suggests substantial associations between religious and spiritual variables and mental health outcomes (Koenig 1997). Pargament's (1997) review indicated that religious coping plays an important part in the prediction of well-being and that the variance attributed to religious coping extends beyond the effects of nonreligious coping. Pargament et al. (1998) suggest that religious coping cannot be fractured into constituent nonreligious parts.

toward freedom and the current impact of racism within the United States. The impact of the process of resilience in coping with the negative personal and societal effects of stereotyping would be another fascinating avenue of future research.

In this chapter, we reviewed specific domains in which the resilience process operates: physiological, emotional, and spiritual/religious. Specific suggestions for research paths in the areas of physiological resilience include physical and cognitive activity and training interventions to increase physiological potential (Tepe and Lukey 2008). Within the area of emotional resilience, Folkman (2009) has suggested a focus on the multidimensional nature of the stress and coping process, which can only meaningfully be studied longitudinally. Regarding spiritual/religious resilience, future research might examine how religious/spiritual coping methods differ in the resilience process at different ages. Some coping methods may be less effective at creating meaning, attaining positive outcomes, and consequently lowering negative emotional outcomes at different points in the adult lifespan. We believe that longitudinal examination of the resilience process holds promise for guiding research and promoting successful aging.

References

Ai, A., & Park, C. (2005) Possibilities of the positive following violence and trauma: Informing the coming decade of research. *Journal of Interpersonal Violence, 20,* 242–250.

Allen, R.S., Hilgeman, M.M., Ege, M.A., Shuster, J.L., Jr., & Burgio, L.D. (2008) Legacy activities as interventions approaching the end of life. *Journal of Palliative Medicine, 11*(7), 1029–1038.

Arnett, J.J. (2000) Emerging adulthood: A theory of development from the late teens through the 20s. *American Psychologist, 55,* 469–480.

Bartlett, D.W. (1994) On resilience: Questions of validity. In M.C. Wang & E.W. Gordon (Eds.), *Educational resilience in inner-city America: Challenges and prospects* (pp. 97–108). Hillsdale, NJ: Erlbaum.

Becker, G. & Newsom, E. (2005) Resilience in the face of serious illness among chronically ill African Americans in later life. *Journal of Gerontology: Social Sciences, 60B*(4), S214–S223.

Belle, S.H., Burgio, L., Burns, R., Coon, D., Czaja, S.J., Gallagher-Thompson, D., et al. (2006) Enhancing the quality of life of dementia caregivers from different ethnic or racial groups. *Annals of Internal Medicine, 145,* 727–738.

Boyce, W.T., Chesney, M.A., Alkon, A., Tschann, J.M., Adams, S., Chesterman, B., et al. (1995) Psychobiologic reactivity to stress and childhood respiratory illness: Results of two prospective studies. *Psychosomatic Medicine, 57,* 411–422.

Bugental, D.B. (2005) *Risk versus thriving in the face of early medical adversity.* Paper presented at the Meetings of the Western Psychological Association, Portland, OR.

Cacioppo, J.T., Hawkley, L.C., & Berntson, G.G. (2003) The anatomy of loneliness. *Current Directions in Psychological Science, 12*(3), 71–74.

Caregiving in the U.S. (2004) National Alliance for Caregiving and the AARP. April 2004.

Chochinov, H.M., Hack, T., Hassard, T., Kristjanson, L.J., McClement, S., & Harlos, M. (2005) Dignity therapy: A novel psychotherapeutic intervention for patients near the end of life. *Journal of Clinical Oncology, 23,* 5520–5525.

Craig, A.D. (2002) How do you feel? Interoception: The sense of the physiological condition of the body. *Nature Reviews Neuroscience, 3,* 655–666.

Dienstbier, R.A. (1989) Arousal and physiological toughness: Implications for mental and physical health. *Psychological Review, 96*(1), 84–100.

Doll, B., & Lyon, M.A. (1998) Risk and resilience: Implications for the delivery of education and mental health services in schools. *School Psychology Review, 27*(3), 348–364.

Drolet, G., Dumont, E.C., Gosselin, I., Kinkead, R., Laforest, S., Trottier, J.F. (2001) Role of endogenous opioid system in the regulation of the stress response. *Progress in Neuro-Psychopharmacology and Biological Psychiatry, 25*, 729–741.

Erikson, E.H. (1950) *Childhood and society.* Oxford, England: Norton and Co.

Erikson, E.H., & Erikson, J.M. (1997) *The life cycle completed: Extended version.* New York, NY: Norton.

Folkman, S. (1997) Positive psychological states and coping with severe stress. *Social Science and Medicine, 45*, 1207–1221.

Folkman, S. (2008) The case for positive emotions in the stress process. *Anxiety, Stress, & Coping, 21*(1), 3–14.

Folkman, S. (2009) Commentary on the special section "Theory Based Approaches to Stress and Coping": Questions, answers, issues and next steps in stress and coping research. *European Psychologist, 14*(1), 72–77.

Franco, O.H., Karnik, K., Osborne, G., Ordovas, J.M., Catt, M., & van der Ouderaa, F. (2009) Changing course in ageing research: The healthy ageing phenotype. *Maturitas, 63*, 13–19.

Gordon, E.W., & Song, L.D. (1994) Variations in the experience of resilience. In M.C. Wang & E.W. Gordon (Eds.), *Educational resilience in inner-city America: Challenges and prospects* (pp. 27–43). Hillsdale, NJ: Erlbaum.

Hawkley, L.C., Bernston, G.G., Engeland, C.G., Marucha, P.T., Masi, C.M., & Cacioppo, J.T. (2005) Stress, aging, and resilience: Can accrued wear and tear be slowed? *Canadian Psychology, 46*(3), 115–125.

Hawkley, L.C., Preacher, K.J., & Cacioppo, J.T. (2007) Multilevel modeling of social interactions and mood in lonely and socially connected individuals: The MacArthur social neuroscience studies. In A.D. Ong & M. van Dulmen (Eds.), *Oxford handbook of methods in positive psychology* (pp. 559–575). New York: Oxford University Press.

Hilgeman, M.M., Allen, R.S., DeCoster, J., & Burgio, L.D. (2007) Positive aspects of caregiving as a moderator of treatment outcome over 12 months. *Psychology and Aging, 22*, 361–371.

Jabbi, M., Kema, I.P., van der Pompe, G., te Meerman, G.J., Ormel, J., & den Boer, J.A. (2007) Catechol-o-methyltransferase polymorphism and susceptibility to major depressive disorder modulates psychological stress response. *Psychiatric Genetics, 17*(3), 183–193.

Kaplan, H.B. (1999) Toward an understanding of resilience: A critical review of definitions and models. In M.D. Glantz & J.R. Johnson (Eds.), *Resilience and development: Positive life adaptations* (pp. 17–83). New York: Plenum.

Koenig, H.G. (1997) *Is religion good for your health? The effects of religion on physical and mental health.* Binghampton, New York: Haworth Press.

Koenig, H.G. (1998) Religious attitudes and practices of hospitalized medically ill older adults. *International Journal of Geriatric Psychiatry, 13*, 213–224.

Lamond, A.J., Depp, C.A., Allison, M., Langer, R., Reichstadt, J., Moore, D.J., et al. (2009) Measurement and predictors of resilience among community-dwelling older women. *Journal of Psychiatric Research, 43*, 148–154.

Langer, N. (2004) Resiliency and spirituality: Foundations of strengths perspective counseling with the elderly. *Educational Gerontology, 30*, 611–617.

Lazarus, R.S., & Folkman, S. (1984) *Stress, appraisal, and coping.* New York: Springer.

Lichstein, K.L., Durrence, H.H., Riedel, B.W., Taylor, D.J., & Bush, A.J. (2004) *Epidemiology of sleep: Age, gender, and ethnicity.* Mahwah, NJ: Lawrence Erlbaum.

Luthar, S.S., Cicchetti, D., Becker, B. (2000) The construct of resilience: A critical evaluation and guidelines for future work. *Child Development, 71*(3), 543–562.

McAdams, D.P. (2001) The psychology of life stories. *Review of General Psychology, 5*, 100–122.

McAdams, D.P., & Pals, J.L. (2006) A new big five: Fundamental principles for an integrative science of personality. *American Psychologist, 61*, 204–217.

McEwen, B.S. (1998) Stress, adaptation, and disease. Allostasis and allostatic load. *Annals of the New York Academy of Sciences, 840*, 33–44.

McEwen, B.S. (2003) Interacting mediators of allostasis and allostatic load: Towards an understanding of resilience in aging. *Metabolism, 52*(10 Suppl 2), 10–16.

Pampel, F.C., & Rogers, R.G. (2004). Socioeconomic status, smoking, and health: A test of competing theories of cumulative advantage. *Health and Social Behavior, 45*, 306–321.

Pargament, K.I. (1997) *The psychology of religion and coping: Theory, research, practice*. New York: Guilford Publications.

Pargament, K.I., Kennell, J., Hathaway, W., Grevengoed, N., Newman, J., & Jones, W. (1988) Religion and the problem-solving process: Three styles of coping. *Journal for the Scientific Study of Religion, 27*, 90–104.

Pargament, K.I., Koenig, H.G., Perez, L.M. (2000) The many methods of religious coping: Development and initial validation of the RCOPE. *Journal of Clinical Psychology, 56*(4), 519–543.

Pargament, K.I., Smith, B.W., Koenig, H.G., & Perez, L. (1998) Patterns of positive and negative religious coping with major life stressors. *Journal for the Scientific Study of Religion, 37*(4), 710–724.

Pearlin, L.I., & Skaff, M.M. (1996) Stress and the life course: A paradigmatic alliance. *The Gerontologist, 36*, 239–247.

Phillips, R.E., Pargament, K.I., Lynn, Q.K., & Crossley, C.D. (2004) Self-directing religious coping: A deistic God, abandoning God, or no God at all? *Journal for the Scientific Study of Religion, 43*, 409–418.

Pinquart, M., & Sorensen, S. (2003) Predictors of burden and depressive mood: A meta-analysis. *Journals of Gerontology, Series B: Psychological Sciences and Social Sciences, 58*, P112–P128.

Ribeiro, S.C., Kennedy, S.E., Smith, Y.R., Stohler, C.S., Zubieta, J.K. (2005) Interface of physical and emotional stress regulation through the endogenous opioid system and mu-opioid receptors. *Progress in Neuro-Psychopharmacology and Biological Psychiatry, 29*, 1264–1280.

Richardson, G.E. (2002) The metatheory of resilience and resiliency. *Journal of Clinical Psychology, 58*, 307–321.

Roff, L.L., Klemmack, D.L., Parker, M., Koenig, H.G., Crowther, M., Baker, P.S., & Allman, R.M. (2004) Depression and religiosity in African American and White community-dwelling older adults. *Journal of Human Behavior in the Social Environment 10*(1), 175–189.

Sapolsky, R.M., Romero, L.M., & Munck, A.U. (2000) How do glucocorticoids influence stress responses? Integrating permissive, suppressive, stimulatory, and preparative actions. *Endocrine Review, 21*(1), 55–89.

Sterling, P., & Eyer, J. (1988) Allostasis: A new paradigm to explain arousal pathology. In S. Fisher & J. Reason (Eds.), *Handbook of life stress, cognition, and health* (pp. 629–649). New York, NY: Wiley.

Tepe, V. & Lukey, B.J. (2008) *Biobehavioral resilience to stress*. Boca Raton, FL: Taylor & Francis.

Tolan, P.T. (1996) How resilient is the concept of resilience? *The Community Psychologist 29*, 12–15.

Wagnild, G.M., & Young, H.M. (1993) Development and psychometric evaluation of the resilience scale. *Journal of Nursing Measurement 1*, 165–178.

Wong-McDonald, A., & Gorsuch, R.L. (2000) Surrender to God: An additional coping style? *Journal of Psychology and Theology, 28*, 149–161.

Chapter 2
Successful Aging and Resilience: Applications for Public Health and Health Care

Angela K. Hochhalter, Matthew Lee Smith, and Marcia G. Ory

Last weekend, Albert celebrated his 78th birthday with his children, grandchildren, and a few of his closest friends. Two of his granddaughters presented a moving tribute to Albert and his lifelong friend Patricia, who was also in attendance. Patricia was beloved by Albert's grandchildren; they were planning a big party for Patricia's 80th birthday next year. The tribute of photos and videos set to Albert's and Patricia's favorite songs showed the striking differences in the challenges and successes Albert and Patricia had experienced over their years as friends.

Albert was born in a poor farming community. His father raised Albert and his younger brother on a farm after the death of Albert's mother. Together, the three raised the crops that sustained the family. A few photos and some pencil drawings Albert created as a young boy showed the ups and downs of farm life from year to year; from bumper crops to years of drought. The boys attended school when they could. Albert finished the 11th grade, then enlisted in the Army. His enlistment photo showed a young boy who was proud to serve his country and excited to find a more consistent way of life.

Patricia was raised in a small farming community near Albert's farm and was in school with Albert for the years he attended. Patricia's mother had inherited a large fortune from her parents, and her father was a writer for several newspapers across the state. The family enjoyed living in the rural area, and travelled extensively when Patricia and her siblings were on break from school.

In the summer after their 11th grade year Albert and Patricia took a road trip in Patricia's new car. It was a chance to show Albert part of the country before he reported for duty. A horrible car accident on a country road hundreds of miles from home changed the teenagers' lives forever. Albert nearly lost his left leg, but after months in various hospitals far from home he found himself back on the farm. He was forever thankful to Patricia's family for the visits and support while he was so far from home in hospitals. It was during his long hospital stays that he met his wife, a young nurse. However, the photos of his early 20s and throughout his life showed his continuous need for walking aids – a cane, walker, and now a wheelchair. He was discharged from the Army because of the injury even before be began serving. He always told his grandchildren "this bad leg is the best thing that ever happened to me because it brought me your beautiful Grandmother!"

A.K. Hochhalter (✉)
Scott & White Healthcare, Temple, TX and Texas A&M Health Science Center, College Station, TX, USA
e-mail: ahochhalter@swmail.sw.org

B. Resnick et al. (eds.), *Resilience in Aging: Concepts, Research, and Outcomes*, DOI 10.1007/978-1-4419-0232-0_2, © Springer Science+Business Media, LLC 2011

Patricia was also injured severely in the accident. She remembers almost nothing of her 6 months in the hospital. Her family brought in specialists from around the country, and she was able to recover fully from her injuries. However, she never forgave herself for the car accident that damaged her friend's leg. She saw the accident as her burden to carry, despite Albert's efforts to console her.

Now ages 78 and almost 80, Albert and Patricia were living full but very different lives. Both had married young. Albert lost his family's farm after several years of drought and had to find new work. Patricia followed in her father's footsteps as a newspaper writer. She lost her job due to cutbacks at the paper a few years after Albert lost his job. She decided to spend her time volunteering at a local charity rather than moving away for a new job. Both friends lost their spouses about 10 years ago. Albert relied heavily on Patricia's support and the kindness of his family to help him grieve. He found new hobbies after his wife's death and is enjoying new friendships. Patricia saw her husband's death as punishment for the accident she felt she had caused so many years ago. Since his death she has been more solitary.

Recently Albert and Patricia were dealing with declining health. Albert saw this as an opportunity to teach Patricia the things he had learned throughout his life about dealing with illness and changing abilities. They were becoming closer than ever – attending chronic disease self-management workshops and cooking healthy meals together. Patricia's daughter was thrilled to see how recent videos showed her Mother smiling and enjoying life. Secretly, the party attendees wondered whether the most recent photos showed a budding romance between Albert and Patricia. They were both greeting their newest health challenges as opportunities for a new take on life, and there certainly seemed to be a lot of dancing lately!

The stories of Albert and Patricia are examples of typical older adults in America who have met the challenges of their lives in a variety of ways using their personal and social resources. Older adults like our examples are living longer, yet there is great debate whether extended life expectancies translate into more quality years. Diversity within the aging population is widely recognized (Federal Interagency Forum on Aging-Related Statistics 2008), and scientists are diligently working to identify concepts to help us understand the aging processes and the experiences of older adults in a rapidly aging society. Among the factors contributing to the diversity seen in aging trajectories are patterns of responses to challenges experienced throughout the lifespan. In this chapter, we discuss the concepts of successful aging and resilience using the experiences of our fictitious characters, Albert and Patricia. First, we describe successful aging and the contribution of resilience to the process of successful aging. Second, we give examples of public health and health care interventions that may enhance resilience in ways that promote healthy aging among older adults.

Successful Aging

Successful aging requires adaptation to multifaceted challenges that maximize an individual's capacity to reach his/her own goals (Baltes and Baltes 1980, 1990; Heckhausen and Schultz 1993; Jopp and Smith 2006). Adaptation occurs throughout the lifespan and can be described as *active aging*, defined by the World Health Organization as "the process of optimizing opportunities for health, participation and security in order to enhance quality of life as people age" (WHO 2002, p. 12). When the result of adaptation leaves one ideally positioned to reach his or her goals, we call that type of adaptation *successful aging.*

The concept of successful aging emerged in the late 1980s and early 1990s as a departure from the loss-focused geriatric and gerontological research that preceded the concept. In their groundbreaking 1987 article *Human Aging: Usual and Successful*, Rowe and Kahn argued that the cognitive and physiological losses documented in the literature as age-related changes were mischaracterizations of the natural aging process. "We believe that the role of aging per se in these losses has often been overstated and that a major component of many age-associated declines can be explained in terms of lifestyle, habits, diet, and an array of psychosocial factors extrinsic to the aging process" (p. 143).

Rowe and Kahn (1987) portrayed *normal* aging as a continuum that spanned from "usual" to "successful." The variability in performance differences between younger adults and older adults without pathological conditions fell along this continuum. In other words, older adults as a group may not perform as well as younger adults as a group; however, within the older adult group, one could identify individuals who showed little or no performance difference when compared to younger adults. Performance that was similar to that of the younger group was considered evidence of successful aging. Examples of such atypically high performance were cited in the areas of carbohydrate metabolism, osteoporosis, and cognitive function. The paper set the stage for multidisciplinary explorations of what it means to age successfully.

Soon after Rowe and Kahn paper, several conceptual frameworks and theoretical models were introduced across disciplines to describe a continuum within normal ("nonpathological") aging from what was "usual" to what was particularly "successful" aging. For example, Baltes and Baltes introduced the Selection, Optimization and Compensation Framework (SOC framework), which posits that adaptation to challenges in older age involves systematic reallocation of resources to pursue new goals, maintain functioning, and regain functioning (Baltes and Smith 2003; Heckhausen et al. 1989). When SOC processes are not effective or efficient, they can be maladaptive. The goal, therefore, is to engage the three processes in ways that lead to desired outcomes or "efficacious functioning" (Baltes and Carstensen 1996). Innumerable models of successful aging are now in use, most of which include the following themes (Inui and Frankel 1991; von Faber et al. 2001; Young et al. 2009):

1. Successful aging happens across the lifespan.
2. Successful aging incorporates many domains, including but not limited to health, social, biological, and psychological domains.
3. Successful aging occurs in response to challenges.
4. Successful aging is defined uniquely for each individual to the degree that individual goals and preferences differ.
5. Capacity for successful aging is partially under one's control (e.g. through new learning) and partially predetermined (e.g. genetic predisposition).

As science more fully describes changes that occur over the lifespan, successful aging has become a construct that fits well into our expanding understanding of the aging process. In 2003, Inui described successful aging as "dynamic equilibrium," and argued that the study of successful aging should integrate a multidisciplinary biopsychological approach. The dynamic equilibrium he described involved capacity in multiple domains to function well as the circumstances of one's life changed. Functioning well, for Inui, means performing in domains on which an individual places high value. Despite certain trait-like determinants of one's capacity to adapt, he emphasized the role of the individual in defining what it meant to be successful. Functioning well in a domain that a person assigns little value is not the goal; rather, one who is aging successfully is adapting in ways that promote optimal functioning in domains he or she values most. Domains of functioning may be physiological, psychological, or sociological; ailing health and limited physical function do not preclude successful aging (Young et al. 2009).

In Fig. 2.1, we offer a hypothetical schematic of an individual's performance in three domains. Domain-specific performance varies over time and can be categorized in some cases as successful and as usual or abnormal/pathological in others. This figure represents what Patricia's performance might look like following her husband's death. She had always functioned fairly well physically. Psychologically she had to grieve her husband's death, but found some relief from the grief she carried over her car accident with Albert. Unfortunately, Patricia pulled away from others following her husband's death.

For the most part, theoretical descriptions of successful aging match older adults' perceptions of the concept as it is represented in the literature. Older adults define successful aging as an ongoing multidimensional process that is distinct from chronological age (Reichstadt et al. 2007). They report that successful aging requires having a positive attitude, coping with change, accepting limitations that cannot be overcome, being secure and stable long term (e.g. social support, knowing one would be taken care of in declining health), practicing spiritual beliefs and receiving

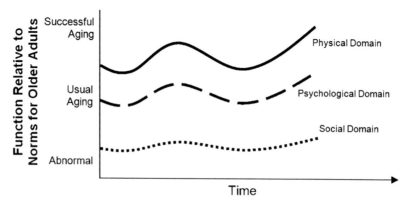

Fig. 2.1 An individual's performance in physical, psychological, and social domains varies in the degree to which successful aging is achieved over time

spiritual blessing, and staying engaged both socially and cognitively (Laditka et al. 2009; Reichstadt et al. 2007). Older adults place high value on maintaining basic physical functioning, being free of major life-threatening disease, engaging in social and recreational activities, and feeling independent (Laditka et al. 2009; von Faber et al. 2001). In the United States, staying cognitively alert and having a good memory is among the most highly valued successes among older adults (Laditka et al. 2009; Sharkey et al. 2009). In interviews, older adults distinguish between successes within (e.g. investments in social contacts) and outside of (e.g. physical health) their control (von Faber et al. 2001). While cognitive health is highly valued, older adults differ in the degree to which they believe that healthy behavior and other factors under their control can promote cognitive health or prevent the onset of cognitive impairment (Logsdon et al. 2009; Wilcox et al. 2009).

Successful Aging and Resilience

How one goes about aging successfully is not fully understood; however, a number of individual characteristics and personality traits have been proposed to contribute to the success with which one adapts to challenges. In addition, the environment in which one ages strongly influences one's ability to adapt to challenges. For example, in Chap. 3 of this volume, Rosowsky considers personality disorders in the context of older age. She points out that the degree to which traits are maladaptive depends in part on the environments in which they are expressed.

Figure 2.2 sets the stage for how we think about the possibility for resilience in the face of given challenges over the course of the lifespan. Challenges faced at different points – Albert's and Patricia's car accident, for example – are labeled at the bottom of the figure. Each challenge impacts domains of functioning to different degrees, represented in the bar graphs. For example, a car accident with associated injury in adolescence may heavily challenge an individual's physical domain when compared to the loss of employment or spouse in mid-life or older adulthood. Conversely, psychological and social domains may be heavily and disproportionately challenged with the death of a spouse in older adulthood. Individuals possess or have access to a wide range of resources with which to meet a challenge. Examples of these resources are represented in pie graphs at the top of the figure. The availability of resources likely changes over time. Here we have represented a growing reserve of resources over the lifespan. Absolute "amount" of resources and types of resources available do not grow linearly across the lifespan – individuals experience differing resources at different times.

For example, we know that Albert had fewer financial resources than Patricia to draw on at the time of their car accident, but Albert may have had more self-efficacy for overcoming challenges and other resources than Patricia had developed at that time. When these two individuals faced job loss, the loss of their spouses, and now new illnesses, the composition of their available resources also likely differed.

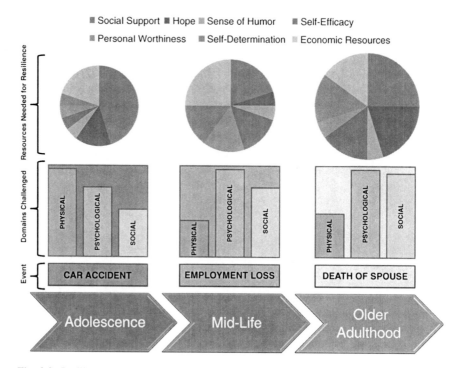

Fig. 2.2 Resilience is possible when one can draw on the appropriate resources to meet the demands of a given challenge

When available resources are sufficient to meet the demands of a new challenge, there is the possibility for resilience.

As the authors note in chapters throughout this book, resilience has been defined in a number of ways and as both a process and a personality trait. The concept of resilience has evolved over time as new applications and evidence have emerged. Initial studies of resilience were limited to childhood; now resilience is applied across the lifespan. In fact, Felten and Hall (2001) have described what they call "resilience in women older than 85" as a distinct concept. They posit that unique experiences of the oldest old women represent unique challenges and that there is great intragroup variability in how particular health stressors are appraised.

Resilience has been described as "bouncing back," "rebounding after a loss," and "reintegration." What is unique about resilience relative to similar concepts (e.g. hardiness) is that resilience is associated with positive growth in addition to overcoming a specific challenge (Earvolino-Ramirez 2007). In other words, through resilience one not only adapts but is also better off, healthier, or has grown after adapting. In our opening example, Albert's positive appraisals of the experiences following his car accident are examples of resilient responses to the circumstance. Patricia's ongoing guilt is an example of a response that is not resilient; she carries her guilt with her throughout her life.

The improvement in the face of challenge that characterizes resilience is particularly relevant to successful aging as defined by Rowe and Kahn (1987) because it explains how one might move beyond usual aging toward the positive extreme of the aging continuum, which they defined as "successful." We argue that resilience is what distinguishes usual responses to everyday stressors and major life events from those that are particularly adaptive or exemplary. Resilience is tied to challenges rather than individuals. For example, Patricia in our example seems to be meeting the onset of new chronic illnesses with resilience even though she has not met other life challenges with resilience.

Psychosocial Factors Associated with Resilience

A number of psychosocial factors have been associated with the emergence of resilience in the face of challenges, including emotional support from others, a sense of personal worthiness, self-efficacy, trust in others, hope for the future, coping by putting things into perspective or appraising things positively, a sense of humor, and having a sense of purpose or self-determination (Earvolino-Ramirez 2007; Garnefski et al. 2008; Thornton and Perez 2006). These predictors or prerequisite conditions (the exact role and necessity has not been fully defined) appear throughout studies of resilience across all ages and are potential targets of intervention when aiming to promote successful aging.

One example of particularly adaptive and exemplary response to adversity is posttraumatic growth following major life events such as heart attack, cancer, violence, or natural disaster (Garnefski et al. 2008; Thornton and Perez 2006). It is noteworthy that resilience can occur over time, with positive adaptation revealed after a period of what initially appears to be maladaptive. Resilience can also fade over time, with negative consequences of trauma emerging after years of successful coping (King et al. 2007). Kleim and Ehlers (2009) conducted two studies of the relationship between posttraumatic growth and psychopathology among adult survivors of physical or sexual assault. In the two studies, approximately 60% of participants reported some degree of growth 6 months after the assault. Higher growth scores were associated with greater posttraumatic stress disorder (PTSD) and/or more severe depressive symptoms; however, the relationships between growth and/or negative symptomotology were curvilinear in both studies. Highest and lowest levels of posttraumatic growth were found when PTSD and/or depressive symptoms were lowest. The greatest posttraumatic growth was observed for participants who reported being more religious and for non-Caucasian participants. The findings exemplify the complexity of human reactions to challenges. One important contribution of the field of successful aging to the field of resilience may therefore be the definition of "success" as at least partially self-defined. Perhaps, in the context of successful aging, the degree to which a resilient response achieves gains depends largely on whether growth is in domains that are most highly valued by the person facing particular challenges.

Lens Metaphor: Successful Aging Through Resilience

In Fig. 2.1, we depict how functioning varies across domains during usual day-to-day experiences. Figure 2.2 illustrated the differences in domains challenged based on adverse life events and possible resources needed for resilience. In Fig. 2.3, we show a schematic of what we call the "lens" through which challenges are experienced. We think of each person's unique resources and perspective on life as a lens through which challenges "pass" The predictors and prerequisite conditions for resilience occur to varying degrees in each person's unique lens, which is framed by one's history and within particular social and environmental contexts (e.g. finances, supportive physical environments). For example, the event of our characters' car accident passed through their very different lenses and produced very different results. Albert's family didn't have the money to travel to see him or bring in specialists to direct his treatment. The result was lasting damage to his leg, but a positive experience in what was gained during the challenge. Perhaps the ups and downs of his childhood helped prepare him for this particular challenge in young adulthood. Patricia, on the other hand, had the advantage of support from her family and specialists to guide her care. Physically she recovered well, but she was plagued by the guilt of the situation for years. Patricia may have been resilient in the physical domain, but psychologically, she was less resilient to the car accident. Individuals may be aging successfully in some domains but not others.

In Fig. 2.4, we introduce the concept of one's unique lens at a time when a major challenge – in this case, a major debilitating event like Albert's leg injury after the car accident – presents itself. After experiencing that event through a unique lens, functioning in various domains may or may not change. Improvements from before to after the event represent resilience in response to personal loss. Figure 2.4 shows

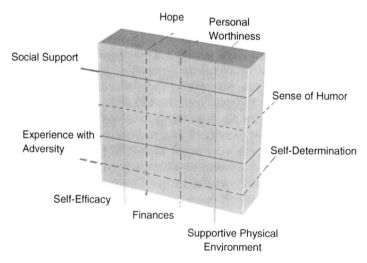

Fig. 2.3 A variety of personal factors interact to create a "lens" through which one experiences and adapts to challenges

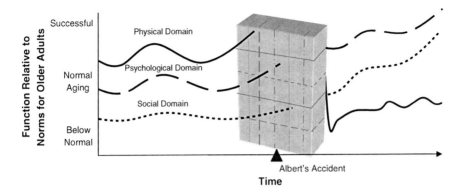

Fig. 2.4 Resilience is demonstrated when performance in one or more domains improves follow-ing adaptation to a challenge such as a major illness. The degree of adaptation achieved depends on the characteristics of the "lens" through which the challenge is experienced

an improvement in the social domain, perhaps due to strengthened relationships with friends and family during a time of great need. Unlike functioning in the social domain, Fig. 2.4 depicts a dramatic decline in physical domain functioning follow-ing the event relative to the physical functioning before the event. This sharp decline may or may not have been preventable; in this case, the initial result is maladaptive.

Possibilities for Promoting Resilience and Successful Aging in Older Adult Health

To some degree, resilience and those conditions that make resilience possible are mutable and therefore lend themselves to interventions that have potential to pro-mote successful aging. In this section we give examples of interventions that can be used to address day-to-day functioning ("everyday interventions") and interven-tions that may help moderate the effects of particular challenges. We have chosen examples that speak to the health of older adults as a population and interventions that are best targeted to individuals. Examples come from the fields of public health and health care.

Everyday interventions. A variety of interventions are available to promote successful aging in the context of challenges posed by what Rowe and Kahn (1987) might have labeled "usual aging." For example, the Active for Life® initiative disseminated two evidence-based physical activity programs for older adults into community settings for the promotion of older adult health (Wilcox et al. 2008). Initiatives like Active for Life® rely on behavioral processes to increase physical activity through goal setting, problem solving, and feedback. Improvements in overall health status, combined with reductions in perceived stress in everyday life, have the potential to (a) improve one's readiness for adapting to physiological challenges like the exposure to an influenza infection or (b) prevent challenges like the exacerbation of existing health conditions. As a result of these programs, participants have reported getting a "new lease on life" as evidenced by delaying or offsetting of age-related health conditions such as progressive heart disease or diabetes.

The *A Matter of Balance* program (Healy 2008; Tennstedt 1998) is an example of a fall prevention intervention that is widely disseminated and extensively evaluated. Falls are a challenge that is associated with a downward spiral of health and well-being. Fear of falling often facilitates behaviors that actually increase the likelihood of falling (e.g. reductions in physical activity, depressive symptomatology, limitations in daily activities). The evidence-based *A Matter of Balance* activity program is intended to diminish the fear of falling and increase physical activity by targeting attitudes and behaviors associated with a predisposition for falls. Participation in the program leads to improved self-efficacy for preventing and managing falls, decreased disruption of daily activities, and improvements in measures of mental health (Ory et al. 2009). Each of these factors is associated with greater likelihood of avoiding future falls or improved managements of the consequences of injurious falls.

There are many opportunities to promote resilience and successful aging in primary care settings such as medical clinics, even in the absence of specific health problems. In the case of geriatric health services, promoting successful aging means that health care is person-centered, focused on quality of care, and aims to improve quality of life rather than cure disease (Kane 2003). Individual practitioners can foster resilience to usual age-related deficits during routine health care encounters by helping older patients select medical devices that are simple to use, encouraging use of organizational tools for medication adherence, providing instructions in well-organized text, encouraging patients to intentionally incorporate behaviors such as glucose monitoring into existing routines, and encouraging participation in decision-making by giving clear choices and adequate time to consider options (Brown and Park 2003).

Health care systems can also deliver care to address the multiple domains of functioning that define successful aging and address patient' goals. The *patient-centered medical home* is a model of care that has been endorsed by a number of leading medical professional organizations (Kellerman and Kirk 2007). Among the principles of care that make this model particularly appropriate for promoting successful aging are establishing a long-term patient–physician relationship, focusing on the whole patient rather than a specific health condition, and actively involving the patient and his or her goals. There is evidence that medical homes contribute to improved health behaviors, health care quality, patient satisfaction, and health outcomes (Rosenthal 2008). Models of care management to support the health of persons with chronic illness incorporate similar patient-centered principles and may also encourage successful aging and/or resilience in the face of everyday challenges posed by chronic illness (Dorr et al. 2008; Wolff et al. 2009). Additional assessments of these patient-centered models of care will reveal the degree to which they promote aspects of successful aging and resilience.

Interventions in response to specific challenges. When challenges do occur, timely interventions can promote resilient responses. The relationships between physiological and psychological responses to challenges or stressors are inextricable. To some degree, resilience is "hard-wired." For example, as the brain ages, areas of the brain lose volume and dopaminergic receptors, connections among neurons become less efficient, and white matter integrity is degraded (Jessberger and Gage 2008; Park and Reuter-Lorenz 2009). However, additional changes occur in the brain that are hypothesized to partially compensate for the age-related cognitive decline that may be caused by loss of brain structure and functioning. There is evidence that neurogenesis occurs in areas important for cognitive functioning (Jessberger and Gage 2008; Lee and Son 2009). When cognitive function is affected by deterioration in some areas of the brain, other areas may be recruited to help compensate for loss in function. Park and Reuter-Lorenz (2009) propose that certain healthy behaviors like exercise, engaging in stimulating cognitive activity like learning new things, and targeted training can enhance the ability for compensatory activity and therefore enhance one's cognitive function.

Our knowledge of brain plasticity is growing rapidly. For now, there is evidence that human capacity for resilience exists across the lifespan in multiple domains, including the domains of our physiological and physical make-up in addition to domains such as personality, coping style or coping skills, psychological health, and social functioning (Garnefski et al. 2008; Young et al. 2009). Exactly how resilience might look at the level of brain anatomy or function is still unknown, but the complexity of our reactions to challenges as we age cannot be overstated. Interventions for major neurological events like stroke currently tap into the brain's natural resilience to help persons regain some of the physical functioning that is sometimes lost after a stroke (Langhorne et al. 2009). New interventions for other neurological events are likely to emerge as the complexities of our brain's natural resilience are revealed.

In addition to intervening at the level of individual persons, system-level interventions are available to support resilience and successful aging. For older adults, most of whom are living with one or more chronic illnesses (e.g. Avendano et al. 2009; Thorpe and Howard 2006), the challenges of transitioning from the hospital back home further complicate disease management for a period of time. It is important that patients and their caregivers play an active role throughout hospital-to-home transitions (Snow et al. 2009). When transitions are unsuccessful, serious events such as adverse drug reactions and falls can and often do occur (Tsilimingras and Bates 2008). Health care interventions that are initiated at the time of hospital-to-home transitions can help older adults transition home safely and prevent complications that lead to additional hospitalizations. Most interventions for hospital-to-home transitions call for nurses or nonclinical coaches to make in-person visits and/or telephone calls to provide supportive care and/or clinical guidance and to empower patients to perform necessary self-care tasks (Coleman et al. 2006; Harrison et al. 2002; Naylor et al. 1999). These interventions have been shown to improve health-related quality of life and reduce rates of rehospitalization for older adults (Coleman et al. 2004; Harrison et al. 2002; Naylor et al. 1999).

Family caregiver interventions and chronic disease self-management programs like those our characters Albert and Patricia attended are designed for longer term challenges. Interventions that provide skills training and ongoing peer or professional support for persons facing illnesses (e.g. diabetes or heart disease) and those facing the stressors involved in caring for a loved one bring about measurable improvements in health behaviors, health-related outcomes, and health care utilization (Chodosh et al. 2005; Warsi et al. 2004). In addition to teaching what one needs to know to meet daily challenges, education and skills training boost motivation and self-efficacy for carrying out recommended tasks (Bodenheimer et al. 2006; Chodosh et al. 2005; Lorig and Holman 2003). As a whole, family caregiver interventions can improve general well-being, depression, and caregiving burden (Belle et al. 2006; Knight et al. 1993; Mittelman et al. 1995, 2004; Sorensen et al. 2002; Toseland et al. 1989).

Conclusion

Resilience is an extraordinary and positive response to a challenge or stressor. Rather than merely "getting through" a hard time, the resilient response is one that adapts so well to the challenge that functioning in one or more domain is better after adapting than before the challenge occurred. When the growth produced by resilience leaves one functioning better than expected in a domain that he or she deems important, resilience can produce successful aging. Quantitative evidence and the qualitative reports of older adults point to a number of individual characteristics that set the stage for resilient responses. As we have seen in the example of Albert and Patricia, physical, psychological, social, and environmental characteristics show promise to either facilitate or impede such adaptive responses. These characteristics are appropriate targets for public health and health care interventions that aim to foster optimal functioning in domains that are highly valued by persons of any age.

References

Avendano, M., Glymour, M. M., Banks, J., & Mackenbach, J. P. (2009) Health disadvantage in US adults aged 50 to 74 years: A comparison of the health of rich and poor Americans with that of Europeans. *American Journal of Public Health, 99*(3), 540–548.

Baltes, P. B., & Baltes, M. M. (1980) Plasticity and variability in psychological aging: Methodological and theoretical issues. In G. E. Gurski (Ed.), *Determining the Effects of Aging on the Central Nervous System* (pp. 41–66). Berlin: Schering.

Baltes, P. B., & Baltes, M. M. (1990) Psychological perspectives on successful aging: The model of selective optimization with compensation. In P. B. Baltes & M. M. Baltes (Eds.), *Successful Aging: Perspectives from the Behavioral Sciences* (pp. 1–34). New York: Cambridge University Press.

Baltes, M. M., & Carstensen, L. L. (1996) The process of successful ageing. *Ageing and Society, 16*, 397–422.

Baltes, P. B., & Smith, J. (2003) New frontiers in the future of aging: From successful aging of the young old to the dilemmas of the fourth age. *Gerontology, 49*(2), 123–135.

Belle, S. H., Burgio, L., Burns, R., Coon, D., Czaja, S. J., Gallagher-Thompson, D., et al. (2006) Enhancing the quality of life of dementia caregivers from different ethnic or racial groups: A randomized controlled trial. *Annals of Internal Medicine, 145*(10), 727–738.

Bodenheimer, T., Lorig, K., Holman, H., & Grumabach, K. (2006) Patient self-management of chronic disease in primary care. *JAMA, 288*(19), 2469–2475.

Brown, S. C., & Park, D. C. (2003) Theoretical models of cognitive aging and implications for translational research in medicine. *Gerontologist,* 43 Spec No 1(1), 57–67.

Chodosh, J., Morton, S. C., Mojica, W., Maglione, M., Suttorp, M. J., Hilton, L., et al. (2005) Meta-analysis: Chronic disease self-management programs for older adults. *Annals of Internal Medicine, 143*, 427–438.

Coleman, E. A., Smith, J. D., Frank, J. C., Min, S., Parry, C., & Kramer, A. (2004) Preparing patients and caregivers to participate in care delivered across settings: The care transitions intervention. *Journal of the American Geriatrics Society, 52*, 1817–1825.

Coleman, E. A., Parry, C., Chalmers, S., & Min, S. J. (2006) The care transitions intervention: Results of a randomized controlled trial. *Archives of Internal Medicine, 166*(17), 1822–1828.

Dorr, D. A., Wilcox, A. B., Brunker, C. P., Burdon, R. E., & Donnelly, S. M. (2008) The effect of technology-supported, multidisease care management on the mortality and hospitalization of seniors. *Journal of the American Geriatrics Society, 56*, 2195–2202.

Earvolino-Ramirez, M. (2007) Resilience: A concept analysis. *Nursing Forum, 42*(2), 73–82.

Federal Interagency Forum on Aging-Related Statistics. (2008) *Older Americans 2008: Key indicators of well-being*. Washington, DC: U.S. Government Printing Office. Document Number.

Felten, B. S., & Hall, J. M. (2001) Conceptualizing resilience in women older than 85: Overcoming adversity from illness or loss. *Journal of Gerontological Nursing, 27*(11), 46–53.

Garnefski, N., Kraaij, V., Schroevers, M. J., & Somsen, G. A. (2008) Post-traumatic growth after a myocardial infarction: A matter of personality, psychological health, or cognitive coping? *Journal of Clinical Psychology in Medical Settings, 15*(4), 270–277.

Harrison, M. B., Browne, G. B., Roberts, J., Tugwell, P., Gafni, A., & Graham, I. D. (2002) Quality of life of individuals with heart failure: A randomized trial of the effectiveness of two models of hospital-to-home transition. *Medical Care, 40*(4), 271–282.

Healy, T. C. (2008) The feasibility and effectiveness of translating a matter of balance into a volunteer lay leader model. *Journal of Applied Gerontology, 27*(1), 34–51.

Heckhausen, J., & Schultz, R. (1993) Optimisation by selection and compensation: Balancing primary and secondary control in life span development. *International Journal of Behavioral Development, 16*(2), 287–303.

Heckhausen, J., Dixon, R. A., & Baltes, P. B. (1989) Gains and losses in development throughout adulthood as perceived by different adult age groups. *Developmental Psychology, 25*(1), 109–121.

Inui, T. S., & Frankel, R. M. (1991) Evaluating the quality of qualitative research: A proposal pro tem. *Journal of General Internal Medicine, 6*(5), 485–486.

Jessberger, S., & Gage, F. H. (2008) Stem-cell-associated structural and functional plasticity in the aging hippocampus. *Psychology and Aging, 23*(4), 684–691.

Jopp, D., & Smith, J. (2006) Resources and life-management strategies as determinants of successful aging: On the protective effect of selection, optimization and compensation. *Psychology and Aging, 21*(2), 253–265.

Kane, R. L. (2003) The contribution of geriatric health services research to successful aging. *Annals of Internal Medicine, 139*(5 Pt 2), 460–462.

Kellerman, R., & Kirk, L. (2007) Principles of the patient-centered medical home. *American Family Physician, 76*(6), 774–775.

King, L. A., King, D. W., Vickers, K., Davison, E. H., & Spiro, A., 3rd. (2007) Assessing late-onset stress symptomatology among aging male combat veterans. *Aging and Mental Health, 11*(2), 175–191.

Kleim, B., & Ehlers, A. (2009) Evidence for a curvilinear relationship between posttraumatic growth and posttrauma depression and PTSD in assault survivors. *Journal of Traumatic Stress, 22*(1), 45–52.

Knight, B. G., Lutzky, S. M., & Macofsky-Urban, F. (1993) A meta-analytic review of interventions for caregiver distress: Recommendations for future research. *Gerontologist, 33,* 240–248.

Laditka, S. B., Corwin, S. J., Laditka, J. N., Liu, R., Tseng, W., Wu, B., et al. (2009) Attitudes about aging well among a diverse group of older Americans: Implications for promoting cognitive health. *Gerontologist,* 49 Suppl 1(1), S30–39.

Langhorne, P., Coupar, F., & Pollock, A. (2009) Motor recovery after stroke: A systematic review. *Lancet Neurology, 8*(8), 741–754.

Lee, E., & Son, H. (2009) Adult hippocampal neurogenesis and related neurotrophic factors. *BMB Reports, 42*(5), 239–244.

Logsdon, R. G., Hochhalter, A. K., & Sharkey, J. R. (2009) From message to motivation: Where the rubber meets the road. *Gerontologist,* 49 Suppl 1(1), S108–111.

Lorig, K., & Holman, H. (2003) Self-management education: History, definition, outcomes, and mechanisms. *Annals of Behavioral Med, 26*(1), 1–7.

Mittelman, M. S., Ferris, S. H., & Shulman, E. (1995) A comprehensive support program: Effect on depression in spouse-caregivers of AD patients. *Gerontologist, 35,* 92–802.

Mittelman, M. S., Roth, D. L., Coon, D., & Haley, W. (2004) Sustained benefit of supportive intervention for depressive symptoms in caregivers of patients with Alzheimer's disease. *American Journal of Psychiatry, 161*(5), 850–856.

Naylor, M. D., Brooten, D., Campbell, R., Jacobsen, B. S., Mezey, M. D., Pauly, M. V., et al. (1999) Comprehensive discharge planning and home follow-up of hospitalized elders. *JAMA, 281*(7), 613–620.

Ory, M. G., Smith, M. L., Wade, A. F., Mounce, C., Larsen, R. A. A., & Parrish, R. (2009) Falls prevention as a pathway to healthy aging: Statewide implementation and dissemination of an evidence-based program. Texas A&M Health Science Center.

Park, D. C., & Reuter-Lorenz, P. (2009) The adaptive brain: Aging and neurocognitive scaffolding. *Annual Review of Psychology, 60*(1), 173–196.

Reichstadt, J., Depp, C. A., Palinkas, L. A., Folsom, D. P., & Jeste, D. V. (2007) Building blocks of successful aging: A focus group study of older adults' perceived contributors to successful aging. *American Journal of Geriatriatric Psychiatry, 15*(3), 194–201.

Rosenthal, T. C. (2008) The medical home: Growing evidence to support a new approach to primary care. *Journal of the American Board of Family Medicine, 21*(5), 427–440.

Rowe, J. W., & Kahn, R. L. (1987) Human aging: Usual and successful. *Science, 237*(4811), 143–149.

Sharkey, J. R., Sharf, B. F., & St John, J. A. (2009) "Una persona derechita (staying right in the mind)": Perceptions of Spanish-speaking Mexican American older adults in South Texas colonias. *Gerontologist,* 49 Suppl 1(1), S79–85.

Snow, V., Beck, D., Budnitz, T., Miller, D. C., Potter, J., Wears, R. L., et al. (2009) Transitions of Care Consensus Policy Statement American College of Physicians-Society of General Internal Medicine-Society of Hospital Medicine-American Geriatrics Society-American College of Emergency Physicians-Society of Academic Emergency Medicine. *Journal of General Internal Medicine, 24*(8), 971–976.

Sorensen, S., Pinquart, M., & Duberstein, P. (2002) How effective are interventions with caregivers? An updated meta-analysis. *Gerontologist, 42*(3), 356–372.

Tennstedt, S. (1998) A randomized, controlled trial of a group intervention to reduce fear of falling and associated activity restriction in older adults. *Journals of Gerontology Series B: Psychological Sciences & Social Sciences, 1998*(6), P384–392.

Thornton, A. A., & Perez, M. A. (2006) Posttraumatic growth in prostate cancer survivors and their partners. *Psychooncology, 15*(4), 285–296.

Thorpe, K. E., & Howard, D. H. (2006) The rise in spending among Medicare beneficiaries: The role of chronic disease prevalence and changes in treatment intensity. *Health Affairs,* W378–388.

Toseland, R. W., Rossiter, C. M., & Labrecque, M. S. (1989) The effectiveness of three group intervention strategies to support family caregivers. *American Journal of Orthopsychiatry*, 59(3), 420–429.

Tsilimingras, D., & Bates, D. W. (2008) Addressing postdischarge adverse events: A neglected area. *Joint Commission Journal on Quality and Patient Safety*, 34(2), 85–97.

von Faber, M., Bootsma-van der Wiel, A., van Exel, E., Gussekloo, J., Lagaay, A. M., van Dongen, E., et al. (2001) Successful aging in the oldest old: Who can be characterized as successfully aged? *Archives of Internal Medicine*, 161(22), 2694–2700.

Warsi, A., Wang, P. S., LaValley, M. P., Avorn, J., & Solomon, D. H. (2004) Self-management education programs in chronic disease: A systematic review and methodological critique of the literature. *Archives of Internal Medicine*, 164(15), 1641–1649.

Wilcox, S., Dowda, M., Leviton, L. C., Bartlett-Prescott, J., Bazzarre, T., Campbell-Voytal, K., et al. (2008) Active for Life: Final results from the translation of two physical activity programs. *American Journal of Preventive Medicine*, 35(4), 340–351.

Wilcox, S., Sharkey, J. R., Mathews, A. E., Laditka, J. N., Laditka, S. B., Logsdon, R. G., et al. (2009) Perceptions and beliefs about the role of physical activity and nutrition on brain health in older adults. *Gerontologist*, 49 Suppl 1(1), S61–71.

Wolff, J. L., Giovannetti, E. R., Boyd, C. M., Reider, L., Palmer, S., Scharfstein, D., et al. (2009) Effects of guided care on family caregivers. *Gerontologist*, 26, 26.

World Health Organization. (2002) *The World Health Report 2002: Reducing Risks, Promoting Healthy Life*. Retrieved from http://www.who.int/whr/2002.

Young, Y., Frick, K. D., & Phelan, E. A. (2009) Can successful aging and chronic illness coexist in the same individual? A multidimensional concept of successful aging. *Journal of the American Medical Directors Association*, 10(2), 87–92.

Chapter 3
Resilience and Personality Disorders in Older Age

Erlene Rosowsky

This entire volume is dedicated to understanding what is meant by the concept of resilience and how it applies to old age. This chapter focuses on that group of older adults who have struggled with life all their life and who are especially poorly equipped to meet the challenges of aging. They are in many ways the antithesis of resilient individuals. They are addressed in the clinical literature as having a personality disorder.

The chapter begins with an overview of what is meant by "personality disorder" and how it is diagnosed according to the *Diagnostic and Statistical Manual of Mental Disorders (DSM-IV-TR)*. This is followed by a discussion of the aging of personality disorders including a description of what can be expected to change and perhaps more relevantly what can be expected to remain the same throughout the course of sentient life. The next section discusses the functions of resilience and challenges to resilience for those with personality disorders. This leads to the final section on implications for treatment.

What Do We Mean by "Personality Disorder?"

Personality defines us as individuals. It encompasses the ways we typically think, feel, and behave. It enables us to identify those whom we know and to reasonably predict how they might be expected to behave under given circumstances. There is comfort in this predictability. Conversely, it is disquieting when someone presents in a way that is markedly different from his or her usual way of being. We count on a level of constancy of presented or manifested self in relationships with others, especially in intimate relationships. The reciprocal of manifest self is internal self-constancy. This refers to the individual's customary inner experiences of thought,

E. Rosowsky (✉)
Harvard Medical School and Massachusetts School of Professional Psychology,
Boston, MA, USA
e-mail: erosowsk@bidmc.harvard.edu

B. Resnick et al. (eds.), *Resilience in Aging: Concepts, Research, and Outcomes*,
DOI 10.1007/978-1-4419-0232-0_3, © Springer Science+Business Media, LLC 2011

affectivity, and impulse regulation, which then give rise to behavior. A major press throughout life is to "feel like me." This press or drive commands behavior, even if this is not useful or adaptive.

Personality is in the main impressively stable (Costa and McCrae 1988) but not immutable. Some people do evidence significant change in some personality domains over time (Valliant 2002; Small et al. 2003). For all, over the life course, the personality is required to interface with different challenges and expectations so that even stability embraces degrees of freedom, or flexibility, in order to remain recognizably "stable." There is thus requisite change in constancy. The personality is ever involved in the complex process of adaptation. This incorporates the processes of assimilation and accommodation (Kegan 1982). Assimilation refers to what the individual brings in to his evolving self from the experience, and accommodation to what he brings to the experience from his present self. Both of these functions are in the service of "being the same." These processes depend upon intrapsychic flexibility, ability to regulate emotions, a repertoire of responses, and access to external resources, including those of others with whom one is in relationship. These requirements are precisely those that are most challenging to individuals with personality disorders who, de facto, are rigid (versus flexible); have problems with affect regulation; are limited to a narrow repertoire of affective, cognitive, and behavioral responses; and have a history marked by complex and dysfunctional relationships (Segal et al. 2006).

The DSM IV-TR requires for a diagnosis of personality disorder that the clinical presentation includes several key elements: A pattern of inner experience and behavior that deviates significantly from what is expected within the individual's culture; that the pattern is inflexible and pervasive; that the pattern is stable and identifiable in adolescence or by early adulthood; and that the pattern leads to the experience of significant distress or to impairment in important areas of functioning. There appear to be fundamental conceptual problems in how we choose to understand, and thus clinically identify, personality disorders. The DSM approach respects a categorical model, wherein the individual either does or does not meet criteria for the diagnosis of a personality disorder. A dimensional perspective appears to have greater relevance with respect to clinical utility, perhaps most especially when applied to older adults, and is anticipated to be reflected in the upcoming DSM-V (Svrakic et al. 2008). Empirical studies strongly support a dimensional as opposed to a categorical perspective. This perspective posits that there is nothing inherently pathological about the personality traits manifested by the individual and that the traits themselves do not distinguish between the normal and the pathological personality, but rather that the disorder reflects an extreme presentation of normal personality function (Jang et al. 2006). However, even this dimensional perspective does not precisely get at what a personality disorder is. Extreme traits do not per se define the disorder (Wakefield 2008), but what does define it is how these traits interfere with impaired social or goal-focused functioning or provoke the experience of distress. The functional relevance of the disorder depends on the roles of adjudicator and referents, and how these relate to the core concept of dysfunction. In addition to the personality traits, cognitive structures and processes need also to be considered

(Livesley and Jang 2000). There is no clear discontinuity between normal and abnormal personality traits. Neither are personality traits per se adaptive or maladaptive. If the traits are judged to be adaptive, they define a personality style. If they are maladaptive, they define a personality disorder. Much of the distinction reflects what is being asked of the personality, where it is being asked to address this, and who is evaluating whether the response/behavior is adaptive or maladaptive. This speaks in part to tolerance and acceptability of individual differences. Svrakic et al. (2008) make a compelling case for the term "personality disorder" to be changed to "disorders of adaptation," which describes what it is they actually are and offers a potential benefit of destigmatizing the diagnosis.

Regardless of the model used, a key concept appears to be the presentation of a maladaptive or inappropriate "pattern." The personality traits taken together comprise the pattern or trait template. While each trait can be viewed as lying along a continuum depicting dimensions of normal, putatively owned by all, it is the pattern and how it is applied which becomes identified as pathology. There are other systems of classification, for example, "structural classification" based on a psychodynamic formulation of personality organization, "protypal classification" (combining the categorical and dimensional classifications), and "relational classification" (including interpersonal and systemic models) (Magnavita 2004). Considered thought about personality disorders has fueled passion and controversy. "No other area in the study of psychopathology is fraught with more controversy than the personality disorders" (Millon and Davis 1996, 485). Personality disorder experts in the main are not satisfied with the current DSM classification system and marked changes in the DSM-V are recommended (Balsis et al. in press) and anticipated (Tackett et al. 2008; Widiger and Lowe 2008; Bernstein et al. 2007; Svrakic et al. 2008).

The DSM IV-TR presents ten specific disorders included in Axis II and these are each dependent upon specific diagnostic criteria. The ten personality disorders are organized into three clusters based upon common themes. Cluster A, "odd and eccentric," includes the paranoid, schizoid, and schizotypal personality disorders. Cluster B, "dramatic and erratic," includes the antisocial, borderline, histrionic, and narcissistic personality disorders. Cluster C, "anxious and fearful," includes the avoidant, dependent, and obsessive compulsive personality disorders. It is inferred that the specific personality disorders within each cluster share not only common themes and etiology, but also that the clusters are significantly distinct from one another, thus establishing valid and reliable diagnostic boundaries.

That the classification system affects the assessment of personality disorders is self-evident. Following this logic, assessment identifies cases, providing what we know of the incidence and prevalence of personality disorders. The prevalence of personality disorders in old age is reported as 2.8–13% in the community, 5–33% among mental health out-patients, and 7–61.5% among inpatients (VanAlphen et al. 2006; Ames and Molinari 1994; Cohen et al. 1994). The broad ranges clearly reflect the challenges to case identification. It is apparent that the current diagnostic criteria in the DSM and ICD do not adequately capture the ways that personality disorders present in old age or reflect how this "shows up" in response to the challenges facing older adults and within the venues in which they are diagnosed (Rosowsky and Gurian 1992).

Personality Disorders in Older Age

What is the effect of aging on personality disorders? We know by definition that personality disorders cannot appear de novo in old age. When it appears that they do, this generally implicates that another process, for example, organic brain disease, is behind the appearance of dramatic changes in personality functioning. An alternative explanation is that we have not taken an adequate, long enough or deep enough, clinical history, as it is the history that will reveal a pattern. It is not unusual for the major manifestations of personality disorder to become relatively quiescent in mid-life, only to re-emerge in older age, exacerbated by the many stage-related challenges or by co-morbid medical illnesses (Segal et al. 2006). To complicate the diagnostic picture, there is impressive co-morbidity for personality disorders with Axis I disorders at all ages. Zweig and Agronin (2006) present co-morbidity as one of several major challenges to making the diagnosis of personality disorder in old age. For example, the Cluster C personality disorders are notably associated with depression in old age (Schneider et al. 1992). Other challenges include differentiating it from personality change due to a medical condition or reaction to medications, or from an underlying organic process, or from regressive behaviors developed in reaction to changes in the environment, or to physical illnesses that have become chronic. There is some anecdotal and empirical support for the more florid symptoms of Cluster B personality disorders to "burn out" with age (Stevenson et al. 2003). In their study of people diagnosed with borderline personality disorder, Stevenson et al. (2003) found that what did appear to "burn out" was their impulsivity. The other symptom categories (interpersonal difficulties, cognitive disturbance, affective disturbance) appeared to remain relatively untouched by age. It needs to be noted, however, that their oldest subject was 52. In a recent study of people diagnosed with borderline personality disorder (in their 30s and 40s), overall improvement as a function of age was not found. At the other extreme, personality disorder has been shown to be markedly associated with suicide in older adults (Harwood et al. 2001).

It is beyond the scope of this chapter to discuss the genesis of personality disorders. This is a complex topic including psychological, biological, and sociological contributions, including a very strong influence by genetic effects, perhaps more than for almost any Axis I disorder (Torgersen et al. 2000; Lautenschlager and Forstl 2007). Often, there has been the experience of trauma in childhood (Goodman et al. 2003; Shea et al. 2000) that can cause or worsen psychological vulnerabilities of the victim. There are those who are more vulnerable and those who are more protected. Those who are more privileged have advantages that accrue over the life course which color the aging process and support resilience, enabling thriving in later life (Collins and Smyer 2005; Schooler and Caplan 2009). Conversely, those who have struggled throughout life often continue to struggle.

Bernice Neugarten, a matriarch in the field of personality and aging, wrote "As individuals age they become increasingly like themselves…the personality structure stands more clearly revealed in an old than in a younger person"(Neugarten

1964, 198). She was referring to "ordered" personalities, but might this hold true for "disordered" personalities as well?

Are personality disorders more "clearly revealed?" Do they become worse in old age? Do they get better? Or, in terms of degree of pathology or PDism, do they remain fairly constant? The empirical literature responding to these questions is sparse and equivocal. It has been reported that with age there occurs a reduction in extraversion and in conscientiousness along with an increase in harm avoidance (Lautenschlager and Förstl 2007). The more dramatic manifestations of the Cluster B psychopathologies are reported to decrease (Lautenschlager and Förstl 2007), as do schizotypal characteristics, whereas the schizoid and obsessive-compulsive characteristics may become more evident (Engels et al. 2003; Coolidge and Merwin 1992). While clinical lore holds that the more florid symptoms of Cluster B personality disorders remit, or quiet, with age, some researchers have suggested otherwise, that personality disorders can worsen with age, including those in Cluster B (Rosowsky and Gurian 1992; Segal et al. 2001); however, the specific expression may morph into more "age-appropriate" expressions, thus denying a diagnosis according to the DSM (Rosowsky and Gurian 1992). For example, a risk-taking behavior in young adulthood could be driving fast on motorcycles without wearing a helmet. In old age, a risk-taking behavior could be smoking cigarettes while attached to an oxygen canister as a treatment for obstructive pulmonary disease.

The themes of the disorders, or at least the personality disorder clusters, also appear to be robust. For those in Cluster A, the central themes are "distant and arelational." For these types of individuals, there is a paucity of relationships in their social field which is perceived by them as being ego-syntonic. They do not yearn for connection, which distinguishes them from the avoidant personality disordered individual in Cluster C. For those in Cluster B, the themes are "erratic and chaotic." They dearly need others, indeed often have trouble tolerating being alone, but their history is marked by stormy relationships, especially intimate relationships. Cluster C themes are "dependent and needy" requiring excessive help in making decisions, reassurance, and direction. While their history may be relational, these relationships are typically difficult due to their overdependence on and clingy neediness of others.

Overall, while stability trumps change, it appears that the more "mature" personality disorders (the ones in Cluster A and obsessive-compulsive personality disorder in Cluster C) remain the most stable. The "immature" personality disorders [Cluster B personality disorders, other than antisocial personality disorder, and passive-aggressive personality disorder (removed from Cluster C in DSM IV and assigned to the Appendix awaiting further consideration)], in contrast, do appear to moderate somewhat by mid-adulthood, consistent with a "maturation hypothesis" (Tyrer 1998).

The DSM does not adequately reflect the ways clinicians identify personality disorders, especially in older adults. The DSM system was derived mostly from observations of younger adults. What is needed to make a formal diagnosis depends on a strong clinical interview, the establishment of a detailed history, including reports from multiple informants who knew the person at different stages of their life (to help identify a pattern), as well as a dimensional assessment of personality and a measure of functional impairment. As yet we do not have a valid instrument to adequately capture the geriatric presentation of personality pathology. We also do not have a clear gold standard for making the diagnosis of personality disorder in old age. In addition, there is resistance by clinicians to assign a diagnosis of personality disorder (Hillman et al. 1997). Even so, these individuals remain clinically recognizable.

Personality Disorders: Enduring Characteristics

There persists, unfortunately, reluctance on the part of clinicians to want to work with older adults, this despite the increasing need and established efficacy of treatment (Smyer et al. 1990; Joska and Fisher 2005; Rosowsky 2005). Adding to this general reluctance, those individuals with personality disorders are notorious for being especially difficult to work with, live with, and be with. In Groves' classic article, "Taking care of the hateful patient" (Groves 1978), he describes several types of patients whom physicians dread seeing. These stereotypes include "dependent clingers," "entitled demanders," "manipulative help-rejecters," and "self-destructive deniers." It is an easy reach to apply DSM personality disorder diagnoses to these types.

There are certain features of personality disorders that appear to remain essentially the same throughout sentient life. These "robust features" are what allow us to continue to recognize the disorders even where the more prototypical presentations may be altered. Before Axis II was created (DSM-III 1980), a core pattern was succinctly described by Bergmann (1978), which included the individuals' life histories, their interaction with and relationship to others, and their attitude to their current problems and challenges. This pattern remains relevant and at the heart of personality disorders at any age. What is of special significance is the effect these "disordered personalities" has on others. This is one of the central and most robust features of personality disorders throughout life. Their powerful and generally negative effect on others with whom they are in close relationship is pathognomonic of the psychopathology (Segal et al. 2006).

Other robust features are the core vulnerabilities of those with personality disorders. These include fear of fusion or abandonment, labile or inappropriate affect or affective dyscontrol (Kessler and Staudinger 2009), and a tendency to idealize or devalue others in relation to the self. Affective control is generally greater in old age (Magai and Passman 1997); there appears to be a natural limiting of arousal in the service of energy conservation and reflecting survivorship of life. Those with personality disorders, however, continue to struggle with affect modulation. The elderly individual with a personality disorder remains highly vulnerable and reactive to stress and distress (Glaser et al. 2007).

Their core vulnerabilities provide a diathesis to distress and are responded to by reliance on a repertoire of primitive defenses, such as denial, projection, reaction formation, and acting out. This is in contrast to the utilization of more mature defenses in the repertoire of resilient individuals (Simeon et al. 2007).

Individuals with personality disorders infrequently employ the loftiest defenses, for example, humor and altruism. Additionally (and a real challenge to psychotherapy), they have great difficulty with self-reflection, the ability to look back at their own behaviors and see a pattern (Yates et al. 2003). To be self-reflective and take one's self as object leaves the individual with a personality disorder open to becoming flooded with anxiety. It may be safer not to look back and see a pattern. Rather, for them, each unique event leads to new distress for which they assume little direct responsibility. This is especially difficult in old age as we recognize a universal tendency to reminisce in the service of self-continuity (and perhaps the development of wisdom). For those in Cluster B, who often suffer from a lifelong identify disturbance, this process of reminiscence (frequently encouraged in therapy) often serves to increase their despair.

Their cognitions are also often distorted and are not immune from being affected by the synergistic effects of age-related cognitive changes. Analysis of these distorted cognitions is likely to revel that they serve, albeit in a maladaptive way, either during periods of instability or following them, the individual's attempt to achieve a new balance in order to regain psychological equilibrium. The healthy, resilient, individual is able to put his energies into growing from experiences, subtly changing, as he copes with, endures and survives (self intact) the stress (or press for change). The individual with a personality disorder (i.e. the nonresilient individual), in contrast, will put his energies into resisting change, doing whatever it takes to avoid being changed by experience. As a clinician, I get concerned when an older adult announces to me at age 80, let's say, "I am exactly the same person I was at age thirty." I have to wonder what he has been doing the last 50 years! To support self-continuity, the press to "feel like me" is lifelong and exerts a powerful resistance to change, even where change is adaptive and healthy, and not to change is maladaptive and leads to distress.

Concept of Maladaptiveness

Evolutionary psychologists invite us to consider that traits or trait patterns presenting as maladaptive may have been, at some point in time, cultivated for being adaptive. In consideration of "evolutionary stable strategies" (Segal et al. 2006, 211), these traits can be understood to have enabled individuals to elevate their position in the status hierarchy and thus their reproductive status. These same principles considered at the macro level can also be considered at the micro level. For example, the excessively emotional pattern often displayed by Cluster B individuals can serve to access resources that would protect, or even elevate, their status in a given hierarchy. Consider, for example, the elderly Cluster C individual receiving rehabilitation services at home who keeps meticulous records of every therapy session, does the program precisely as ordered and exactly at the preferred time and interval. In another context, say a rehabilitation facility, his insistence on this degree of precision would likely lower his status.

Of essential consideration is that the notion of maladaptiveness, or adaptiveness, is not an independent construct solely dependent on the individual. Whether a core trait or trait pattern is adaptive or maladaptive depends on factors outside the individual, including referents and adjudicators. Svrakic et al. (2008) in suggesting that the clinical category "disorders of adaptation" replace "personality disorders" notes that the "disorder" is not wholly subscribable to the individual, but rather the context, or environment, plays a role in the expressed behavior being adaptive or not. In addition, there is the need of "someone" to identify and label (adjudicate) the behavior as adaptive or maladaptive, and this is cohort, stage, and context informed as well as what the individual presents. This concept has been described as a model of "goodness of fit" between the "personality" and tasks (what is being asked of it), and contexts (where) [see a full discussion in Segal et al. (2006)]. Following this concept, core personality traits that were once adaptive now, in old age, may be maladaptive or, conversely, that were once maladaptive may now be adaptive.

While well-being and happiness have been shown to be quite stable in old age (Collins and Smyer 2005), and most adults, quite wonderfully, adapt well to the challenges of late life, those with personality disorders do not. Commonly occurring stressors, for example, include the need to rely on strangers for care (whether this be temporary or permanent), to relocate to a new environment (whether this be "elected" or "mandated"), to experience the loss of social supports (whether by death, relocation, or lack of access), and loss of power and control. The experience of stress reflects to a significant degree, how the stressor is perceived and appraised as to how well the individual anticipate he can cope with it (Rossi et al. 2007). Specific personality disorders can be expected to have more trouble with some stressors than with others. For example, "reliance on strangers for care" is especially onerous to the individual with schizoid, paranoid, schizotypal, or avoidant personality disorder. The key is that the particular challenge, or accrual of challenges, overwhelms their ability to cope, exceeding the resources, internal and external, that they can bring to bear.

Table 3.1 presents several challenges often faced by older adults and how certain core personality traits and trait patterns can be expected to be adaptive or maladaptive.

Extraversion: A moderate degree of extraversion in old age appears to be optimal. Too much and the usual aloneness that accompanies old age is experienced as loneliness, as stressful, and often intolerable. Too little and the requisite ability to relate to others is compromised. The talents of many in Cluster B in terms of extraversion can be used adaptively to engage others to help; a charming, colorful interactional style can be used as a highly adaptive coping style. Introversion marks the opposite end of the trait continuum.

Dependence: While dependence is often less valued during the industrious midlife years, it appears to increase in value, and is often actually quite adaptive, in old age. Autonomy, dependency, and reciprocity all relate to resilience, especially in older age. What is most adaptive is that the individual be able to tolerate a reasonable degree of dependence, where appropriate, and to be able to reciprocate, thus converting the dependent relationship into one of mutual interdependence.

Table 3.1 Table of frequent challenges in old age and adaptive/maladaptive core personality traits

Challenge/demand	Adaptive trait(s)	Maladaptive trait(s)
Relocation to new environment	Openness, conscientiousness	Extraversion, introversion
Required changes in self-care	Conscientiousness	Dramatic/histrionic
Reliance on strangers for care	Dramatic/histrionic extraversion	Dependent, arelational (Cluster A), avoidant
Lessening of control/power	Dependent	Narcissistic
More time spent alone	Introversion, conscientiousness	Extraversion, narcissistic, borderline, histrionic
Loss of support	Cluster A	Clusters B and C

Some individuals with personality disorder (notably Cluster A) cannot relate to others and engage them to help. Some (notably Cluster C) are overly dependent and prone to regress in terms of functional ability when they become even more dependent on others (this is not unusual to observe following admission to a nursing home). Some individuals with Cluster B personality disorders, most notably borderline personality disorder, have extreme difficulty tolerating the closeness that comes with needing others and depending on them, often rejecting the person and pushing them too far away, only to be dissatisfied with that option too.

Narcissism: Healthy narcissism is critical to maintaining a sense of self-continuity, especially when, as in old age so much conspires to challenge this. However, extreme narcissistic traits and the manifest behaviors are off-putting and come to deny the care and caring of others. It is not the healthy narcissism, which, in the service of shoring up the battered ego, is problematic. Rather it is that the person goes about securing the necessary nutrients to shore up the self in a way that is practically guaranteed to have the opposite effect. In contrast, the resilient individual would be able to shift approaches in order to secure what he needs from another individual or from systems of care. The individual with a personality disorder continues to do the same maladaptive song and dance, only doing it louder and stronger when it does not have the desired effect.

Conscientiousness: This refers to achievement- or goal-direction and organization. It is manifested through self-discipline, self-control, and perseverance versus laissez-faire behavior and impulsivity. In the extreme, this pattern describes the classic workaholic. In moderation (or a bit more), it is often highly adaptive. (Consider trying to get through graduate school without being high in conscientiousness.) However, also consider what might happen when an older highly conscientious individual comes to need to rely on others who may not be as conscientious? How does she secure the requisite level of care to meet her own conscientiousness needs? The way this is done, and the result of this, comes to define whether her efforts are adaptive or maladaptive.

Openness: This refers to the individual's receptiveness to new ideas, experiences, and approaches. This receptivity is applied to creating ways to address challenges in novel but appropriate ways (*aka* adaptive). The individual with a personality disorder embraces a very narrow repertoire of responses, cognitively, affectively and behaviorally; stereotypically a "Johnny-one-note." If the response "fits" in terms of the challenge and context of the challenge it is adaptive, if not then it is maladaptive. The old adage "a little goes a long way" can be applied to personality traits. It is the extreme traits (Svrakic et al. 2008) or inappropriately applied traits that come to define what is maladaptive.

Resilience: Features and Challenges

This entire volume is devoted to a review of what we know about resilience in old age and what questions are raised. Many academicians have addressed, in work theoretically and empirically based, the concept of resilience in old age (Bergeman and Wallace 1999; Staudinger and Fleeson 1996; Windle et al. 2008). There have emerged significant, creative and well-considered differences of course, but there does appear an apparent consensus as well and that is this: the resilient older adult is able tolerate the vicissitudes of aging, defray the overhead of growing old, better than others, from whom these extract far greater cost. Those with personality disorders pay the most dearly.

We recognize that there are biological, psychological, and social contributions to resilience whether these are considered as a style of adaptation (Yates et al. 2003), explanatory processes, competencies or outcomes, and that resilience is often defined by how it is operationalized (Svrakic et al. 2008; Leipold and Werner 2009). The concept of psychological resilience suggests that resilience directly reflects a pattern of personality traits, which are mainly stable (Asendorpf and van Aken 1999; Weed et al. 2006; Windle et al. 2008). Most define resilience as the ability to bounce back and recover after a major stress or negative life event (Tugade et al. 2004; Windle et al. 2008; Smith et al. 2008; Rossi et al. 2007). The aspects within a whole construction of resilience, assessed by measures developed to do so, include many "items" relating to personality traits (Smith et al. 2008; Bartone et al. 1989). Often considered, for example, are self-efficacy, self-esteem, self-confidence, self-discipline, self-control, and self-acceptance (Rutter 1987; Masten 1999; Ryff and Singer 1996). A common substrate or core appears to be a gestalt incorporating personal competence, self-esteem, and interpersonal control (Windle et al. 2008); in older age, resilient individuals have access to psychological resources, which allow and enable these. As we have discussed, those with a personality disorder are among the least resilient, the least hardy, the least able to handle the challenges of aging.

Resilience in older adults may be different than in younger adults, and not only because of differences in what is being *asked* of the individual. Lamond et al. (2008) studied predictors of resilience in older women using the Connor–Davidson Resilience Scale (CD-RISC) and reported somewhat different findings than those previously reported for younger adults using this scale. For both populations, the CD-RISC scores were positively correlated with task-focused coping strategies and negatively with emotion-focused coping. However, with older women the scores were also associated with *tolerance for negative affect* and *adaptability*, the lack of which are hallmarks of personality disorders. Kessler and Staudinger (2009) found that negative arousal decreased from middle age to older age and that older subjects evidenced advantage in perceived affect regulation.

Three Major Functions of Resilience (and How These Relate to Personality Disorders)

Aging is accompanied by many losses: health, financial security, functional abilities, roles, and relationships. Psychologically healthy older adults manage these losses well (Collins and Smyer 2005). In contrast, older adults with personality disorders do not manage losses well. For example, loss of personal control can be expected to be especially difficult for those in Cluster B who also may have extreme difficulty tolerating negative affect. Those personality disorders marked by chronic anger, hostility, and suspiciousness evidence impaired physical resilience (Smith 2006) as well as impaired psychological resilience.

Personality has been clearly shown to relate to exposure and reactivity to stressors (Stawski et al. 2008). As noted, individuals with personality disorders are inherently more vulnerable to stress than are other individuals. As such, their reserves of resources (internal and external) for coping are tapped more frequently and more extensively. In contrast, the resilient individual is able to (1) avoid avoidable stressors, (2) cope with stressors that are not avoidable, and (3) equilibrate or "bounce back" from stressors that have been experienced.

Avoidance

The ability to avoid stressors is less frequently discussed as an aspect of resilience in the literature than is coping or re-equilibrating, but it may have special relevance to the individual with a personality disorder. Consider that the core of these disorders is vulnerability of the self. Therefore, all aspects that resilience depends upon will be vulnerable. This essential vulnerability is what is measured by the Neuroticism (N) factor of the Big Five (McCrae and Costa 1990); a high N is a marker of a vulnerable personality. Consider also that self-efficacy, self-esteem, self-confidence, self-discipline, self-control, self-acceptance, all depend upon a reasonably intact and integrated self. Some types of personality disorder are known for not only avoiding stress where possible, but rather their lives reflect a history of having courted stress and chaos. The borderline personality disorder quickly comes to mind, but also consider the individual with avoidant personality disorder. She or he has suffered distress by being arelational while yearning for relationality, thereby increasing the experience of stress (this is in contrast to the individual in

Cluster A for whom the arelational experience is ego-syntonic). In a discussion of the mechanisms of association between personality and physical health, one of the models proposed by Smith (2006) is the "transactional stress moderation model" which posits that personality influences, not only reactions to stresses, but also exposure to stresses "through decisions to enter or avoid situations, unintentional evocation of responses from other persons, and intentional impacts on others" (p. 225). Those with personality disorders cannot save themselves nor can they stay away from deep and troubled waters.

Coping

There are also protective resources that serve to mediate between the stressor and what is done to regulate the stress, including both internal and external resources (Pearlin and Skaff 1995). With age, such protective resources become ever more important (Rossi et al. 2007). One such internal source of mediation is the way in which the individual is prone to appraise stressors (Rossi et al. 2007), whether these are as challenges, hassles, or threats. Nonresilient responses to stressors have been demonstrated to describe more severe stressors than those demonstrating resilient responses (Hildon et al. 2008). The way the individual responds reflects the individual's prior history with coping in general, coping with like events, a felt sense of current vulnerability (which can be impacted by current health status), as well as what resources he believes he can bring to meet the demand. This is consistent with the "interactional stress moderation model" (Smith 2006), which suggests that personality influences both the appraisal of and coping responses to stressful experiences.

Resources the resilient individual brings to dealing with the challenge rely upon their internal and external resources (Hildon et al. 2008). Some ways of coping are strictly cognitive, for example, constructing a narrative that allows them to revisit and reconstruct previous experiences in ways that can guide and support their ability to deal with current ones. While well-being is generally stable in old age, self-esteem has been shown to be more variable (Collins and Smyer 2005). A more highly developed cognitive structure can be important in the maintenance of support of self-esteem. In addition, keeping up with one's usual social activities and continuing one's social roles can be useful. Facing challenges, individuals often rely on ongoing relationships, including spiritual relationships; being able to lean on others for guidance and strength during times of adversity and stress. The individual with a personality disorder will likely have an impoverished, chaotic, and conflicted social network, people unavailable or unwilling to be relied upon to help.

Re-equilibration ("Bouncing Back" and "Re-centering")

Recovery from stress involves a self-regulation process which incorporates the abilities to control emotions and to "choose" (volition, motivation, cognition)

(Beckmann and Kellmann 2004) to re-center after the event has been experienced. It also incorporates the (now past) experience in such a way as to reinforce self-continuity and a sense of survivorship. These processes, culminating in the integration of the experience or re-centering, depend in large measure upon the individual's abilities to reflect, observe a pattern, take this pattern as object for evaluation, and acknowledge one's role in it. Being able to do so further defines the resilient individual. This also defines where the individual with a personality disorder is likely to fail. In their consideration of the concept of resilience as a critical aspect of a conceptual bridge between coping and development, Leipold and Werner (2009) suggest that the process of coping, coming through life experiences, contributes to the individual's development even without outward manifestations of change; the individual has arrived at a new centered state.

Clinical Utility: Implications for Treatment

Personality disorders do not in the main "go away" in old age. They continue to affect treatment, albeit while the disorder is often left unaddressed in a treatment plan. This omission is likely to result in significant challenges to the treatment, compromising its efficacy or outright dooming it to failure (Devanand et al. 2000). Those with personality disorders in general have difficulty creating a therapeutic alliance, are prone to terminate treatment prematurely, and are less compliant with treatment protocols than are those without personality disorder.

In addition, the individual with a personality disorder functions "as if" in accordance with certain rules which contribute to making any treatment in the service of change very difficult. These putative rules operate to direct or govern his thoughts, feelings, and behaviors. One rule is that the personality traits are, even when causing or contributing to his distress, ego-syntonic. To him, whether or not they are maladaptive is not the issue. Rather, the issue is to maintain his center "as is." This is the press for "feel like me-ness," and, even if frankly counter-productive, he will do what needs to be done to get the response he needs (from others, from the system, the environment) in order to restore or reinforce this position. This "rule" is behind a question I've often heard in consultation: "If he knows this makes people so angry at him, why does he continue to do it?" He continues to "do it" because the response he gets confirms his center and, to him, "feels like me." In addition, he has limited flexibility to shift his responses, a limited repertoire of responses to call upon, and limited ability to accommodate and integrate what change that does occur. He is, the elderly individual with a personality disorder, nonresilient.

Another "rule" is that the press for change is externalized, characterized by the perception: "I'm not the problem. The problem is out there." Yet another rule is that what problems, issues, or stressors occur are, each one, unique; there is no pattern to the individual's involvement in them. She feels that what she does is the only right response possible, so is closed to the possibility of change. And finally, personality disorder respects a rule of an illusion of uniqueness. This defines a major distinction between the Axis I and I disorder. Personality disorders are not experienced by the individual as episodic or adventitious, as is the case with other clinical conditions. Rather, they *are* the individuals, and this includes how they are reacted to. As noted earlier in the chapter, the effect (and thus responses to the effect) they have on others is a central and robust feature of personality disorder throughout life (Segal et al. 2006).

How might this concept of personality disorders behaving "as if" rule-governed guide or inform treatment? Are there ways in which resilience might be trained or enhanced? To begin, the requirements for treatment or intervention would need to respect these rules. In addition, as consistent with any offer of treatment with older adults, what is offered needs to be clearly relevant to what the individual comes to treatment for, to respect the individual's self-resources (time, money, energy), to appear doable, and to predict a positive effort/benefit balance.

Treatment involving the older individual with a lifelong personality disorder may in addition have special goals.

Relief of symptoms: A study by assessed the congruence between dyads of experienced mental health clinicians and their older adult patients with personality disorders regarding the symptoms presented and distress caused by these symptoms. They found that the patients reported greater distress from their symptoms than what was attributed to them by their clinicians. Above all, any treatment offered must first address the relief of symptoms experienced by the patient. While pharmacological treatment is not designed to address the personality disorder itself, it is often a reasonable first line of treatment to address manifest symptoms and relieve distress from frequent co-morbid conditions, primarily anxiety and mood disorders but also transient psychosis, agitation, and impulsivity. Psychological treatment, in addition, has the goal of helping the individual accommodate what change is necessary and helping him to adjust to a new reality without (to the extent possible) forcing upon him a new, unrecognizable sense of self. The ideal intervention, of course, would be effortless, seamless, and invisible. Alas!

While it would be cruel (and perhaps unethical) to compel an individual to see the pattern that *is* his personality has lead to his misery, how he has been responsible for this, and how this pattern has caused misery and pain throughout his life, it is a goal of treatment to give the individual tools to reduce "excess misery" in the future. Consider this in terms of the functions of resilience discussed.

Avoidance: Can she be led to see "trouble down the road"? Can she be helped to use past experiences to think about/talk about how she could be able to see this? Can she brainstorm ways she might be able to avoid trouble? This approach does not require that she shift her attribution of the source of the trouble, or force ownership of it, but it focuses rather on empowering her ability to have some control over the situation; that trouble often just does not "happen." If she can *see* it she might be able to *avoid* it, even if she attributes the cause to being "out there."

Coping: The vicissitudes of aging are legend; some "troubles" cannot be avoided. A guided review of how he has coped in the past is a good place to begin. The next step could be identifying what has worked and what has not worked. A more refined next step could be identifying what has worked for specific challenges, in specific contexts, etc. A psychoeducational piece can be helpful by setting out a smorgasbord of coping options; identifying which ones have been considered and tried before and which have not. A skill-building piece can follow this nicely. The therapy has now served to expand the repertoire of coping/responding to stressors. For example, for those with affective dyscontrol, the role play can be used to intensify the affect while simple behavioral techniques for stress reduction can be used to reduce the affect.

It is beyond the scope of this chapter to discuss specific psychotherapies, but the use of the therapeutic encounter as a microcosm of the real world of the patient has special relevance for the patient with a personality disorder. The clinician's response to the patient, in psychoanalytic parlance the countertransference, is, as has been noted, a core and robust feature of the disorder. This can be used to understand the patient's experience of the world and the world's experience of the patient. This helps illuminate what is maladaptive. The countertransferential response can be positive or negative. For example, feelings of heightened protectiveness are often in response to someone with a dependent personality disorder. Feelings of intimidation or conversely of omnipotence can be in reaction to the individual with a narcissistic personality disorder. A response of extreme frustration, a feeling of being manipulated, might be in response to the borderline character. The essential point is that the reaction is not just ambient noise in the treatment but rather can be used to understand the phenomenology of the patient and guide the treatment.

There are certain recommendations, which can be made whatever specific psychotherapy is used. The therapy should be focused, directive, active, cooperative, engaging, supportive, and encouraging of self-efficacy and responsibility. The common goals are to address the specific (here and now) problem(s), improve essential interpersonal relations (those relevant to the problem), limit maladaptive responses, expand the response repertoire, and coach the selection of responses to improve the probability of their being adaptive.

Re-centering: This phase or function incorporates a number of aspects including reviewing the experience ("What occurred?"); reviewing the response ("What did you think? Feel? Do?"); and evaluating the response ("What happened?" "Did it work for you? Did you get what you needed or wanted?"). If "yes," then the next phase is to reinforce the response as under her control and as adaptive. If "no," then the next phase is to generate alternative responses, which might have been more adaptive. The goal of the final phase is to help the patient integrate and assimilate the experience, achieving a new center. This defines the processes of "working through" and effecting closure. An ideal outcome would be that the individual comes to trust that, as life continues on, one can change *and* remain the same.

Conclusion

There are numerous challenges inherent to growing older, to becoming old. It is the resilient individual who can survive what are often frank assaults on one's integrity and sense of self. The individual with a lifelong personality disorder is less equipped to handle life at any stage, but perhaps especially in old age which is a stage defined by having inexorably run out of time to do it over again. For all of us our personalities are ego-syntonic, and actually may define this. For the individual whose way of being in the world has repeatedly caused distress and impaired successful functioning in important life spheres, it is still ego-syntonic. Adaptive or maladaptive, there is a fierce press to remain our essential selves throughout life. It is hard to change. It becomes even more difficult to change with advanced age. For those who are historically change aversive, those whom we recognize as being more rigid than flexible, the need for change, indeed multiple changes, in late life can be experienced as intolerable. In addition, for those with a lifelong personality disorder, their relationships with others are often the source and focus of their distress. At a time in life when the ability to secure and tolerate mutual interdependence becomes the coin of the realm, they are impoverished. Limited external resources mirror their limited internal resources.

Old age is also a time in life marked by uncertainty, both concrete and existential. Uncertainty itself is a handmaiden of old age, and for the individual with a personality disorder, uncertainties are experienced as distress and pain.

As we understand personality disorders, we recognize that they reflect biological irregularities, and are shaped by the environment, life experiences, and the process of aging. The particular interaction of innate and external factors conspires to lead to maladaptive manifestations of the personality traits, be they affective, cognitive, or behavioral. These then contribute to impaired functioning and the experience of distress.

Changes with advancing age include biological changes, and the accrual of challenges and losses, including the loss of roles and relationships, which had, earlier, in life, served to contain, mediate, and attenuate the expressions of the psychopathology. The synergistic effect of aging and a personality disorder serves organically to intensify the rigidity of the affects, cognitions, and behaviors even as the lifelong press for self-continuity goes on (Hooker 2000).

What is adaptive in old age is the ability to achieve a balance between maintaining one's antonymous functional integrity, where reasonably able, and effecting mutual independence with others, where reasonably necessary. It is of course at this juncture of interpersonal relationships where the older adult with a personality disorder can be expected to have the greatest difficulty.

Resilience in old age can continue to be operationalized as the ability to avoid avoidable stressors, cope with those that cannot be avoided, and be able to bounce back to a prior level of functioning but with a new, more evolved center of self. A resilient old dog can learn new tricks and be able to use them adaptively. In old age, resilience often means calling in all of one's chips to shore up overly challenged internal resources. The good news, as the research informs us, is that psychologically healthy older adults, even in advanced old age, are able to fare remarkably well.

References

American Psychiatric Association (APA). (1980). Diagnostic and statistical manual of mental disorders (3rd ed.). Washington, DC: American Psychiatric Association.

Ames, A., & Molinari, V. (1994) Prevalence of personality disorder in community-living elderly. *Journal of Geriatric Psychiatry and Neurology*, 7, 189–194.

Asendorph, J., & van Aken, M. (1999) Resilient, overcontrolled, and undercontrolled personality prototypes in childhood: Replicabilty, predictive power, and the trait-type issue. *Journal of Personality and* Social Psychology, 77, 815–832.

Balsis, S., Segal, D., & Donahue, C. (in press) Revising the personality disorder criteria for DSM-V: Considering the later life context. *American Journal of Orthopsychiatry*.

Bartone, P., Ursano, R., Wright, K., & Ingraham, L. (1989) The impact of a military air disaster on the health of assistance workers: A prospective study. *Journal of Nervous and Mental Disease*, 177, 317–327.

Beckmann, J., & Kellmann, M. (2004) Self-regulation and recovery: Approaching an understanding of the process of recovery from stress. *Psychological Reports*, 95, 1135–1153.

Bergeman, C., & Wallace, K. (1999) Resiliency in later life. In T. Whitman, T. Merluzzi, & R. White (Eds.), *Life-span perspectives on heath and Illness* (pp. 207–223). Mahwah, NJ: Lawrence Erlbaum Associates.

Bernstein, D., Iscan, C., & Maser, J. (2007) Opinions of personality disorder experts regarding the DSM-IV personality disorders classification system. *Journal of Personality Disorders*, 21(5), 536–551.

Cohen, B., Nestadt, G., Samuels, J., Romanoski, A., McHugh, P., & Rabins, P. (1994) Personality disorder in later life: A community study. *British Journal of Psychiatry*, 165, 493–499.

Collins, A., & Smyer, M. (2005) The resilience of self-esteem in late adulthood. *Journal of Aging and Health*, 17(4), 471–489.

Coolidge, F., & Merwin, M. (1992) Reliability and validity of the Coolidge Axis II Inventory: A new inventory for the assessment of personality disorders. *Journal of Personality Assessment*, 59, 223–238.

Costa, P., & McCrae, R. (1988) Personality in adulthood: A 6-year longitudinal study of self-reports and spouse ratings on the NEO personality inventory. *Journal of Personality and Social Psychology*, 54(5), 853–863.

Devanand, D., Turret, N., Moody, B., Fitzsimmons, L., Peyser, S., Mickle, K., et al. (2000) Personality disorders in elderly patients with dysthymic disorders. *American Journal of Geriatric Psychiatry*, 8, 188–195.

Engels, G., Duijsens, I., Haringsma, R., & van Putten, R. (2003) Personality disorders in the elderly compared to four younger age groups: A cross-sectional study of community residents and mental heath patients. *Journal of Personality Disorders*, 17(5), 447–459.

Glaser, J., Van Os, J., Mengehers, R., & Myin-Germeys, I. (2007) A momentary assessment study of the reported emotional phenotype associated with borderline personality disorder. *Psychological Medicine*, 38(9), 1231–1239.

Goodman, M., Weiss, D., Koenigsberg, H., Kotlyarevsky, V., Neu, A., Mitropoulou, V., et al. (2003) The role of childhood trauma in differences in *affective* instability in those with personality disorders. *CNS Spectrums*, 8(10), 763–770.

Groves, J. (1978) Taking care of the hateful patient. *New England Journal of Medicine*, 298(16), 883–887.

Harwood, D., Hawton, K., Hope, T., & Jacoby, R. (2001) Psychiatric disorder and personality factors associated with suicide in older people: A descriptive and case-control study. *International Journal of Geriatric Psychiatry*, 16(2), 155–165.

Hildon, Z., Smith, G., Netaveli, G., & Blane, D. (2008) Understanding adversity and resilience at older ages. *Sociology of Health and Illness*, 30(5), 726–740.

Hillman, J., Stricker, G., & Zweig, R. (1997) Clinical psychologists' judgments of older adult patients with character pathology: Implications for practice. *Professional Psychology: Research and Practice*, 28(2), 179–183.

Hooker, K. (2000) New directions for research in personality and aging: A comprehensive model for linking levels, structures and processes. Paper presented at the Annual Meeting of the Gerontological Society of America, Washington, DC.

Jang, K., Taylor, S., & Livesley, W.J. (2006) The University of British Columbia twin project: Personality is something and personality does something. *Twin Research and Human Genetics*, 9(6), 739–742.

Joska, J., & Fisher, A. (2005) The assessment of need for mental health services. *Social Psychiatry and Psychiatric Epidemiology*, 40, 529–539.

Kegan, R. (1982) *The evolving self*. Cambridge, MA: Harvard University Press.

Kessler, E.M., & Staudinger, U. (2009) Affective experience in adulthood and old-age: The role of affective arousal and perceived affect regulation. *Psychology and Aging*, 24(2), 349–362.

Lamond, A., Depp, C., Allison, M., Langer, R., Reichstadt, J., Moore, D., et al. (2008) Measurement and predictors of resilience among community-dwelling older women. *Journal of Psychiatric Research*, 43(2), 148–154.

Lautenschlager, N., & Förstl, H. (2007) Personality change in old age. *Current Opinions in Psychiatry*, 20, 62–66.

Leipold, B., & Werner, G. (2009) Resilience: A conceptual bridge between coping and development. *European Psychologist*, 14(1), 44–50.

Magai, C., & Passman, V. (1997) The interpersonal basis of emotional behavior and emotion regulation in adulthood. *Annual Review of Geriatrics and Gerontology*, 17, 104–137.

Magnavita, J. (2004) Classification, prevalence, and etiology of personality disorders: Related issues and controversy. In J. Magnavita (Ed.), *Handbook of personality disorders: Theory and practice* (pp. 3–23). Hoboken, NJ: Wiley.

Masten, A. (1999) Resilience comes of age: Reflections on the past and outlook for the next generation of research. In M. Glantz & L. Jeanette (Eds.), *Resilience and development: Positive life adaptations. Longitudinal research in the social and behavioral sciences* (pp. 281–296). Dordrecht, Netherlands: Kluwer-Academic.

McCrae, R., & Costa, P. (1990) *Personality in adulthood*. New York: Guilford.

Neugarten, B. (1964) *Personality in middle and late life: Empirical studies*. Oxford: Atherton Press.

Pearlin, L., & Skaff, M. (1995) Stressors and adaptation in late life. In M. Gatz (Ed.), *Emerging issues in mental health and aging* (pp. 97–123). Washington, DC: American Psychological Association.

Rosowsky, E. (2005) Ageism and professional training in aging: Who will be there to help? *Generations*, 29, 55–58.

Rosowsky, E., & Gurian, B. (1992) Impact of borderline personality disorder in late life on systems of care. *Hospital and Community Psychiatry*, 43, 386–389.

Rossi, N., Bisconti, T., & Bergeman, C. (2007) The role of dispositional resilience in regaining life satisfaction after the loss of a spouse. *Death Studies*, 31, 863–883.

Rutter, M. (1987) Psychosocial resilience and protective mechanisms. *American Journal of Orthopsychiatry*, 57(3), 316–331.

Ryff, C., & Singer B. (1996) Psychological well-being: Meaning, measurement and implications for psychotherapy research. *Psychotherapy and Psychosomatics*, 65, 14–23.

Schneider, L., Zemansky, M., Berden, M., & Sloane, R. (1992) Personality in recovered depressed elderly. *International Psychiatry*, 4, 177–185.

Schooler, C., & Caplan, L. (2009) How those who have, thrive: Mechanisms underlying the well-being of the advantaged in later life. In H. Bosworth & C. Hertzog (Eds.), *Aging and cognition: Research methodologies and empirical advances* (pp. 121–141). Washington, DC: APA.

Segal, D., Hook, J., & Coolidge, F. (2001) Personality dysfunction, coping style and clinical symptoms in younger and older adults. *Journal of Clinical Geropsychology*, 7, 201–212.

Shea, M., Zlotnick, C., Dolan, R., Warshaw, M., Phillips, K., Brown et al. (2000) Personality disorders, history of trauma, and posttraumatic stress disorder in subjects with anxiety disorders. *Comprehensive Psychiatry*, 41(5), 315–325.

Simeon, D., Yehuda, R., Cunill, R., Knutelska, M., Putnam, F., & Smith, L. (2007) Factors associated with resilience in healthy adults. *Psychoneuroendocrinology*, 32(8–10), 1149–1152.

Small, B., Hertzog, C., Hultsch, D., & Dixon, R. (2003) Stability and change in adult personality over 6 years: Findings from the Victoria Longitudinal Study. *Journal of Gerontology: Psychological Sciences*, 58B(3), 166–176.

Smith, T. (2006) Personality as risk and resilience in physical health. *Current Directions in Psychological Science*, 15(5), 222–231.

Smith, B., Dalen, J., Wiggins, K., Tooley, E., Christopher, P., & Bernard, J. (2008) The brief resilience scale: assessing the ability to bounce back. *International Journal of Behavioral Medicine*, 15(3), 194–200.

Smyer, M., Zarit, S., & Qualls, S. (1990) Psychological intervention with the aging individual. In J. Birren & K. Schaie (Eds.), *Handbook of the psychology of aging*, 3rd ed. (pp. 373–40). San Diego, CA: Academic.

Staudinger, U., & Fleeson, W. (1996) Self and personality in old and very old age: A sample case of resilience? *Development and Psychopathology*, 8(4), 867–885.

Stawski, R., Sliwinski, M., Almeida, D., & Smyth, J. (2008) Reported exposure and emotional reactivity to daily stressors: The roles of adult age and global perceived stress. *Psychology and Aging*, 23(1), 52–61.

Stevenson, J., Meares, R., & Comerford, A. (2003) Diminished impulsivity in older patients with borderline personality disorder. *American Journal of Psychiatry*, 160, 165–166.

Svanborg, P., Gustavsson, P., Mattila-Evenden, M., & Asberg, M. (1999) Assessment of maladaptiveness: A core issue in the diagnosing of personality disorders. *Journal of Personality Disorders*, 13(3), 241–256.

Svrakic, D., Lecic-Toseviski, D., & Divac-Janovic, M. (2008) DSM Axis II: Personality disorders or adaptation disorders? *Current Opinion in Psychiatry*, 22, 111–117.

Tackett, J., Quilty, L., Sellbom, M., Rector, N., & Bagby, M. (2008) Additional evidence for a quantitative hierarchical model of mood and anxiety disorders for DSM-V: The context of personality structure. *Journal of Abnormal Psychology*, 4, 812–825.

Torgersen, S., Lygren, S., Quien, P., Ingunh, S., Onstad, S., Evardsen, J., et al. (2000) A twin study of personality disorders. *Comprehensive Psychiatry*, 41, 416–425.

Tyrer, P. (1998) Feedback for the personality disordered. *Journal of Forensic Psychiatry*, 9, 1–4.

Tugade, M., Fredrickson, B., & Barrett, L. (2004) Psychological resilience and positive *emotional granularity*: examining the benefits of positive emotions on coping and health. *Journal of Personality*, 77(6), 1161–1190.

Valliant, G. (2002) Aging well. Boston: Little, Brown.

Van Alphen, S., Engelen, G., Kuin, Y., & Derksen, J. (2006) The relevance of a geriatric sub-classification of personality disorders in the DSM-V. *International Journal of Geriatric Psychiatry*, 21, 205–209.

Wakefield, J. (2008) The perils of dimensionalization: Challenges in distinguishing negative traits from personality disorders. *Psychiatric Clinics of North America*, 31(3), 379–393.

Wallace, K., Bisconti, T., & Bergeman, C. (2001) The mediational effect of hardiness on social support and optimal outcomes in later life. *Basic and Applied Social Psychology*, 23, 267–279.

Weed, K., Keough, D., & Borkowski, P. (2006) Stability of resilience in children of adolescent mothers. *Journal of Applied Developmental Psychology*, 27, 60–77.

Widiger, T., & Lowe, J. (2008) A dimensional model of personality disorder: Proposal for DSM-V. *Psychiatric Clinics of North America*, 31(3), 363–378.

Windle, G., Markland, D., & Woods, R. (2008) Examination of a theoretical model of psychological resilience in older age. *Aging & Mental Health*, 12(3), 285–292.

Yates, T., Egeland, B., & Sroufe, L. (2003) Rethinking resilience: A developmental process perspective. In S. Luthar (Ed.), *Resilience and vulnerability: Adaptation in the context of childhood adversities* (pp. 243–266). New York: Cambridge University Press.

Zautra, A., Finch, J., Reich, J., & Guarnaccia, C. (1991) Predicting the everyday life events of older adults. *Journal of Personality*, 59(3): 507–538.

Zivian, M., Larsen, W., Knox, J., Gekoski, W., & Hatchette, V. (1992) Psychotherapy for the elderly: Psychotherapists' preferences. *Psychotherapy: Theory, Research, Practice, Training*, 29(2), 668–674.

Zweig, R., & Agronin, M. (2006) Personality disorders in late life. In M. Agronin & G Maletta (Eds.), *Principles and practice of geriatric psychiatry*, (pp. 449–446). Philadelphia: Lippincott, Williams & Wilkins.

Chapter 4
What Do We Know About Resilience in Older Adults? An Exploration of Some Facts, Factors, and Facets

Phillip G. Clark, Patricia M. Burbank, Geoffrey Greene,
Norma Owens, and Deborah Riebe

Introduction

As the field of gerontology has become better established and developed more historical perspective and interdisciplinary depth, we can note a progression in thinking about concepts and theories of aging, what the experience of getting older means, and how it can be shaped as a process (e.g. Bengtson et al. 2008). Conceptual theses generate antitheses resulting in syntheses and new directions for research. So it is with the development of the concept of resilience with respect to older adults. Just as early research characterizing "normal" aging led to the excitement and enthusiasm surrounding the concept of "successful" aging, so, too, has this latter concept given way to the more recent concept of "resilience" in aging.

Similarly, conceptualizing the concept itself has presented unique potentials and pitfalls, as has been examined in the earlier chapters in this handbook. Is resilience a personality trait, a process, or both? Is it a single trait or actually part of a larger constellation of related personal characteristics? Does it remain constant or change over time? Seeking answers to these questions is both complicated and facilitated by the use of different disciplines and research methodologies to study the concept of resilience. This research effort has recently generated statements about the pressing need to deconstruct the essence of resilience and "interrogate the social, cultural, and economic dimensions that shape it" (Becker and Newsom 2005, 221).

As mentioned, in this context it is interesting to note how the early and subsequent articulation of the concept of "successful aging" (Rowe and Kahn 1987, 1997) gave way to criticism of its highly individualistic biases and disregard of the broader social, economic, political, and environmental dimensions and determinants of health in old age (Holstein and Minkler 2003). Some researchers now suggest that resilience might be a preferable concept to the more well-established one of successful aging, because it represents a more reasonable and attainable goal for most older adults (Hildon et al. 2010). The biopsychosocial approach to research

P.G. Clark (✉)
University of Rhode Island, Kingston, RI, USA
e-mail: aging@uri.edu

B. Resnick et al. (eds.), *Resilience in Aging: Concepts, Research, and Outcomes,*
DOI 10.1007/978-1-4419-0232-0_4, © Springer Science+Business Media, LLC 2011

on successful aging suggested by Inui (2003) includes studies of resilience and generativity.

Additionally, factors that influence or are, in turn, affected by resilience are also subjects for study and research. For example, what is the relationship between resilience and psychological well-being, physical health, social support, and economic resources? Additionally, how is our interpretation of resilience shaped by our understanding of factors both internal and external to the individual, as studied by different research traditions in gerontology (e.g. qualitative vs. quantitative)? It has been said that, "we don't see things as they are; we see things as we are" [Anaïs Nin, as cited in Baldwin (2000, xii)], and so it is with the concept of resilience and its interrelated facets.

The purpose of this chapter is to provide a framework for sorting out these complex and sometimes conflicting relationships, in a way that both broadens and deepens our understanding of the factors associated with resilience and its importance for older adults. In particular, we employ an interdisciplinary approach, highlighting the important contributions that different fields of study make to an understanding of the facts, factors, and facets surrounding this emerging concept. If, as suggested above, "we see things as we are," then differing views and perspectives are needed to assemble a complete and accurate understanding of any multifaceted and multidimensional concept.

Developing a Metaphor

Thinking metaphorically can be helpful in furthering our understanding of, and insights into, complex and complicated concepts. A metaphorical representation can provide new avenues of understanding to guide both research and application. Metaphor-based approaches may be particularly useful in gerontology, shedding new light on interdisciplinary correlations and connections (Kenyon et al. 1991).

Buffers of Old Age

Early research on resilience as a general concept suggested that it be thought of as a "buffer" between adversity and negative outcomes (Rutter 1987), a term that had already been used previously in epidemiological research in gerontology to interpret some significant health-related outcomes from the involuntary relocation of older adults in the community (Kasl et al. 1980; Ostfeld 1985). In this research, the "buffers of old age" included such external factors as social support (having a child living within a 50-mile radius) and internal factors as life meaning (having a sense of oneself as a religious person).

The concept of "buffers of old age" has reappeared again more recently in the gerontological literature (e.g. Wagnild 2003; Wagnild and Young 1993; Windle et al. 2008) to describe protective factors that seem to mediate between stressful or adverse events and consequent behaviors or protective responses. This concept may be considered to capture both "intrinsic" factors, such as personality traits of flexibility, and "extrinsic" elements, such as social support. In terms based on Bourdieu's (1986) capital framework, resilience includes elements of both human capital (i.e. resources within the person) and social capital (e.g. social networks and support) that can be used to convert resources into adaptive responses (Harris 2008; Netuveli et al. 2008).

Resilience Repertoire

The metaphor we would like to propose in this chapter as a framework for exploring factors related to resilience in older adults is that of a "resilience repertoire," i.e. a supply of skills and resources that can be used to moderate "the bad things that happen" in the lives of older adults to reduce or blunt the negative consequences of those events, or even in some cases to lead to positive growth and development (Hardy et al. 2002). Individuals may have a variety of factors or elements in their repertoire and use them in differing ways at different times and in varying circumstances. There is thus a contextual and dynamic aspect to resilience over time and across an individual's lifespan (Kinsel 2005).

In addition, there can be cumulative or additive effects involved, such as when adverse events or challenges become compounded or chronic and create a greater element of risk for negative outcomes (Hildon et al. 2008). As Netuveli et al. (2008) suggest, "The resilient [are] ordinary people, without superpowers, as indicated by the fact that as adversities add up the probability of resilience decreases; resilience does not imply invulnerability" (p. 990).

Finally, there is a dimension to resilience suggesting that one's repertoire is a part of their life story or personal narrative, a theme of growing importance and relevance in gerontology generally (Birren et al. 1996; Kenyon et al. 2001, 2010). In this instance, the meaning assigned by individuals to life events and adversity, and how this meaning is incorporated into their ongoing development of self-identity to maintain constancy and continuity across their lifespan, can itself become a resource in the face of life's adversity (Collins and Smyer 2005; Hildon et al. 2010). As Windle et al. (2008) point out in the area of psychological resilience, such divergent theorists of aging as Erikson et al. (1986) and Kaufman (1986) both underscore the importance of the continuing development of the self across the life span and the emergence of life themes and wisdom as a key component of resilience in old age.

Meaning in life has been identified as an important dimension of resilience among adults and older adults in several studies. For example, Heisel and Flett (2008) identified perceived meaning in life as a factor related to resilience, and found that it explained significant variation in suicide ideation over and above physical and mental health problems. Having meaning and meaningful relationships was identified as a theme in an exploratory study of resilience among adults who have experienced mental illness (Edward et al. 2009). Meaning-making was also found to be essential to resilience in Greene and Graham's (2009) study of Nazi Holocaust survivors, and in Gosselink and Myllykangas' (2007) research on older women living with HIV/AIDS. Overcoming loneliness through maintaining connections to others was found to be key to resilience for older widowers after the death of their spouses (Crummy 2002). Taken together, these studies support the earlier work by Burbank (1992) that meaning in life – especially meaning in relationships with others, spirituality, and activities – is key to health and resilience.

Research on the related and earlier concept of "stamina" by Colerick (1985) reinforces the importance of understanding an older individual's life history and how adversity has been addressed previously and incorporated into current experience. In this research, stamina is characterized by five different dimensions, based on the analysis of extensive interview data: (1) capacity for growth, (2) personal insight, (3) life perspective, (4) likelihood of functional breakdown, and (5) general competence. Both good physical health over the entire life history and greater levels of educational attainment were related to higher stamina. These findings are significant, because they emphasize the need for a life course perspective on resilience and suggest the possibility of a resilience "trajectory" in old age based on previous experiences of coping with challenges in one's life. Cumulatively, these life experiences may enrich and enhance one's repertoire for dealing with continued adversity as one grows older and faces the likelihood of increasing losses associated with advancing age.

These aspects of the "resilience repertoire" can be used as a conceptual framework for understanding the factors linked by research to an understanding of the adaptive responses to adversity that may help to protect adults from some of the losses and challenges of growing older.

Stressors and Adversities

Perhaps not unexpectedly, the research on resilience seems to emphasize the responses by older adults to life events more than the specific, in-depth understanding of the dimensions of these events themselves. This may not be surprising, given the fact that research on stress has suggested that it is not so much the event itself that may be stressful, as the meaning or significance of the event to the individual and the larger context in which it occurs (Hardy et al. 2002; Masuda and Holmes 1978).

Ryff et al. (1998) have suggested that resilience in later life be focused on the potential of older adults to maintain their mental health in the face of threat or risk. Some gerontological research has specifically been directed toward determining the types of adversities that can be expected with increasing age and that therefore may serve as the basis for stressors. For example, Hildon et al. (2008) suggest that "adversity [centers] on limited circumstances and opportunities brought about by physical, mental, or social losses" (p. 737), which are most often related to the death or illness of a loved one, one's own poor health, or circumstances in retirement. They also propose a temporal dimension to understanding adversity, and recommend capturing changes in these domains over multiple years and based on deteriorating health, increased stress, and worsening life circumstances. There is some suggestion that resilience may be more prevalent among the old–old than among young–old adults (Mehta et al. 2008; Seplaki et al. 2006).

In this research in particular, health issues play a central role. For example, Netuveli et al. (2005, 2006) have reported that poor or declining health reduces the quality of life of older adults, particularly when it results in physical impairment or functional limitation. Hildon et al. (2010) extend this insight by demonstrating that the experience of adversity is magnified by the more limiting effects of health problems, such as impacts on activities of daily living (ADL). In addition, they may be less easily managed and be experienced as problems that have become compounded and gotten worse over time.

Hardy et al.'s (2002) research specifically assessed stressful life events among community-dwelling older adults, and it was found that among their subjects 18% identified a personal illness or injury, 42% the death of a family member or friend, 23% the illness or injury of a family member or friend, and 17% a nonmedical event over the previous 5 years. The last category included such events as victimization and changing residence, as well as events affecting another family member (such as divorce or the unemployment of a child). A significant finding from this research is that medical and nonmedical events may be of equal importance in their impact on the lives of older adults.

More recent research by Hildon et al. (2010) defined the adversities examined as "being limited by ill health or (in the past 5 years) deteriorating health, having more stress, changing life circumstances, being worse off financially, and experiencing a negative or difficult event such as bereavement" (p. 39). Importantly, they also suggested that negative life events, including both bereavement and retirement, may be acute or chronic. For example, the death of a spouse can continue to interfere with the daily routine of the survivor, serving as a constant and ongoing reminder of the loss. In their research, they found that 34.5% of respondents had experienced worse health, 33.3% more stress, 23% worse life circumstances, 40.8% limiting illness, 19.5% worse finances, and 71.3% had had a negative life event in the past 5 years.

Enriching these results and insights into the circumstances of adversity are studies focusing on specific types of stressors. For example, the experience of illness has been explored in the context of dementia (Harris 2008) and serious chronic conditions (Becker and Newsom 2005). Importantly, the latter study added the dimension of ethnicity to the need for a complete understanding of the role of a life course perspective within the broader cultural, social, and economic context of adversity, a theme also captured in other research (e.g. Felten 2000). Still other studies have gone into more depth in exploring the circumstances surrounding adversity in bereavement and widowhood (e.g. Bonanno et al. 2004).

The collective importance of these studies is that they draw attention to questions about the nature or types of stressors, the possibility of additive or cumulative effects of adversity, and its duration and whether it is acute or chronic. Each of these aspects may create very different and challenging experiences for older adults, depending on their total set of life circumstances and resources for coping.

Specific Components of the Resilience Repertoire

The focus of this discussion will not include the personality- or trait-related factors in one's resilience repertoire, as these are topics considered by other authors in this book. Rather, this chapter focuses on those elements related to the two broad categories of health and social and economic factors that can be characterized as part of the individual's personal supply of resources for coping with adversity.

Health Resources

There are five aspects of health that are relevant to a discussion of resilience: (1) health status, (2) health promotion, (3) physical activity, (4) nutrition, and (5) medication compliance and personal medicine.

Health Status

Older adults are sometimes quoted as saying, "if you have your health in old age, you have everything," based on the insight that good health is a major instrumental resource in achieving other important life goals and outcomes. Poor health and resultant functional limitations can, indeed, become a barrier and a challenge in reaching a whole host of other objectives in one's life as an older adult.

Consequently, in much of the current resilience research, (poor) health tends to be addressed more as a factor in causing adversity than as a response to it. An exception is the early research on stamina by Colerick (1985), suggesting that high levels of self-reported physical health that extend back over one's life history are correlated with increased levels of stamina in old age. A "life pattern" of self-perceived good health seems to equip an individual with important resources for facing some of the potential challenges of growing older.

Additional studies extend this insight by suggesting that it is not so much the level of health status or absence of health problems, but rather how health is defined and viewed by the individual that is important. This finding is consistent with the now widely recognized phenomenon that older adults "overestimate" their self-reported health compared to "objective" measures of their health status. Even under these circumstances, however, there does not seem to be a clear-cut correlation between resilience and self-reported or perceived health.

For example, Nygren et al. (2005) found that there was no correlation between scores on a variety of psychological measures of resilience, sense of coherence, purpose in life, and self-transcendence in relation to perceived physical health. In contrast, Hardy et al. (2004) determined that good to excellent self-rated health was associated with high resilience. Interestingly, in their study Hildon et al. (2008) found that participants with resilient outcomes rarely talked about health-related limitations and did not dwell on them.

In summary, it seems not to be the case in every instance that health status constitutes a major resource in an older adult's resilience repertoire; rather, it is the way in which health problems are viewed and given meaning by the individual that is important. More research is certainly needed here to clarify apparent opposite findings and to shed more light on the role that health plays as a component of the resilience repertoire.

Health Promotion

A focus not found in the previous research literature on resilience, yet one having increasing importance for the future in terms of reducing the prevalence of chronic disease and functional impairment, is that of health promotion with older adults and its interrelationship with reducing risk and increasing resilience (Smith et al. 2004). This topic draws on a life course perspective, suggesting the importance of a long history of established healthy behaviors, a point emphasized earlier in the literature on stamina (Colerick 1985). An emphasis on health promotion is based on the assumption that appropriately designed interventions can improve or maintain health status and thereby enhance resilience in older adults (Luthar and Cicchetti 2000).

For example, pilot research by Clark et al. (2009) suggests that interventions may be successfully developed for older adults to maintain key elements of healthy lifestyle – such as exercise and diet – and thereby buffer them from "going off track" in these behaviors in response to a range of setbacks associated with aging. Anchored in the concepts and methods of selective optimization with compensation (Schulz and Heckhausen 1996) and goal-setting (Gebhardt and Maes 2001), such interventions may promote and support the internal processes used by individuals to acquire or maintain healthy behaviors (Prochaska et al. 1992; Prochaska and Velicer 1997).

Initial findings from this intervention research suggest that there may be different types of trajectories of maintaining positive behavioral patterns in the face of risks for "going off track" (followed by their relative proportions in the participant pool): (1) those older adults readily maintaining behaviors (50%), (2) those benefiting from guidance in coping with adversity (25%), (3) those stymied by adversity (15%), and (4) those with low motivation to maintain behaviors or participate in the intervention (10%). Identifying those vulnerable individuals for whom resilience to adverse events might be strengthened has important implications for targeting future interventions.

Physical Activity

A geriatrician colleague of the authors talks to his patients about the importance of their "making daily deposits into their exercise account" to build up their physical reserve capacity upon which to draw if they become sick or hospitalized – much like financial deposits in a bank account provide needed resources in an economic downturn. This expression captures the importance of physical activity in one's resilience repertoire.

A lifetime of regular physical activity strengthens a broad range of physiological systems in older adults, which influence health and well-being, chronic disease development, and functional capacity. Regular physical activity provides many health benefits, including reduced coronary risk, higher bone density, greater muscle mass, lower risk of falls, less body fat, and slower development of disability in old age (American College of Sports Medicine 2009). Research also suggests that physical activity levels are associated with cognitive resilience, including faster reaction times, improved psychological well-being, and reduced risk of cognitive decline and dementia (Hogan 2005).

With regard to the effects of acute care, hospital stays impose a degree of immobility on patients, often resulting in functional decline that begins as early as the second day (Hirsh et al. 1990). In a study of over 1,200 community-dwelling older adults hospitalized for acute illnesses, 31% experienced a decline in their ability to perform ADL between preadmission and time of hospital discharge (Sager et al. 1996). During hospitalization, those with the greatest loss in ADL are most likely to be admitted to a nursing home (Rudberg et al. 1999). Individuals who are physically active have higher levels of functional ability and may be better able to tolerate a hospital stay with no loss in the ability to perform ADL.

Indeed, research findings suggest that "prehabilitation," a program to enhance functional exercise capacity in older adults before surgery to minimize postoperative morbidity, is feasible (Carli and Zavorsky 2005). Moreover, other research indicates that walking more than four hours per week is associated with a significantly reduced risk of hospitalization for cardiovascular disease in older men and women, allowing individuals to avoid the negative functional outcomes of hospital stays (LaCroix et al. 1996).

Physical activity also contributes to resilience via psychosocial pathways. It is associated with improvements in psychological health and well-being, including reduced levels of perceived stress and a lower risk of depression and anxiety (American College of Sports Medicine 2009; Starkweather 2007; Taylor-Piliae et al. 2005). Social support may also play an important role in improvements in overall well-being. In one study, improved social relations were related to increased satisfaction with life and reductions in loneliness in sedentary older adults who participated in an exercise program (McAuley et al. 2000). In another study of community-dwelling older adults by Talsma (1995), physical function, psychological function, and well-being were all supported as dimensions of resilience. Physical activity, aerobic exercise, and community involvement were significantly related to resilience and moderated the effects of chronic conditions on resilience.

Finally, the relationship between physical activity and self-efficacy is also well established. In a literature review, McAuley and Katula (1998) concluded that most exercise intervention studies in older adults result in improvements in both self-efficacy for physical activity and physical fitness. Self-efficacy contributes to the maintenance of physical activity and physical function, particularly in those who are at risk for functional decline, allowing them to carry out basic self-care activities when their ability to do so is challenged (Mendes de Leon et al. 1996).

Nutrition

Healthful dietary and activity patterns have been associated with a reduction in mortality among the elderly as well as a reduction in the rate of cognitive decline (Feart et al. 2009; Knoops et al. 2004; Mitrou et al. 2007). Dietary patterns characterized by consumption of a variety of such nutrient-dense foods as fruits and vegetables appear to be most protective. This pattern could be conceptualized as building up a "nutritional bank account." The 2005 Dietary Guidelines for Americans (USDHHS/USDA 2005) recommend that older adults select a variety of nutrient-dense foods. On the other hand, inadequate dietary intake (protein-energy undernutrition) can lead to a loss of muscle mass with a negative effect on the performance of ADL (Sharkey et al. 2004) as well as an increased risk of mortality (Mahan and Escott-Stump 2008). Age-related loss of taste sensitivity (Shaffer and Tepper 1994), depression, lack of access to food, social isolation, and bereavement are other factors associated with inadequate intake (Mahan and Escott-Stump 2008). Simple interventions such as providing an additional meal or a companion at meals have been effective in increasing intake in homebound older adults (Locher et al. 2005).

Another factor is the presence of chronic diseases leading to dietary restrictions often related to inadequate dietary guidance provided by health care providers (Shatenstein 2008). The dietary pattern associated with inadequate intake is one of low dietary variety and limited consumption of nutrient-dense foods (Roberts et al. 2005). Although there has been little research focusing on nutrition-related resilience in older adults, a qualitative study by Greaney and colleagues found that disruption in routine, illness, and loss were cited as reasons for relapse. Those who were resilient cited determination and willpower as important in returning to healthful eating patterns (Greaney et al. 2004).

Medication Compliance and Personal Medicine

For older adults, the analysis of medications taken to manage chronic illnesses can serve as a proxy measure of complex and overlapping medical conditions that threaten independence. Adherence to complex medication regimens is presumed to be all-important to managing a person's chronic conditions, causing recovery or stabilization from disease symptoms and helping to promote well-being. However, an approach to a patient with a chronic illness that focuses on sickness alone will oftentimes miss adaptive strategies that individuals use to maintain good health.

The adaptive steps individuals take to maintain health and well-being have been referred to as "personal medicine" (Deegan 2005). Personal medicine includes activity that gives meaning and purpose to one's life, such as participating in hobbies, helping others, and performing one's work and family role. Personal medicine is also a self-care strategy when individuals perform activities, such as exercise or socializing, that they recognize help them to feel better.

The concept of personal medicine also includes noncompliance to medication when the person believes that the medication interferes with life activities that are meaningful. For instance, a medication used to treat hypertension that causes dizziness and impairs mobility so that an individual can no longer complete a meaningful activity in his or her life may not be accepted. Medication nonadherence, as a coping skill and a component of self-efficacy, is an important example of resilience in adults. Unfortunately, the concept of individual nonadherence to medications that is consistent with health promotion is not well developed or well studied. Health care providers must try to incorporate a person's treatment and health goals into the medical care plan. Understanding activities that individuals value, as well as self-initiated interventions that people use to control disease and disease symptoms, will identify important outcomes of treatment.

Social and Economic Resources

There are three aspects of social and economic resources that are relevant to a discussion of resilience: (1) social support, (2) activities, and (3) finances.

Social Support

Social support has emerged consistently as a major component of resilience. The term "social capital" has been used to describe the resources involving social support and networks that can be employed to buffer older adults from adversity (Netuveli et al. 2008). For example, these same researchers found that, "The only variable that was consistently related to resilience was social support, measured in terms of having people who can be trusted and who will offer help, comfort, and appreciation, especially in a crisis" (p. 989). Importantly, it appeared that support before and during adversity, rather than after and in response to it, was the important factor. Earlier research on stamina has also highlighted the importance of support available from close family members, such as spouses and confidants (Colerick 1985).

The specific element of personal relationships as a factor in social support has also been highlighted. Hildon et al. (2008) suggest that a key factor in weathering life events is the recognition of the availability of help and those who can be relied on for it. In their study both resilient and nonresilient groups, in fact, relied on family, friends, and neighbors for socializing and sometimes practical support.

The key difference between the groups was related to the nature of the impacts of the loss of a loved one or the consequences of health problems.

In addition to relationships, integration into the community, suggesting placement of the older adult within a web of supportive relationships, has emerged as an important variable. In the research by Hildon et al. (2010), a good sense of community was related to "having a lot of friendly neighbors," "people looking out for each other," "a good community spirit," and "having a good mix of people." Community integration was also captured through involvement in paid employment, voluntary work, or community organizations. Expanding on the theme of webs and networks, Netuveli et al. (2008) state that, "resilience is to be found in the warp and woof of family and civic society" (p. 990), suggesting through a weaving metaphor the importance for resilience of an integrated and interwoven set of relationships that make up the very fabric of a community.

Activities

In addition to social support, the concept of activities in which older adults may be engaged seems relevant to resilient responses to adversity. For example, using activities diaries, Hildon et al. (2008) found that study participants with resilient outcomes reported nearly twice as much involvement in leisure or household activities that took place alone than those in the vulnerable outcome group. In related research on successful aging, a higher level of daily activity (e.g. reading, listening to the radio, and visiting with family) was associated with greater self-reported levels of successful aging (Montross et al. 2006), and ultimately with increased happiness, better functioning, and lower mortality (Menec 2003).

Finances

Hildon et al. (2010) specifically studied the role that financial or economic resources (including home ownership) might play in moderating adversity or enhancing quality of life among older adults. Somewhat paradoxically, their research determined that worsening financial circumstances were not significantly related to negative changes in quality of life in their older adult cohort, nor were adequate or more than adequate financial resources considered a protective factor in facing adversity. Their conclusion was that "insufficient income may not be as threatening and indeed sufficient income may not be as protective as other, perhaps less tangible, circumstances" (p. 9), such as social support.

Discussion and Conclusions

It is clear that the concept of resilience is multifaceted and multidimensional, a dynamic relationship between, on the one hand, stressors and adversities in the environment and, on the other, responses and reactions to them from an older adult. In understanding this complex interplay of factors and forces, it is essential that we approach the topic of resilience from an integrative and interdisciplinary perspective, much as the field of gerontology in general deals with the issues of aging.

Research on the stress and adversity side of the equation includes consideration of health and mental health status and maintenance, and includes losses and changes in these factors over time. In particular, impacts creating impairment and functional limitation in ADL are important. Additionally, such losses as those associated with bereavement and relocation represent nonmedical factors that may be as important as those related to health. In all these stressors, it is essential that we consider the broader social, cultural, and economic contexts represented by gender, ethnicity, and class. Additive or cumulative effects over time, as well as acute vs. chronic conditions, are also aspects that must be taken into account. Finally, resilience has temporal and developmental aspects, and depends on the individual's interpretation of his or her life situation, experience, and resources.

On the other side of the resilience equation, the metaphor of resilience "repertoire" has been suggested as a way to understand the supply of skills and resources that can be used to moderate the impacts of stressors and adversities on the individual, and even lead to positive growth and development. The emergence of the meaning of life events for the individual, set against the backdrop of their own personal story or narrative that gives life continuity and meaning, is especially relevant here. In this regard, the skills and resources in one's repertoire are organized, selected, and wielded in unique ways that depend on the individual's values and themes that give his or her life integrity and meaning in a very personal way.

As an element in the resilience repertoire, health status may be important as a factor filtered through the individual's perception, but the research on its importance seems to be mixed in understanding its relationship to resilience. However, a life course perspective on healthy behaviors and health promotion does seem to be relevant to reducing risk and increasing resilience, suggesting a way of examining the concept through a life trajectory approach introducing the possibility of intervention to change its slope and even direction. In particular, physical activity and nutrition have a strong research base of evidence linking these two health behaviors to the development of a "reserve account" upon which the individual may draw when such health-related events as illness or hospitalization occur. In addition, the concept of "personal medicine" as an extension of individual health behavior captures elements of activities that give one's life meaning and purpose, linked to self-efficacy and self-care, in support of feeling well.

Finally, there is a substantial and well-documented literature on the importance of social support for an individual's ability to weather life's crises. Turning to friends, family, neighbors, and others during such times has consistently been shown to provide critical resources for an older adult in coping with life's adversities. In a larger sense, being part of a community, of a web of supportive relationships, is the essential ingredient in support. Having meaningful activities on a daily basis, whether pursued alone or with others, is another facet of the psychosocial factors related to resilience.

In conclusion, investing in one's human and social capital may be seen as a critical element in supporting an individual's ability to weather life's crises and to cope with adversities. An understanding of the different factors that go into one's resilience repertoire can suggest areas for potential interventions to support and enhance it. In this sense, examining the facts, factors, and facets of resilience in older adults can lead to designing ways to develop and enhance it to promote an individual's quality of life into old age – a worthy goal, indeed!

References

American College of Sports Medicine (2009) Exercise and physical activity for older adults. *Medicine and Science in Sports and Exercise, 41,* 1510–1530.

Baldwin, D. C. (2000) Foreword. In T. J. K. Drinka & P. G. Clark, *Health care teamwork: Interdisciplinary practice and teaching.* Westport, CT: Auburn House/Greenwood.

Becker, G., & Newsom, E. (2005) Resilience in the face of serious illness among chronically ill African Americans in later life. *Journals of Gerontology: Social Sciences, 60B,* S214–S223.

Bengtson, V. L., Gans, D., Putney, N., & Silverstein, M. (Eds.) (2008) *Handbook of theories of aging* (2nd Edition). New York: Springer.

Birren, J. E., Kenyon, G. M., Ruth, J.-E., Schroots, J. J. F., & Svensson, T. (Eds.) (1996) *Aging and biography: Explorations in adult development.* New York: Springer.

Bonanno, G. A., Wortman, C. B., & Nesse, R. M. (2004) Prospective patterns of resilience and maladjustment during widowhood. *Psychology and Aging, 19,* 260–271.

Bourdieu, P. (1986) The forms of capital. In J. G. Richardson (Ed.), *The handbook of theory and research for the sociology of education* (pp. 241–258). New York: Greenwood Press.

Burbank, P. M. (1992) Meaning in life among older adults: An exploratory study. *Journal of Gerontological Nursing, 18*(9), 19–28.

Carli, F., & Zavorsky, G. S. (2005) Optimizing functional exercise capacity in the elderly surgical population. *Current Opinions in Clinical Nutrition and Metabolic Care, 8,* 23–32.

Clark, P. G., Riebe, D., Greene, G., & Mlinac, M. (November 2009). Active maintenance of healthy lifestyles: Understanding and promoting resilience in the face of aging's challenges. Symposium presented at the 62nd Annual Scientific Meeting of the Gerontological Society of America, Atlanta, GA.

Colerick, E. J. (1985) Stamina in later life. *Social Science and Medicine, 21,* 997–1006.

Collins, A. L., & Smyer, M. A. (2005) The resilience of self-esteem in late adulthood. *Journal of Aging and Health, 17,* 471–489.

Crummy, D. B. (2002) *Resilience: The lived experience of elderly widowers following the death of a spouse.* Unpublished doctoral dissertation, University of San Diego.

Deegan, P. E. (2005) The importance of personal medicine: A qualitative study of resilience in people with psychiatric disabilities. *Scandinavian Journal of Public Health, 33*(Suppl. 66), 29–35.

Edward, K., Welch, A., & Chater, K. (2009) The phenomenon of resilience as described by adults who have experienced mental illness. *Journal of Advanced Nursing, 65,* 587–595.

Erikson, E. H., Erikson, J. M., & Kivnick, H. Q. (1986) *Vital involvement in old age.* New York: W. W. Norton.

Feart, C., Samieri, C., Rondeau, V., Amieva, H., Portet, F., Dartigues, J. F., Scarmeas, N., & Barberger-Gateau, P. (2009) Adherence to a Mediterranean diet, cognitive decline, and risk of dementia. *Journal of the American Medical Association, 302,* 638–648.

Felten, B. S. (2000) Resilience in a multicultural sample of community-dwelling women older than age 85. *Clinical Nursing Research, 9,* 102–123.

Gebhardt, W. A., & Maes, S. (2001) Integrating social-psychological frameworks for health behavior research. *American Journal of Health Behavior, 25*, 528–536.

Gosselink, C. A., & Myllykangas, S. A. (2007) The leisure experiences of older U.S. women living with HIV/AIDS. *Health Care for Women International, 28*, 3–20.

Greaney, M. L., Lees, F. D., Greene, G. W., Clark, P. G. (2004) What older adults find useful for maintaining healthy eating and exercise habits. *Journal of Nutrition and the Elderly, 24*, 19–35.

Greene, R. R., & Graham, S. A. (2009) Role of resilience among Nazi Holocaust survivors: A strength-based paradigm for understanding survivorship. *Family and Community Health, 32*(15 Suppl. 1), S75–S82.

Hardy, S. E., Concato, J., & Gill, T. M. (2002) Stressful life events among community- living older persons. *Journal of General Internal Medicine, 17*, 841–847.

Hardy, S. E., Concato, J., & Gill, T. M. (2004) Resilience of community-dwelling older persons. *Journal of the American Geriatrics Society, 52*, 257–262.

Harris, P. B. (2008) Another wrinkle in the debate about successful aging: The undervalued concept of resilience and the lived experience of dementia. *International Journal of Aging and Human Development, 67*, 43–61.

Heisel, M. J., & Flett, G. L. (2008) Psychological resilience to suicide ideation among older adults. *Clinical Gerontologist, 31*(4), 51–70.

Hildon, Z., Montgomery, S. M., Blane, D., Wiggins, R. D., & Netuveli, G. (2010) Examining resilience of quality of life in the face of health-related and psychosocial adversity at older ages: What is "right" about the way we age? *Gerontologist. 50*, 36–47.

Hildon, Z., Smith, G., Netuveli, G., & Blane, D. (2008) Understanding adversity and resilience at older ages. *Sociology of Health and Illness, 30*, 726–740.

Hirsh, C. H., Simmers, L., Mullen, L., & Winograd, C. H. (1990) The natural history of functional morbidity in hospitalized older patients. *Journal of the American Geriatrics Society, 38*, 1296–1303.

Hogan, M. (2005) Physical and cognitive activity and exercise for older adults. *International Journal of Aging and Human Development, 60*, 95–126.

Holstein, M. B., & Minkler, M. (2003) Self, society, and the "new gerontology." *Gerontologist, 43*, 787–796.

Inui, T. S. (2003) The need for an integrated biopsychosocial approach to research on successful aging. *Annals of Internal Medicine, 139*(5) (Part 2), 391–394.

Kasl, S. V., Ostfeld, A. M., Brody, G. M., Snell, L., & Price, C. A. (1980) Effects of 'involuntary' relocation on the health and behavior of the elderly. In S. G. Haynes & M. Feinleib (Eds.), *Second conference on the epidemiology of aging* (pp. 211–232). NIH Publication No. 80-969. Bethesda, MD: National Institutes of Health.

Kaufman, S. R. (1986) *The ageless self: Sources of meaning in late life.* Madison, WI: University of Wisconsin Press.

Kenyon, G., Birren, J., & Schroots, J. J. F. (Eds.) (1991) *Metaphors of aging in science and the humanities.* New York: Springer.

Kenyon, G., Bohlmeijer, E., & Randall, W. (Eds.) (2010) *Storying later life: Issues, investigations, and interventions in narrative gerontology.* New York: Oxford University Press.

Kenyon, G., Clark, P., & de Vries, B. (Eds.) (2001) *Narrative gerontology: Theory, research, and practice.* New York: Springer.

Kinsel, B. (2005) Resilience as adaptation in older women. *Journal of Women and Aging, 17*, 23–39.

Knoops, K. T., de Groot, L. C., Kromhout, D., Perrin, A. E., Moreiras-Varela, O., Menotti, A., & van Staveren, W. A. (2004) Mediterranean diet, lifestyle factors, and 10-year mortality in elderly European men and women. *Journal of the American Medical Association, 292*, 1433–1439.

LaCroix, A. Z., Leveille, S. G., Hecht, J.A., Grothaus, L. C., & Wagner, E. H. (1996) Does walking decrease the risk of cardiovascular disease hospitalizations and death in older adults? *Journal of the American Geriatrics Society, 44*, 113–120.

Locher, J. L., Robinson, C. O., Roth, D. L., Richie, C. S., & Burgio, K. L. (2005) The effect of the presence of others on caloric intake in homebound older adults. *Journals of Gerontology: Medical Sciences, 60A*, M1475–M1478.

Luthar, S. S., & Cicchetti, D. (2000) The construct of resilience: Implications for interventions and social policies. *Development and Psychopathology, 12*, 857–885.

Mahan, L. K., & Escott-Stump, S. (2008) *Krause's food and nutrition therapy* (12th Ed.). St. Louis, MO: Elsevier.

Masuda, M., & Holmes, T. H. (1978) Life events: Perceptions and frequencies. *Psychosomatic Medicine, 40*, 236–261.

McAuley, E., Blissmer, B., Marquez, D. X., Jerome, G. J., Kramer, A. F. & Katula, J. (2000) Social relations, physical activity and well-being in older adults. *Preventive Medicine, 31*, 608–617.

McAuley, E., & Katula, J. (1998) Physical activity interventions in the elderly: Influence on physical health and psychological function. In M. P. Schultz & L. R. Maddox (Eds.) *Annual review of gerontology and geriatrics* (pp. 115–154). New York: Springer.

Mehta, M., Whyte, E., Lenze, E., Hardy, S. A., Roumani, Y., Subashan, P., Huang, W., & Studenski, S. (2008) Depressive symptoms in later life: Associations with apathy, resilience, and disability vary between young-old and old-old. *International Journal of Geriatric Psychiatry, 23*, 238–243.

Mendes de Leon, C. F., Seeman, T. E., Baker, D. I., Richardson, E. D. & Tinetti, M. E. (1996) Self-efficacy, physical decline, and change in functioning in community-living elders: A prospective study. *Journals of Gerontology: Social Sciences, 51B*, S183–S190.

Menec, V. H. (2003) The relation between everyday activities and successful aging: A 6-year longitudinal study. *Journals of Gerontology: Social Sciences, 58B*, S74–S82.

Mitrou, P. N., Kipnis, V., Thiebault, A. C., Reedy, J., Subar, A. F., Wirfalt, E., Flood, A., Mouw, T., Hollenbeck, A. R., Leitzmann, M. F., & Schatzkin, A. (2007) Mediterranean dietary pattern and prediction of all-cause mortality in a U.S. population. *Archives of Internal Medicine, 167*, 2461–2468.

Montross, L. P., Depp, C., Daly, J., Reichstadt, J., Golsban, S., Moore, D., Sitzer, D., & Jeste, D. (2006) Correlates of self-rated successful aging among community-dwelling older adults. *American Journal of Geriatric Psychiatry, 14*, 43–51.

Netuveli, G., Blane, D., Hildon, Z., Montgomery, S. M., & Wiggins, R. D. (2006) Quality of life at older ages: Evidence from the English Longitudinal Study of Ageing (Wave 1). *Journal of Epidemiology and Community Health, 60*, 357–363.

Netuveli, G., Wiggins, R. D., Hildon, Z., Montgomery, S. M., & Blane, D. (2005) Functional limitation in long standing illness and quality of life: Evidence from a national survey. *British Medical Journal, 331*, 1382–1383.

Netuveli, G., Wiggins, R. D., Montgomery, S. M., Hildon, Z., & Blane, D. (2008) Mental health and resilience at older ages: Bouncing back after adversity in the British Household Panel Survey. *Journal of Epidemiology and Community Health, 62*, 987–991.

Nygren, B., Alex, L., Jonsen, E., Gustafson, Y., Norberg, A., & Lundman, B. (2005) Resilience, sense of coherence, purpose in life, and self-transcendence in relation to perceived physical and mental health among the oldest old. *Aging and Mental Health, 9*, 354–362.

Ostfeld, A. (1985) *Between disease and death: The buffers of older age.* Paper presented in a symposium on old age and freedom. Providence, RI: Brown University.

Prochaska, J. O., DiClemente, C. C., & Norcross, J. C. (1992) In search of how people change: Applications to addictive behavior. *American Psychologist, 47*, 1102–1114.

Prochaska, J. O., & Velicer, W. F. (1997) The transtheoretical model of health behavior change. *American Journal of Health Promotion, 12*, 38–48.

Roberts, S. B., Hajduk, C. L., Howarth, N. C., Russell, R., McCroy, M. A. (2005) Dietary variety predicts low body mass index and inadequate macronutrient and micronutrient intakes in community-dwelling older adults. *Journals of Gerontology: Medical Sciences, 60A*, M613–M621.

Rowe, J. W., & Kahn, R. L. (1987) Human aging: Usual and successful. *Science, 237*, 143–149.

Rowe, J. W., & Kahn, R. L. (1997) Successful aging. *Gerontologist*, *37*, 433–440.

Rudberg, M. A., Sager, M. A., & Zhang J. (1999) Risk factors for nursing home use after hospitalization for medical illness. *Journals of Gerontology: Medical Sciences*, *51A*, M189–M194.

Rutter, M. (1987) Psychosocial resilience and protective mechanisms. *American Journal of Orthopsychiatry*, *57*, 316–331.

Ryff, C. D., Singer, B., Love, G. D., & Essex, M. J. (1998) Resilience in adulthood and later life: Defining features and dynamic processes. In J. Lomrantz (Ed.), *Handbook of aging and mental health* (pp. 69–96). New York: Plenum Press.

Sager, M. A., Franke, T., Inouye, S. K. Landefeld, C. S., Morgan, T. M., Rudberg, M. A., Sebens, H., & Winograd, C. H. (1996) Functional outcomes of acute medical illness and hospitalization in older persons. *Archives of Internal Medicine*, *156*, 645–652.

Schulz, R., & Heckhausen, J. (1996) A life span model of successful aging. *American Psychologist*, *51*, 702–714.

Seplaki, C. L., Goldman, N., Weinstein, M., & Lin, Y. H. (2006) Before and after the 1999 Chi-Chi earthquake: Traumatic events and depressive symptoms in an older population. *Social Science and Medicine*, *61*, 3121–3132.

Shaffer, S. E., & Tepper, B. J. (1994) Effects of learned flavor cues on single meal and daily food intake in humans. *Physiology and Behavior*, *55*, 979–986.

Sharkey, J. R., Branch, L. G., Giuliani, C., Zohoori, M., & Haines, P. S. (2004) Nutrient intake and BMI as predictors of severity of ADL disability over 1 year in homebound elders. *Journal of Nutrition and Healthy Aging*, *8*, 131–139.

Shatenstein, B. (2008) Impact of health conditions on food intakes among older adults. *Journal of Nutrition for the Elderly*, *27*, 333–361.

Smith, T. W., Orleans, C. T., & Jenkins, C. D. (2004) Prevention and health promotion: Decades of progress, new challenges, and an emerging agenda. *Health Psychology*, *23*, 126–131.

Starkweather, A. R. (2007) The effects of exercise on perceived stress and IL-6 levels among older adults. *Biological Research for Nursing*, *8*, 186–194.

Talsma, A. N. (1995) *Evaluation of a theoretical model of resilience and select predictors of resilience in a sample of community-based elderly*. Unpublished doctoral dissertation, University of Michigan.

Taylor-Piliae, R. E., Haskell, W. L., Waters, C. M., & Froelicher, E. S. (2005) Change in perceived psychosocial status following a 12-week Tai Chi exercise programme. *Journal of Advanced Nursing*, *54*, 313–329.

U.S. Department of Health and Human Services (USDHHS)/U.S. Department of Agriculture (USDA), Dietary Guidelines Advisory Committee (2005) *Dietary guidelines for Americans* (6th Edition). Washington, DC: U.S. Government Printing Office.

Wagnild, G. (2003) Resilience and successful aging: Comparison among low and high income older adults. *Journal of Gerontological Nursing*, *29*, 42–49.

Wagnild, G. M., & Young, H. M. (1993) Development and psychometric evaluation of the resilience scale. *Journal of Nursing Measurement*, *1*, 165–178.

Windle, G., Markland, D. A., & Woods, R. T. (2008) Examination of a theoretical model of psychological resilience in older age. *Aging and Mental Health*, *12*, 285–292.

Chapter 5
Psychological Resilience

Michelle E. Mlinac, Tom H. Sheeran, Bryan Blissmer, Faith Lees, and Diane Martins

Aging successfully has been held as a goal for older adults (Bowling 2007), yet late life brings its share of troubles that do not always lend themselves to this ideal (Harris 2008). For many elders, simply maintaining stability despite loss is the more achievable aim. Resilience in late life can be conceptualized as the maintenance of physical and psychological health in the face of risk or threats (Mehta et al. 2008). The study of resilience originally developed from the literature on psychopathology (Staudinger et al. 1995), and has grown to incorporate a diverse literature base that includes positive psychology, adult development, and stress and coping. The process of aging itself can lead to development of adaptive coping mechanisms and wisdom, allowing one to meet the demands of later life with strength (Foster 1997). Resilience may well be possible for all older adults, including those with cognitive or emotional impairments.

Factors Affecting Psychological Resilience

In contrast to the focus on personality variables such as hardiness that may make one resilient (Funk 1992), often known as the "first wave" of resilience theory, or to the processes that result in resilience after a loss or threat ("second wave"), later researchers began asking by presuming that given the right context of interpersonal and social variables, resiliency is more likely to occur, the third wave of resiliency inquiry (Richardson 2002). In a review of the literature on the first two waves, Jacelon (1997) described the traits associated with resilience in adulthood including self-reliance as well as equanimity and outlined a possible two-step path to the process of resilience: disruption and reintegration. The third wave of research poses the question of what is innate that drives resilience to occur, perhaps a more existential line of inquiry than the preceding waves, incorporating theories from such

M.E. Mlinac (✉)
Boston Healthcare System, Harvard Medical School, Boston, MA, USA
e-mail: michellemlinac@yahoo.com

B. Resnick et al. (eds.), *Resilience in Aging: Concepts, Research, and Outcomes*,
DOI 10.1007/978-1-4419-0232-0_5, © Springer Science+Business Media, LLC 2011

diverse disciplines as physics, Eastern medicine, and psychoneuroimmunology (Richardson 2002). The application of these waves of research to late-life development is varied. Leipold and Greve (2009) argue that the debate between resilience as a trait or a process is ultimately circular, and resilience should instead be seen as part of a broader model of coping and development. They have proposed a model attempting to incorporate resilience as the activation of coping processes successfully utilized across time to maintain stability or growth. These coping processes may include assimilation and accommodation which foster stability and growth.

There is a debate in the resilience literature as to whether the term "resilience" implies simply a recovery to stability, or if it may also include the concept of growth or evolution following a disruptive event, termed "adversarial growth" (Richardson 2002; Linley and Joseph 2005; Bonanno 2005). Resiliency itself implies that there is something to overcome or bounce back from, though previous methodology has not always identified what older adults are resilient to, besides late life itself. Using a stratified subsample of a longitudinal study (Boyd Orr cohort aged 62–82 years), Hildon et al. (2009) captured acute and chronic effects of various adverse events, including bereavement, deteriorating health, and financial woes. The effect of multiple adversities was also investigated, as most individuals in reality do not confront just one difficulty at a time. In this study, resilience was operationalized by having a better than average quality of life. Results suggested that while those who were resilient had experienced adversity, they also displayed use of resources. Psychological resilience was correlated with an adaptive coping style, marked by problem-solving and learning from experience. Those with less resilience (termed vulnerable) tended to use an avoidant style of coping. Access to social support (with emphasis on useful and meaningful assistance) was also an important component of resilience.

In a companion study utilizing both quantitative and qualitative data from focus groups of the Boyd Orr cohort, specific means of coping were elicited from participants in their own words (Hildon et al. 2008). Adversity was correlated with rigid, inflexible ways of coping. Resilient focus group members also emphasized a sense of stability that (along with social support and positive coping skills) resulted in their being able to weather problems over time. Researchers recommended that interventions to promote resilience be made on both an individual level (engaging in reminiscence or life review therapy to provide a sense of meaning and coherence in the face of adversity) and a community level (improving access to social supports to alleviate burden).

Self-Esteem

The maintenance of self-esteem into later-life may shore up individuals against adversity. Two waves of data from a larger study (Collins and Smyer 2005) were used to explore the trajectory of self-esteem across time (a 3-year period), in the context of typical stresses of late life (e.g. financial burden). Participants were over 60, with an average of a tenth grade education. They completed measures of self-esteem, values, and loss. Results indicated little deterioration in self-esteem across time, even in the face of loss. Further, when individuals experienced a loss in a domain tied to their sense of self, such a blow did not diminish their self-esteem; despite identifying oneself as a healthy person, having later illness did not result in a substantial shift in self-esteem. Older adults in this study were seen as able to absorb the losses of later life and maintain a stable self.

A theory of psychological resilience in older people was recently proposed to incorporate a variety of related constructs including self-esteem and control (Judge et al. 2002; Windle et al. 2008). Utilizing a stratified localized (to the UK) sample from a larger European study of adult wellbeing, researchers obtained data on 1,853 adults aged 50–90. Self-report measures of resilience, self-control, and self-esteem were administered to participants. While the model that was derived was suggestive of a common factor relating to self-esteem, competence, and self-control, the construct of resilience itself was not fully validated in this study. Researchers suggested that there may be a number of theoretical models of psychological resilience in late life, and suggested that further research into the presentation of these constructs in late life is needed.

Social Support

Social support has often been correlated with resilience (Hildon et al. 2009; Maddi et al. 2006). Other studies have found that resilience and emotional support (but not instrumental support) yield higher quality of life for older adults (Netuveli and Blane 2008). In a study of older HIV-positive New Yorkers, Poindexter and Shippy (2008) identified unique social support networks contributing to the resilience of their members. Researchers conducted focus groups with five informal support networks comprised of mostly HIV-positive individuals. Despite their avenues for social support shrinking due to fear and stigma, these individuals were able to reallocate their resources and replenish their support networks via the HIV-positive resources in their community. Participants indicated that the loss of a group member to illness or death provided an opportunity for members to strengthen their bonds of support.

Socioemotional selectivity theory – in which older adults sensitized to their own mortality select to maintain only those relationships which they find emotionally supportive – has found empirical support in the literature (Adams et al. 2004; Charles and Carstensen 2009). This theory holds that as time passes, older adults aware of fewer resources and greater demands prioritize emotional connections that are worthwhile to them and shed those that are not. Thus, it may be that older adults do not find new relationships as emotionally satisfying as longer-standing ones. Further, it provides evidence that older adults are able to regulate their emotions and social networks to allow for the best possible outcome for themselves; they are able to prioritize needs in a way that preserves the self.

Spirituality

In addition to social support, other factors have been identified that promote resilience against mental strain and distress including hardiness and religiousness, and their overlap, spirituality (Maddi et al. 2006). Spirituality entails a search for meaning in the universe, a view that the world is larger than oneself, irrespective of the adherence to a specific doctrine. An investigation of hardiness, religiousness, and spirituality concluded that these qualities allowed individuals to cope with life stresses and provided protection against depression and stress (Maddi et al. 2006). Positive aspects of spirituality may serve to restore a sense of control following illness and foster adaptation to chronic illness and disability (Crowther et al. 2002). Spirituality was linked to resilience in cancer survivors; though these individuals are more at risk of developing depression and anxiety, their levels of spirituality and personal growth improved post-cancer recovery (Costanzo et al. 2009). Older cancer survivors also indicated an improved outlook on self and society.

Positive Emotions

Reacting with positive emotions in times of crisis may be a way to diminish stress response and cope more effectively (Davis et al. 2007). Further, the experience of positive emotions may provide a protective effect against threats to the ego. The broaden-and-build theory set forth by Fredrickson (1998) postulates that as humans have evolved, positive emotions have assisted with adaptation to stressful situations. Specifically, while negative responses to stress (e.g. fight or flight response) are inherently limited, employing positive emotions during stressful times allows for a wider variety of responses. In a series of studies, Tugade and Fredrickson (2004) found that employing positive emotions in times of stress correlated with a return to baseline of physiological arousal, supporting a mind–body connection. Similarly, coping was found to be improved when individuals were instructed to see stressful situations as a challenge they could grow from rather than a threat to harm them. This cognitive reframing may be a way to improve resiliency. The third portion of the study provided evidence for a link between positive emotions and positive appraisal of a situation. Across studies, support was found for the broaden-and-build theory, indicating that those with greater resilience were more likely to experience positive emotions and utilize them to cope with stress.

Cohn et al. (2009) utilized Fredrickson's broaden-and-build theory to test how happiness relates to resilience. In this study, ego resilience and life satisfaction were measured before and after participants tracked their daily emotions for a month. Those who experienced more frequent positive emotions were also those with more growth in resilience and improved life satisfaction. Negative emotional experiences were not directly related to resilience or life satisfaction, or with the experience of positive emotions. Experiencing frequent pleasant emotions was theorized to improve resiliency, and those who were more resilient were thought to be more likely to feel positive emotions. Positive emotions have also been thought to lead to greater spirituality (Saroglou et al. 2008) and improved health (Fredrickson and Levenson 1998).

To better determine how positive affective experiences buffer against stress, researchers have proposed that emotional memory plays a role in how individuals react to negative events. Emotional memories are powerful and are easily triggered, so might be recruited to assist in cognitive processing of a stressor. Philippe et al. (2009) examined the relationship between these memories and how people reacted to sadness and anxiety. They hypothesized that more resilient responses would entail activation of positive emotional memory networks. Psychological resilience against sadness and anxiety was found to be associated with positive emotional experiences. From these findings, researchers speculated that people might deal with a difficult event by accessing positive emotional memories, which can help them to cope in the moment and later process the experience more positively. Given the lifetime of pleasant emotional experiences upon which older adults can draw, the applicability of this research to late life has promise.

Perceived affect regulation has recently been suspected to be an aspect of resilience in old age. The emotional experience of older adults is important in determining how they navigate life's challenges. Positive and negative emotions can differ in the amount of energy invested in expressing them. For example, low-arousal positive emotions include feeling serene and at ease. In contrast, euphoria and delight are high-arousal positive emotions. Similarly, low-arousal negative emotions (e.g. lethargy) can be contrasted with high-arousal negative emotions (e.g. annoyance). Older adults have been found to differ both in the strength and direction of their affective experiences in comparison to younger adults. Kessler and Staudinger (2009) investigated how older adults perceive the effort they put forth in expressing positive and negative emotions, known as "affective arousal." When compared with younger and middle-aged adults across four quadrants of emotional expression (arousal × valence), older adults more frequently displayed positive, low-arousal emotions, remaining fairly unruffled by the losses and changes experienced in late life. Elders also displayed fewer negative emotions of either high or low arousal, suggesting that they appeared to take the developmental challenges of the later years in stride. These findings also suggest that older adults may be better able to regulate their emotions over time, and that this improved regulation (whether due to neurophysiology or personal experience) allows them to better adapt to negative life events.

In a review of the literature on depression and aging (Karel 1997), helplessness was identified as a factor that contributes to depression, and despite the many losses of late life, older adults do not demonstrate a diminished sense of control. Further, they display strengths such as more nuanced understanding of emotion, better ability to regulate that emotion, and are more likely to accept circumstances as being out of their personal control. These developmental processes may be similar to Erikson's view of achieving wisdom and gerotranscendence (a shift in perspective from the personal and rational to the cosmic and spiritual accompanied by an increase in life satisfaction) as the last stages of ego development (Erikson 1998). The ninth stage has been empirically tested in the literature, suggesting the potential for continued psychosocial growth across the end of the lifespan (Brown and Lowis 2003). Transcendence and resilience were examined in a community-dwelling sample of the oldest old (85+), along with other existential aspects of aging: sense of coherence and purpose in life (Nygren et al. 2005). Significant correlations were found among the four constructs, and higher levels corresponded to better mental health (but were unrelated to physical health, suggesting that for this cohort, health issues do not directly bear on existential concerns and wellbeing). The oldest old were found to have greater levels of resilience and sense of coherence than have been reported for younger samples.

Although the oldest old are potentially the most resilient of all, an age limit on psychological resilience has been questioned (Baltes and Smith 2003). In a study of centenarians, found evidence against this assumption. Using data from the Heidelberg Centenarian Study, they completed face-to-face interviews with 91 centenarians who had been participants in the longitudinal study. They assessed participants' functional health and cognitive status as well as self-ratings of happiness. Centenarians in this study displayed happiness at or greater than younger- or middle-aged adults, though many areas of their functioning were compromised. Factors predicting happiness included social support, extraversion, optimism, and self-efficacy, which were potent even at very late life. For this group of mostly female centenarians (89%), having had job training negatively correlated with happiness, which may be due to other factors (e.g. those with job training were less likely to have had families). Happiness was not correlated with health status. Researchers suggested that centenarians may have accepted the inevitable declines in functioning and health and instead find happiness for reasons other than physical abilities.

Empirical Measures of Resilience

Resilience measures have primarily been developed with children and adolescents, as this has been the primary population for resilience work over the years (Ahern et al. 2006). Most commonly used has been the Resilience Scale (Wagnild and Young 1993; Jacelon 1997), a 25-item scale that has been used with a variety of age groups, and was originally normed on a sample of 810 older women (Ahern et al. 2006; Windle et al. 2008). The scale was conceptualized on five components of resilience: equanimity, self-reliance, existential aloneness, perseverance and meaningfulness (Wagnild and Young 1993). Further factor analysis has yielded personal competence and acceptance of self and life as constructs captured by the scale (Ahern et al. 2006). This scale has subsequently been used with other elderly samples (Lamet et al. 2009; Nygren et al. 2005).

The Connor–Davidson Resilience Scale (CD-RISC), also a 25-item instrument, has yielded good validity and reliability across community, primary care, and psychiatric populations (Connor and Davidson 2003; Ahern et al. 2006). The scale has been utilized with older adults and reflects characteristics of resilience such as optimism (Montross et al. 2006). Analysis found factors comprising resilience for a group of community-dwelling older women included: personal control and goal orientation, adaptation and tolerance for negative affect, leadership and trust in instincts, and spiritual coping (Lamond et al. 2008). As the relative strength of the factors in this sample differed from that of younger samples, researchers proposed that resilience for older women may be a different psychological process than it is for younger people. Alternately, it may be that older woman utilize (or have available) different resources than younger people do to face the particular developmental challenges of late life. They further suggested that while many of the elements of resilience (e.g. optimism) are associated with successful aging, it is not only those aging successfully who can be resilient. There is evidence for a correlation between successful aging and resilience but how the two may impact each other remains to be determined (Wagnild 2003).

In a study examining resilience in community-dwelling elders, Hardy et al. (2004) developed a 14-item scale to detect factors that allowed elders to maintain stability after a stressful life event. They asked older adults to rate how stressful a specific life event was, and to identify how the event impacted their lives. Events rated included their own health concerns, the illness or death of a family member or friend, or a non-medical life event. The scale used was derived from a larger health questionnaire based on Rowe and Kahn's construct of resilience (Rowe and Kahn 1997). For older adults, results indicated that the more stressful the life event, the lower their resilience. This measure has subsequently been utilized to examine resilience to late-life disability.

Caregiving

Because of its demanding nature, caregiving has been conceptualized as a "career" (Haley et al. 2008), encompassing many stressors including emotional, financial, and physical. Often, caregivers of those with dementia or other chronic illness and disability are elders themselves (Schulz et al. 2003; Garand et al. 2005). Caregiving for a person with a fatal illness or disability can take a toll on physical and mental health (Flaskerud and Lee 2001). In a study on patients with amyotrophic lateral sclerosis (ALS) and their caregivers, a blend of qualitative interviews and self-report measures was administered to determine the prevalence of depression among patients and caregivers, how closely symptoms were tied to disease course, and any correlations between caregiver and patient level of distress (Rabkin et al. 2000). Results indicated a high correlation between depressive symptoms in caregivers and patients. Both groups evidenced positive coping mechanisms. For caregivers, those with higher burden also were more likely to see positive meaning in their caregiving experience.

Racial differences in resilience to caregiver stress have been examined, with social support being identified as a protective factor. A longitudinal study of African-American and White dementia caregivers measured levels of social support, life satisfaction, and depressive symptoms across 5 years (Clay et al. 2008). On a self-rated measure of social support, the African-American caregivers reported a higher level of satisfaction with their level of social support than what their White counterparts reported, and in turn White caregivers reported higher levels of depressive symptoms than what the African-American caregivers reported. Both groups reported that, across time, they had fewer supportive individuals to rely on. Satisfaction with social support was found to correlate with life satisfaction and possibly protect against depressive symptoms. Researchers suggested that caregivers' coping could be improved by targeting interventions to improve their satisfaction with social support.

Gaugler et al. (2007) examined resilience throughout the course and end of the caregiving career, here operationalized as perceived emotional burden in the context of caregiving demands. High levels of resilience are thus associated with low burden despite high demands, also conceptualized as "stress resistance." The sample included nearly 2,000 caregivers from the Medicare Alzheimer's Disease Demonstration Evaluation (MADDE) study, which was a randomized trial of case management for dementia caregivers. Among the factors indentified to correlate with resilience include longer duration of caregiving role and access to available resources (such as respite or home care). An important finding of this study was that higher caregiver resilience was correlated with less frequent institutionalization; those who displayed better coping and support were able to keep their loved one at home for a longer period of time. Authors suggested that future research on caregiving incorporate resilience as a variable for identifying appropriate intervention, rather than a one size fits all approach to providing support.

Bereavement

The course of caregiving in dementia or chronic illness often leads to the death of the individual being cared for, and caregivers have been shown to experience grief symptoms prior to and after the death of their loved ones (Schulz et al. 2003; Bonanno et al. 2004). People handle the death of their loved ones in different ways; the emotions felt after such a loss can vary across individuals. Conventional wisdom has held that the optimal way of coping with grief is to process the loss in a timely manner, lest suppressed negative emotions overwhelm the grieving individual (Bonanno & Field 2001). That assumption has been challenged by recent research, suggesting that losses can be dealt with in a healthy manner without significant turmoil. There is a significant empirical evidence for resiliency following the loss of a loved one (Rossi et al. 2007; Bonanno et al. 2002; Ott et al. 2007). Researchers have consistently found that older adults are capable of responding resiliently to a loss, and do so fairly commonly, with many empirical studies approaching a rate of 50% among subjects (Bonanno 2004).

Bonanno et al. (2004) identified five trajectories of coping in bereaved older widows (normal grief, resiliency, chronic grief, chronic depression, and depressed-improved). Normal or common grief refers to the brief episode of depressive symptoms, distress, and disruption in normal functioning that are typically thought of as the normative response to a loss. This response also known as "recovery" (Ott et al. 2007) differs from the resilient response to loss and also from chronic grief which occurs in 10–20% of individuals (Bonanno et al. 2002). Chronic grievers began with a non-depressed presentation prior to the death of their loved ones and exhibited similar levels of functional impairment as the common grief group did, though their functioning did not return to baseline after 18 months. The group of individuals who have depression prior to a loss can remain depressed following the loss (chronic depression), but also have potential to recover to non-pathological levels of functioning 6–18 months after the loss of their loved one (depressed-improved). Relief of caregiver burden, which had likely been a chronic stressor, may account for this improvement. This group was found to be similar to the resilient group in terms of exhibiting a minimal grief response (Bonanno et al. 2002), suggesting that there may be more than one pathway to resilience (Bonanno 2004). A minimal grief response has in the past been thought to be pathological.

Resilience has been shown to play a significant role in adjustment to widowhood. Rossi et al. (2007) identified "dispositional resilience" as a protective factor in helping older women to cope with the stress of widowhood. Dispositional resilience is analogous to hardiness, which is a personality characteristic that can enhance resilience (Maddi 2005). In study, dispositional resilience was comprised of three personal characteristics: control (believing one has power over outcomes), commitment (maintaining connection with others), and challenge (approaching obstacles and learning from experience). Those high on dispositional resilience were found to perceive the stress of widowhood differently than those who were less resilient, and in turn had a higher degree of life satisfaction. Researchers also suggested that resilient individuals might perceive and cope with stress more effectively by drawing on social support, feeling more empowered, and directly confronting their stressors.

Sense of control and social support were also identified as correlating to resilience in another study of older widowed persons (Ott et al. 2007). In this study, 37% of participants fell into the resilient group, while approximately 50% were in the normal grieving group and the remaining individuals were identified as chronic grievers. Researchers suggested that relying on social support may have helped the resilient individuals to maintain their stability and sense of personal control following the death of a spouse, change in role status, and other losses associated with widowhood.

The complex feelings that one faces after a loss may include the buffering effect of positive emotions. Utilizing daily diaries to track emotional constellations of the recently widowed, Ong et al. (2004) identified that the greater the number of positive emotions experienced by widows, the less potent were levels of stress and depressive symptoms. In addition, the use of humor was found to be a possible resilient coping style; those who utilized it were better able to capitalize on positive emotions and keep depression from taking hold.

Interventions that target coping across pre- and post-loss time periods (both caregiver and bereavement interventions) have been examined. In a study of caregivers whose spouses had Alzheimer's disease, support interventions were administered both before and after the death of their spouses (Haley et al. 2008). When compared to usual care controls, a pattern of resilience was found to be more common in those who received enhanced counseling and support (60% resilient with intervention, 42.9% resilient without intervention). This study lends support to resiliency being a common response in the face of chronic stress and loss, and indicates that interventions can be undertaken to further enhance such resiliency before and after loss.

Depression

In considering the myriad losses older adults confront, it is presumed that they may be at greater risk of depression. Health and functional declines are more common in late life contributing to greater vulnerability for depressive symptoms (Karel 1997; Lyness et al. 2006), though old age in and of itself does not cause depression (Rothermund and Brandtstädter 2003). Depression is characterized by cognitive symptoms (sadness, apathy, anhedonia) and somatic symptoms (sleep disturbance, weight gain or loss). Physical health symptoms such as sleep quality can have an impact on psychological resilience (Motivala et al. 2006). Depressed older adults have been found to display a greater number of somatic symptoms than cognitive symptoms when compared to depressed younger adults, though this may be confounded by the increase in physical health problems in late life (Balsis and Cully 2008; Karel 1997).

In older adults, fewer depressive symptoms correlate with higher resilience (Hardy et al. 2004). Depressive symptoms (e.g. withdrawal, loss of motivation) may interfere with resilient processes in individuals, particularly as resources diminish in later life. In a cohort-sequential study, Rothermund and Brandtstädter (2003) compared six cohorts (representing age groups from 54 to 77) over 8 years on measures of depression, health status and impairment, socioeconomic resources, coping styles, and time perspectives (such as future-orientation and feelings of obsolescence). They found that depressive symptoms in the younger cohorts remained relatively stable over time. Above a certain age (~70), depressive symptoms increase and resiliency, while still present, tends to diminish. The researchers correlate this phase change with the average life expectancy of their participants, suggesting that older adults may cease viewing stressors as normal parts of aging and begin anticipating end-of-life.

Further evidence of age-related changes in resilience to depression was found by Mehta et al. (2008). Presuming that physical disability and apathy might interfere with resilience in depressed older adults (and that interference would increase at later ages), they compared young–old (<80) and old–old (>80) patients visiting community-dwelling geriatric clinics on measures of depression, disability, apathy, and resilience. Their results also corroborated resilience's waning protective effects on depression in later life. Researchers suggested that the old–old may have fewer external resources on which to draw to help them cope with stressors and declines. Internal resources may also be compromised; at later ages, apathy also appeared to drive depression.

Depression in older adults can lead to suicidal ideation (Karel 1997; Alexopoulos et al. 2009). Identifying resilience in those at risk for suicide may support prevention efforts. McLaren et al. (2007) hypothesized that sense of belonging (feeling valued by others and part of a community) was a protective factor buffering against suicidality in depression. To investigate this, they asked 351 retired Australians to complete depression, suicide, and belongingness measures. They compared results with four resiliency models: (1) compensatory model (depression will increase risk of suicidality while sense of belongingness will decrease that risk), (2) risk-protective model (as sense of belongingness increases, depression will have less effect on suicidality), (3) challenge model (only high levels of depression will have an effect on suicidality, at lesser levels of depression people will activate their resources), (4) protective–protective model (the greater the number of protective factors such as sense of belonging, the less suicidality would be present. Although these models have been studied with children and adolescents, they have not often been applied to older adults (Fergus and Zimmerman 2005; McLaren et al. 2007). As expected, sense of belonging was found to be a protective factor against suicidal ideation, whereas depression was a risk factor. These factors lent support to the risk-protective model; the more people feel accepted and valued, the less likely they are to be affected by depression and suicidal ideation. High levels of depression corresponded with a spike in suicidal ideation, which supported the challenge model. For women, the compensatory model was also supported; depressed women who felt part of a group were less likely to display suicidal ideation. For men, being seen as vital to the community removes depression as risk factor for suicidal ideation. Researchers emphasized that helping older adults feel part of a community may help alleviate depression and suicidal ideation, but cautioned that mere proximity to others is insufficient.

This caveat was supported by Adams et al. (2004) in a study of older adults living independently in retirement communities. The benefit of living in such communities as opposed to say single-family homes in the community is the built-in network of resources, activities, and nearby peers. Despite these available resources, loneliness was still prevalent in these communities. Loneliness was found to be an independent risk factor for depression, corresponding with having had a recent loss, narrower social network, and less frequent visits from friends. Although depression may preclude individuals from accessing available social resources (due to apathy, fatigue, or withdrawal), loneliness can be more easily treated. Researchers suggest that psychosocial interventions to help older adults connect with others within the community may prevent mental health problems secondary to loneliness and depression.

Schizophrenia

Compared to elders without severe mental illness, individuals aging with schizophrenia typically have additional barriers to overcome including: being more likely to be institutionalized (Andrews et al. 2009; Manderscheid et al. 2009), experiencing stigma and the emotional effects of living with the illness (Seeman 2005), exhibiting greater incidence of comorbid depression (Diwan et al. 2007), receiving less aggressive medical care (Vahia et al. 2008), and coping with the side-effects of long-term antipsychotic use (Karim et al. 2005; Berry and Barrowclough 2009). Insight into symptoms and a stubborn, determined personality style are qualities of those who may be more likely to improve over time (Torrey 2005). Symptom remission is a realistic goal for older adults with schizophrenia (Bankole et al. 2008), but remission of symptoms alone may not lead to successful aging (Cohen et al. 2009).

Investigations into psychological resilience in older adults with schizophrenia are few (Berry and Barrowclough 2009). In a review of the course of the disease across time, identified several factors promoting recovery in schizophrenia, including neural plasticity, engaging in a variety of treatment modalities, and an optimistic outlook, bolstered by positive appraisals from others. Across time, social functioning may be restored and allow for the social support that promote resilience in elders with schizophrenia (Karim et al. 2005). These findings are contrary to the long-held view of schizophrenia being chronic and deteriorating. Argues that assumptions and predictions regarding outcomes for older adults with schizophrenia are inadequate, citing data from several longitudinal studies which revealed significant recovery in many functional areas for these patients. Interventions which focus on building coping skills and treatment adherence can help those with schizophrenia weather transitory stressors (Yanos and Moos 2007). Specific coping strategies that have been correlated with age include refocusing attention from unwanted thoughts and acceptance of symptoms.

Trauma

Adapting to the losses associated with later life is an expected part of the aging process. Coping with sudden and severe trauma by contrast may not result in the same levels of resilience that have been demonstrated by bereavement researchers (Litz 2005), but others have argued that resilience is a common human response to both significant loss and significant trauma (Bonanno 2004; Kelley 2005). Frequent indicators of resilience, specifically religiousness, hardiness, positive emotional experiences, and social support, have also been found to be protective factors for those who have been exposed to trauma (Bonanno 2004; Maddi 2005; Nemeroff et al. 2006). In contrast, predictors of PTSD include poor social support, limited education, and history of mental health problems (Bonanno 2004). Litz (2005) suggested that in addition to the absence of psychopathology as an outcome measure following trauma, researchers and clinicians should also consider functional resilience, the ability to retain day-to-day functional abilities with little disruption.

Trauma and Neurobiology

The way in which people cope with a stressful event varies, based not only on personal characteristics and situational factors, but also on unique physiological responses. Researchers are hopeful that a broadened understanding of psychobiology will allow us to anticipate how people react to traumatic events and prevent or alleviate PTSD symptoms when they occur (Charney 2004). Physical correlates such as hippocampal volume have been found to correlate with specific risk and resilience factors for PTSD. Yehuda et al. (2007) examined the brain imaging, neuropsychological testing, and neuroendocrine assessment on two groups of veterans with and without chronic PTSD, and found that a smaller left hippocampus, a part of the brain associated with memory, was correlated with earlier onset of PTSD. Individuals who developed PTSD following a single traumatic incident had smaller left hippocampal structures than those who developed PTSD only after multiple traumatic events. Interestingly, no overall differences in hippocampal volume were found between the groups of aging veterans with and without PTSD. Researchers hypothesized that these veterans may have reached a point in development where age-related atrophy masked any former differences in hippocampal volume.

Early Trauma Exposure and Late-Life Resilience

The interplay between long-standing trauma, stressors experienced in late life, and resilience is complex. In a study comparing Holocaust survivors to non-Holocaust surviving older adults in the wake of 9/11, Holocaust survivors exhibited a higher number of post-traumatic symptoms than did their counterparts (Lamet et al. 2009). Of note, they also displayed higher levels of resilience, suggesting a nonlinear relationship between distress and coping. Older adults may be resilient in some ways but not in others. In this study, despite being more likely to experience post-traumatic symptoms after 9/11, Holocaust survivors continued to function well in other areas of their lives and had greater resilience than the comparison group. One limitation of this study was that this group of Holocaust survivors may have evidenced the same level of symptoms prior to 9/11; findings may simply have reflected the life-course of these survivors in comparison to non-survivors. Unfortunately, non-American Holocaust survivors were not utilized as a second comparison group so that the specific trauma of 9/11 on the American survivors could have been examined.

The effects of trauma such as combat exposure experienced decades earlier can result in resiliency later in life. Elder and Clipp (1989) proposed a model of resilience and risk in aging combat veterans. They demonstrated that the experience of participating in combat produces positive and negative results. Later-life emergence of traumatic symptoms may be a result of an experience similar to what was experienced in combat. For example, the loss of independence through long-term care placement may evoke feelings of helplessness and fear. They utilized a cohort of WWII and Korean veterans who had been enrolled in three longitudinal studies undertaken at the Institute of Human Development at the University of California, Berkeley. At the time of the study, the sample was primarily in their 60s, though data points were also taken from participants pre- and post-service, and mid-life (40s). Veterans were rated on severity of combat exposure (with variables such as exposure to the dead or wounded). They were asked to share their beliefs about how their experience in the military impacted their lives for the better and/or worse. Researchers then examined how these perspectives impacted on the functioning of these veterans from the age of 55 onward, at the time of the study. Those veterans who were exposed to heavier combat were found to be higher on resilient characteristics such as assertiveness. When compared to pre-war levels, ego resilience appeared to be developed in those exposed to heavy combat during and after their war-time experiences. Ego-resilience was not a protection against PTSD. Even those veterans experiencing post-traumatic symptoms were seen as having commensurate ego resilience to those without PTSD symptoms. However, those with lower levels of resilience in adolescence were more likely to have emotional and behavioral problems that endured to later life. Elder and Clipp called for further longitudinal research into the late effects of trauma exposure in combat veterans.

On the basis of Elder and Clipp's model of resilience in aging veterans, Aldwin et al. (1994) examined how combat affected older adults positively and negatively. As part of a longitudinal aging study, they obtained data on 1,287 veterans of primarily WWII and the Korean War, aged 43–91, administering a measure of combat exposure, cognitive appraisal of military service, and scales of PTSD and depression. With regard to resiliency, those who had positive appraisals of their stress and military experience were less likely to be experiencing PTSD symptoms. Many respondents indicated that despite the stresses of combat, their time in the service yielded improved self-esteem, coping, and character development.

Studies of resilience in Vietnam veterans have suggested that hardiness and social support were correlated with resilience to PTSD (King et al. 1999). This broad research included 1,200 male and 432 female veterans from the National Veterans Readjustment Study. Using structural equation modeling, they examined the relationship between pre-war risk factors, stressors during war, post-war resilience and recovery variables, and PTSD for both men and women. They found that for both genders, hardiness and functional social support mitigated PTSD symptoms. Yet as veterans were subjected to greater stress during and after the war, hardiness and functional social support lost their potency, and fewer coping resources were available to access.

Late-Onset Stress Symptomatology

In investigating the course of trauma across the life course, clinical researchers within the Department of Veterans Affairs have encountered the emergence of symptoms in aging combat veterans who had not previously exhibited significant psychopathology (Davison et al. 2006; King et al. 2007). This phenomenon has been termed "late-onset stress symptomatology," or LOSS, and encapsulates intrusive thoughts and feelings related to the combat experience (Davison et al. 2006). These symptoms emerge in concert with the typical challenges of aging, often with retirement, change in health status, or loss of a spouse. LOSS is not necessarily associated with functional decline, and has been considered a normative developmental response not a "disorder" per se (King et al. 2007), in contrast to delayed-onset PTSD which can emerge at midlife and onward (Solomon and Mikulincer 2006). In a study of older combat veterans from several conflicts (WWII, Korea, Vietnam), researchers developing a scale to assess LOSS symptoms found that veterans exhibited resilient characteristics inversely proportional to severity of trauma related symptoms (King et al. 2007). Those exhibiting higher measured LOSS symptoms displayed lower social support, life satisfaction, and sense of personal mastery and higher stressors, pessimism, and negative affect. Resiliency may play a role in helping these veterans cope with combat-related thoughts and feelings that emerge in the course of life review or in reappraisal following a disruptive life event. Appraising participation in combat as an adversity that was overcome may help veterans to confront future challenges with a sense of self-efficacy (Davison et al. 2006). Older veterans may thus navigate the usual stressors of aging with a more complex set of challenges but also a unique constellation of personal resources. Researchers have proposed that these veterans may benefit from interventions such as psychoeducation to shore up their strengths, rather than engaging in a more intensive trauma-focused therapy that may not suitably address their developmental needs (Davison et al. 2006).

Dementia

Psychological resilience in those with cognitive decline is just beginning to be considered in the literature, as the assumption that diminished cognition necessarily negates resilience is changed (Jopp and Rott 2006). A recent editorial by the editors of the journal *Dementia* have argued that studies of dementia should also encompass resiliency, successful aging, and strengths exhibited by those living with the disease (Harris and Keady 2008). This person-centered approach has been advocated to counter the Rowe and Kahn's model of successful aging which may exclude those with functional declines and disabilities (Rowe and Kahn 1997; Harris 2008). The spirit of that model argued by Kahn (2002) may still serve older adults with cognitive impairment, such that they successfully age by doing what they can to maintain or improve their abilities.

To open up this line of research more fully, Harris completed a qualitative study of older adults with early stage dementia (Harris 2008). A portion of the open-ended interviews she utilized asked participants' thoughts on resilience. She presented two case studies, eliciting themes of protection (positive self-concept and religious beliefs) and vulnerability (health concerns and social isolation). While these cases are certainly not representative, the framework utilized in this study may assist clinicians in conceptualizing the experiences of those with cognitive impairment. Further, Harris suggests a resilience perspective allows for being inclusive of the experiences of all older adults.

Another avenue to explore resilience in the context of cognitive decline and psychological health was recently proposed by Forstmeier and Maercker (2008). They identified the concept of "motivational reserve," motivational abilities that have been theorized to provide protection against cognitive decline. These processes include making a decision quickly, preparing to act, and following through with the action, along with self-efficacy, the belief that one can decide on a behavior and see it through. Motivational processes are used in nearly every aspect of life, though like any skill set, some individuals utilize these skills more successfully than others do. Researchers have hypothesized that those who use these skills more effectively throughout the life span develop better neural networks and compensatory mechanisms that may protect against cognitive decline. Further, they questioned whether having better motivational abilities (and in turn better cognitive abilities) might also be better off psychologically.

To test these theories, Forstmeier and Maercker extrapolated motivational abilities from archival occupational data. Cognitive tests included premorbid estimate of intelligence. Those instruments measures along with scales of self-efficacy and activation regulation yielded comprehensive picture of motivation, cognition, and psychological wellbeing across time. Subjects in this study were aged 60–94, living independently or in nursing homes. Results indicated that motivational abilities at midlife (as assessed by subjects' primary occupation) were predictive of cognitive and psychological status in late life. Assuming a good fit between subjects' occupations and their decision-making and motivational skills, feeling effective and capable in the workplace (where good decisions and task follow-through are valued) may predict later cognitive status and psychological health. Conversely, apathy around one's decisions and goals is a negative predictor, and may increase the risk of late life cognitive dysfunction. The model of motivational reserve shows promise in bridging psychological wellness and cognitive ability in late life.

Conclusion

One topic that might be further investigated is whether societal attitudes prevent or inhibit resilience in older adults. The stigma of older adults as feeble, frail, and vulnerable has historically been perpetuated. When social work students were asked to imagine how resilient older adults would be in trying situations, they rated older adults as being less resilient than they themselves would be at that age in the same circumstances (Kane 2008). These students rated themselves as more likely to recover from trauma, more able to work through negative emotions, and less willing to be seen as a victim of circumstance.

The same shift in perspective may be true for older adults. Elders' perceptions of themselves and other peers were measured after they were shown negative stereotypes of aging (Pinquart 2002). Following exposure to these stereotypes, older adults tended to rate their peers more poorly than they had prior to receiving negative information. Yet, their self-perceptions actually improved. Consistent with resiliency theory, these older adults modified their beliefs about themselves in comparison with what their perceptions about other elders (e.g. "Maybe I'm not doing so badly after all, compared with other people"). This mechanism can be seen as a protective factor; older adults reject negative information about aging rather than allowing it to harm their self-perceptions. Later research has suggested that a diagnosis of cognitive impairment or dementia may negate this process and render older adults more vulnerable to negative stereotypes of aging and exacerbate functional declines (Scholl and Sabat 2008).

One definition offered for resilience is surpassing what is expected in spite of great odds (Netuveli and Blane 2008). What constitutes such adversity is subjective and unique to each individual (Van Vliet 2008). The potential for resilience may be in the eye of the beholder, as it ultimately falls on each individual to react to life's challenges, drawing upon available resources to cope as best they are able.

References

Adams, K. B., Sanders, S., and Auth, E. A. (2004) Loneliness and depression in independent living retirement communities: Risk and resilience factors. *Aging and Mental Health, 8,* 475–485.

Ahern, N. R., Kiehl, E. M., Sole, M., and Byers, J. (2006) A review of instruments measuring resilience. *Issues in Comprehensive Pediatric Nursing, 29,* 103–125.

Aldwin, C. M., Levenson, M. R., and Spiro, A. (1994) Vulnerability and resilience to combat exposure: Can stress have lifelong effects? *Psychology and Aging, 9,* 34–44.

Alexopoulos, G. S., Reynolds, C. F., Bruce, M. L., Katz, I. R., Raue, P. J., Muslant, B. H., et al. (2009) Reducing suicidal ideation and depression in older primary care patients: 24-month outcomes of the PROSPECT study. *American Journal of Psychiatry, 166,* 882–890.

Andrews, A. O., Bartles, S. J., Xie, H., and Peacock, W. J. (2009) Increased risk of nursing home admission among middle aged and older adults with schizophrenia. *American Journal of Geriatric Psychiatry, 17,* 697–705.

Balsis, S. and Cully, J. A. (2008) Comparing depression diagnostic symptoms across younger and older adults. *Aging and Mental Health, 12,* 800–806.

Baltes, P. B. and Smith, J. (2003) New frontiers in the future of aging: From successful aging of the young old to the dilemmas of the fourth age. *Gerontology, 49,* 123–135.

Bankole, A., Cohen, C. I., Vahia, I., Diwan, S., Palekar, N., Reyes, P., et al. (2008) Symptomatic remission in a multiracial urban population of older adults with schizophrenia. *American Journal of Geriatric Psychiatry, 16,* 966–973.

Berry, K. and Barrowclough, C. (2009) The needs of older adults with schizophrenia: Implications for psychological interventions. *Clinical Psychology Review, 29,* 68–76.

Bonanno, G. A., & Field, N. P. (2001). Evaluating the delayed grief hypothesis across 5 years of bereavement. American Behavioral Scientist, *44,* 798–816.

Bonanno, G. A. (2004) Loss, trauma, and human resilience: Have we underestimated the human capacity to thrive after extremely aversive events? *American Psychologist, 59,* 20–28.

Bonanno, G. A. (2005) Clarifiying and extending the construct of adult resilience. *American Psychologist, 60,* 265–267.

Bonanno, G. A., Wortman, C. B., and Nesse, R. M. (2004) Prospective patterns of resilience and maladjustment during widowhood. *Psychology and Aging, 19,* 260–271.

Bonanno, G. A., Wortman, C. B., Lehman, D. R., Tweed, R. G., Haring, M., Sonnega, J., et al. (2002) Resiliency to loss and grief: A prospective study from preloss to 18-months postloss. *Journal of Personality and Social Psychology, 83,* 1150–1164.

Bowling, A. (2007) Aspirations for older age in the 21st century: What is successful aging? *International Journal of Aging and Human Development, 64,* 263–297.

Brown, C. and Lowis, M. J. (2003) Psychosocial development in the elderly: An investigation into Erikson's ninth stage. *Journal of Aging Studies, 17,* 415–426.

Charles, L. T. and Carstensen, L. L. (2007) Emotion regulation and aging. In J. J. Gross (Ed.) *Handbook of Emotion Regulation* (pp. 307–327). New York: Guilford Press.

Charles, S.T. & Carstensen, L.L. (2009). Socioemotional selectivity theory. In H. Reis & S. Sprecher (Eds.) Encyclopedia of Human Relationships. Sage Publications.

Charney, D. S. (2004) Psychobiological mechanisms of resilience and vulnerability: Implications for successful adaptation to extreme stress. *American Journal of Psychiatry, 161,* 195–216.

Clay, O. J., Roth, D. L., Wadley, V. G., and Haley, W. E. (2008) Changes in social support and their impact on psychosocial outcome over a 5-year period for African American and White dementia caregivers. *International Journal of Geriatric Psychiatry, 23,* 857–862.

Cohen, C. I., Pathak, R., Ramirez, P. M., Vahia, I. (2009) Outcome among community dwelling older adults with schizophrenia: Results using five conceptual models. *Community Mental Health Journal, 45,*151–156.

Cohn, M. A., Fredrickson, B. L., Brown, S. L, Mikels, J. A., and Conway, A. M. (2009) Happiness unpacked: Positive emotions increase life satisfaction by building resilience. *Emotion, 9,* 361–368.

Collins, A. L., and Smyer, M. A. (2005) The resilience of self-esteem in late adulthood. *Journal of Aging and Health, 17,* 471–489.

Connor, K. M., and Davidson, J. R. T. (2003) Development of a new resilience scale: The Connor-Davidson Resilience Scale (CD-RISC). *Depression and Anxiety, 18,* 76–82.

Costanzo, E. S., Ryff, C. D., and Singer, B. H. (2009) Psychosocial adjustment among cancer survivors: Findings from a national survey of health and well-being. *Health Psychology, 28,* 147–156.

Crowther, M. R., Parker, M. W., Achenbaum, W. A., Larimore, W. L., and Koenig, H. G. (2002) Rowe and Kahn's model of successful aging revisited: Positive spirituality – the forgotten factor. *The Gerontologist, 42,* 613–620.

Davis, M. C., Zautra, A. J., Johnson, L. M., Murray, K. E., and Okvat, H. A. (2007) Psychosocial stress, emotion regulation, and resilience among older adults. In C. M. Aldwin, C. L. Park, and A. Spiro (Eds.), *Handbook of Health Psychology and Aging* (pp. 250–266). New York: Guilford Press.

Davison, E. H., Pless, A. P., Gugliucci, M. R., King, L. A., King, D. W., Salgado, D. M., et al. (2006) Late-life emergence of early-life trauma: The phenomenon of late-onset stress symptomatology among aging combat veterans. *Research on Aging, 28,* 84–114.

Diwan, S., Cohen, C. I., Bankole, A. O., Vahia, I., Kehn, M., and Ramirez, P. M. (2007) Depression in older adults with schizophrenia spectrum disorders: prevalence and associated factors. *American Journal of Geriatric Psychiatry, 15,* 991–998.

Elder, G. H., and Clipp, E. C. (1989) Combat experience and emotional health: Impairment and resilience in later life. *Journal of Personality, 2,* 311–341.

Erikson, E. H. (1998) *The Life Cycle Completed. Extended Version with New Chapters on the Ninth Stage by Joan M. Erikson.* New York: Norton.

Fergus, S. and Zimmerman, M. A. (2005) Adolescent resilience: A framework for understanding healthy development in the face of risk. *Annual Review of Public Health, 26,* 399–419.

Flaskerud, J. H. and Lee, P. (2001) Vulnerability to health problems in female informal caregivers of persons with HIV/AIDS and age-related dementias. *Journal of Advanced Nursing, 33,* 60–68.

Forstmeier, S. and Maercker, A. (2008) Motivational reserve: Lifetime motivational abilities contribute to cognitive and emotional health in old age. *Psychology and Aging, 23,* 886–899.

Foster, J. R. (1997) Successful coping, adaptation and resilience in the elderly: An interpretation of epidemiologic data. *Psychiatric Quarterly, 68,* 189–219.

Fredrickson, B. L. (1998). What good are positive emotions? Review of General Psychology, 2, 300–319.

Fredrickson, B. L. and Levenson, R. (1998) Positive emotions speed recovery from the cardiovascular sequelae of negative emotions. Cognition and Emotion, 12, 191–220.

Funk, S. C. (1992) Hardiness: A review of theory and research. *Health Psychology, 11*, 335–345.

Garand, L., Dew, M. A., Eazor, L. R., DeKosky, S. T., and Reynolds, C. F. (2005) Caregiving burden and psychiatric morbidity in spouses of persons with mild cognitive impairment. *International Journal of Geriatric Psychiatry, 20*, 512–522.

Gaugler, J. E., Kane, R. L., and Newcomer, R. (2007) Resilience and transitions from dementia caregiving. *Journals of Gerontology: Psychological Sciences, 62B*, P38–P44.

Haley, W. E., Bergman, E. J., Roth, D. L., McVie, T., Gaugler, J. E., and Mittelman, M. S. (2008) Long-term effects of bereavement and caregiver intervention on dementia caregiver depressive symptoms. *The Gerontologist, 48*, 732–740.

Hardy, S. E., Concato, J., and Gill, T. M. (2004) Resilience of community-dwelling older persons. *Journal of the American Geriatrics Society, 52*, 257–262.

Harris, P. B. (2008) Another wrinkle in the debate about successful aging: The undervalued concept of resilience and the lived in experience of dementia. *International Journal of Aging and Human Development, 67*, 43–61.

Harris, P. B. and Keady, J. (2008) Wisdom, resilience and successful aging: Changing public discourses on living with dementia. *Dementia*

Hildon, Z., Montgomery, SM., Blane, D., Wiggins, RD., and Netuveli, G. (2010) Examining resilience of quality of life in the face of health-related and psychosocial adversity at older ages: what is "right" about the way we age?. *Gerontologist. 50*, 36–47.

Hildon, Z., Smith, G., Netuveli, G., and Blane, D. (2008) Understanding adversity and resilience at older ages. *Sociology of Health and Illness, 30*, 726–740.

Jacelon, C. S. (1997) The trait and process of resilience. *Journal of Advanced Nursing, 25*, 123–129.

Leipold, B. and Greve, W. (2009) Resilience: A conceptual bridge between coping and development. *European Psychologist, 14*, 40–50.

Judge, T. A., Erez, A., Bono, J. E., and Thoresen, C. J. (2002) Are measures of self-esteem, neuroticism, locus of control and generalized self-efficacy indicators of a common core construct? *Journal of Personality and Social Psychology, 83*, 693–710.

Kahn, R. L. (2002) Guest editorial: On "Successful aging and well-being: Self-rated compared with Rowe and Kahn." *The Gerontologist, 42*, 725–726.

Kane, M. N. (2008) Imagining recovery, resilience, and vulnerability at 75: Perceptions of social work students. *Educational Gerontology, 34*, 30–50.

Karel, M. (1997) Aging and depression: Vulnerability and stress across adulthood. *Clinical Psychology Review, 17*, 847–879.

Karim, S., Overshott, R., and Burns, A. (2005) Older people with schizophrenia. *Aging and Mental Health, 9*, 315–324.

Kelley, T. M. (2005) Natural resilience and innate mental health. *American Psychologist, 60*, 265.

Kessler, E. and Staudinger, U. M. (2009) Affective experience in adulthood and old age: The role of affective arousal and perceived affect regulation. *Psychology and Aging, 24*, 349–362.

King, D. W., King, L. A., Foy, D. W., Keane, T. M., and Fairbank, J. A. (1999) Posttraumatic stress disorder in a national sample of female and male Vietnam veterans: Risk factors, war-zone stressors, and resilience-recovery variables. *Journal of Abnormal Psychology, 108*, 164–170.

King, L. A., King, D. W., Vickers, K., Davison, E. H., and Spiro, A. (2007) Assessing late-onset stress symptomatology among aging male combat veterans. *Aging and Mental Health, 11*, 175–191.

Lamet, A., Szuchman, L., Perkel, L., and Walsh, S. (2009) Risk factors, resilience, and psychological distress among Holocaust and non-Holocaust survivors in the post-9/11 environment. *Educational Gerontology, 35*, 32–46.

Lamond, A. J., Depp, C., Allison, M., Langer, R., Reichstadt, J., Moore, D. J., et al. (2008) Measurement and predictors of resilience among community-dwelling older women. *Journal of Psychiatric Research, 43*, 148–154.

Linley, P. A. and Joseph, S. (2005) The human capacity for growth through adversity. *American Psychologist, 60,* 262–263.

Litz, B. T. (2005) Has resilience to severe trauma been underestimated? *American Psychologist, 60,* 262.

Lyness, J. M., Niculescu, A., Tu, X., Reynolds, C. F., and Caine, E. D. (2006) The relationship of medical comorbidity and depression in older, primary care patients. *Psychosomatics, 47,* 435–439.

Maddi, S. R. (2005) On hardiness and other pathways to resilience. *American Psychologist, 60,* 261–262.

Maddi, S. R., Brow, M., Khoshaba, D. M., and Vaitkus, M. (2006) Relationship of hardiness and religiousness to depression and anger. *Consulting Psychology Journal: Practice and Research, 58,* 148–161.

Manderscheid, R. W., Atay, J. E., and Crider, R. A. (2009) Changing trends in state psychiatric hospital use from 2002 to 2005. *Psychiatric Services, 60,* 29–34.

Mehta, M., Whyte, E., Lenze, E., Hardy, S., Roumani, Y., Subashan, P., et al. (2008) Depressive symptoms in late life: Associations with apathy, resilience and disability vary between young-old and old-old. *International Journal of Geriatric Psychiatry, 23,* 238–243.

McLaren, S., Gomez, R., Bailey, M., and Van Der Horst, K. (2007) The association of depression and sense of belonging with suicidal ideation among older adults: Applicability of resiliency models. *Suicide and Life-Threatening Behavior, 37,* 89–102.

Montross, L. P., Depp, C., Daly, J., Reichstadt, J., Golshan, S., Moore, D., et al. (2006) Correlates of self-rated successful aging among community-dwelling older adults. *American Journal of Geriatric Psychiatry, 14,* 43–51.

Motivala, S. J., Levin, M. J., Oxman, M. N., and Irwin, M. R. (2006) Impairments in health functioning and sleep quality in older adults with a history of depression. *Journal of the American Geriatrics Society, 54,* 1184–1191.

Nemeroff, C. B., Bremner, J. D., Foa, E. B., Mayberg, H. S., North, C. S., and Stein, M. B. (2006) Posttraumatic stress disorder: A state-of-the-science review. *Journal of Psychiatric Research, 40,* 1–21.

Netuveli, G. and Blane, D. (2008) Quality of life in older ages. *British Medical Bulletin, 85,* 113–126.

Nygren, B., Aléx, L., Jonsén, E., Gustafson, Y., Norberg, A., and Lundman, B. (2005) Resilience, sense of coherence, purpose in life and self-transcendence in relation to perceived physical and mental health among the oldest old. *Aging and Mental Health, 9,* 354–362.

Ong, A. D., Bergeman, C. S., and Bisconti, T. L. (2004) The role of daily positive emotions during conjugal bereavement. *Journal of Gerontology: Psychological Sciences, 59B,* P168–P176.

Ott, C. H., Leuger, R. J., Kelber, S. T., and Prigerson, H. G. (2007) Spousal bereavement in older adults. *The Journal of Nervous and Mental Disease, 195,* 332–341.

Philippe, F. L., Lecours, S., and Beaulieu-Pelletier, G. (2009) Resilience and positive emotions: Examining the role of emotional memories. *Journal of Personality, 77,* 139–176.

Pinquart, M. (2002) Good news about the effects of bad old-age stereotypes. *Experimental Aging Research, 28,* 317–336.

Poindexter, C. and Shippy, R. A. (2008) Networks of older New Yorkers with HIV: Fragility, resilience, and transformation. *AIDS, Patient Care, and STDs, 22,* 723–733.

Rabkin, J. G., Wagner, G. J., and Del Bene, M. (2000) Resilience and distress among amyotrophic lateral sclerosis patients and caregivers. *Psychosomatic Medicine, 62,* 271–279.

Richardson, G. E. (2002) The metatheory of resilience and resiliency. *Journal of Clinical Psychology, 58,* 307–321.

Rothermund, K. and Brandtstädter, J. (2003) Depression in later life: Cross-sectional patterns and possible determinants. *Psychology and Aging, 18,* 80–90.

Rossi, N. E., Bisconti, T. L., and Bergeman, C. S. (2007) The role of dispositional resilience in regaining life satisfaction after the loss of a spouse. *Death Studies, 31,* 863–883.

Rowe, J. W. and Kahn, R. L. (1997) Successful aging. *The Gerontologist, 37,* 433–440.

Saroglou, V., Buxant, C., and Tilquin, J. (2008) Positive emotions as leading to religion and spirtuality. *The Journal of Positive Psychology, 3*, 165–173.

Scholl, J. M. and Sabat, S. R. (2008) Stereotypes, stereotype threat and ageing: Implications for understanding and treatment of people with Alzheimer's disease. *Ageing and Society, 28,* 103–130.

Schulz, R., Mendelsohn, A. B., Haley, W. E., Mahoney, D., Allen, R. S., Zhang, S., et al. (2003) End-of-life care and the effects of bereavement on family caregivers of persons with dementia. *New England Journal of Medicine, 349,* 1936–1942.

Seeman, M. V. (2005) Parallels between aging and schizophrenia. *Psychiatry, 68,* 1–8.

Solomon, Z. and Mikulincer, M. (2006) Trajectories of PTSD: A 20-year longitudinal study. *American Journal of Psychiatry, 163,* 659–666.

Staudinger, U. M., Marsiske, M., and Baltes, P. B. (1995) Resilience and reserve capacity in later adulthood: Potentials and limits of development across the life span. In D. Cicchetti and D. J. Cohen (Eds.), *Developmental Psychopathology Vol 2: Risk, Disorder, and Adaptation* (pp. 801–847). New York: Wiley.

Torrey, E. F. (2005) Commentary on "Parallels between aging and schizophrenia": Why some patients succeed. *Psychiatry, 68,* 14–16.

Tugade, M. M. and Fredrickson, B. L. (2004) Resilient individuals use positive emotions to bounce back from negative emotional experiences. *Journal of Personality and Social Psychology, 86,* 320–333.

Vahia, I. V., Shilpa, D., Bankole, A. O., Kehn, M., Nurhussein, M., Ramirez, P., et al. (2008) Adequacy of medical treatment among older persons with schizophrenia. *Psychiatric Services, 59,* 853–859.

Van Vliet, K. J. (2008) Shame and resilience in adulthood: A grounded theory study. *Journal of Counseling Psychology, 55,* 233–245.

Wagnild, G. (2003) Resilience and successful aging: Comparison among low and high income older adults. *Journal of Gerontological Nursing, 29,* 42–49.

Wagnild, G. M. and Young, H. M. (1993) Development and psychometric evaluation of the resilience scale. *Journal of Nursing Measurement, 1,* 165–178.

Windle, G., Markland, D. A., and Woods, R. T. (2008) Examination of a theoretical model of psychological resilience in older age. *Aging and Mental Health, 12,* 285–292.

Yanos, P. T. and Moos, R. H. (2007) Determinants of functioning and well-being among individuals with schizophrenia: An integrated model. *Clinical Psychology Review, 27,* 58–77.

Yehuda, R., Golier, J. A., Tischler, L., Harvey, P. D., Newmark, R., Yang, R. K., and Buschbaum, M. S. (2007) Hippocampal volume in aging combat veterans with and without post-traumatic stress disorder: Relation to risk and resilience factors. *Journal of Psychiatric Research, 41,* 435–445.

Chapter 6
Physiological Resilience

Gregory Hicks and Ram R. Miller

In aging studies, resilience is often used to suggest an ability to recover from stressors and the relative degree of resilience depends on the stressor in question. Individuals may have adequate physiologic reserves to recover from moderate stressors yet lack sufficient resilience to recover from severe stressors. We have examined the recovery process from the relatively significant physiologic stressor of hip fracture. Following a hip fracture, there is a sudden loss of physical function (as measured by ability to walk independently and walking speed) followed by a period of recovery that can continue for a year or more depending on the area of function examined. The trauma of hip fracture and subsequent surgical repair may result in an oxidative stress and inflammatory response that, if excessive, can result in a detrimental effect on muscle strength and function. Antioxidant vitamins, vitamin D, and the statin class of medications and exercise may exert a beneficial effect, in part through a favorable modification of the post-traumatic inflammatory response.

In its most common usage, the term resilience refers to an ability to recover from change. In aging studies, resilience is often used to suggest an ability to recover from stressors. Using this definition it is possible to conceptualize resilience as the opposite of the geriatric syndrome of frailty. Frailty has increasingly been described as a biologic syndrome of, *decreased* reserve and resistance to stressors, resulting from cumulative declines across multiple physiologic systems, and causing vulnerability to adverse outcomes. Although there has been an extensive amount of research that has been recently conducted into the frailty syndrome, significantly less research has been directed toward the concept of resiliency. In contrast to frailty, resilience represents a state of, *adequate* reserve and resistance to stressors.

The relative degree of resilience obviously depends on the stressor in question. Individuals may have adequate reserves to recover from moderate stressors yet lack sufficient resilience to recover from severe stressors. Given the demographic trends in this aging population, older adults will, with increasing frequency, continue to encounter severe stressors (i.e. myocardial infarction, stroke, hip fracture, surgeries)

R.R. Miller (✉)
University of Maryland School of Medicine, Baltimore, MD, USA
e-mail: RRMILLER@epi.umaryland.edu

B. Resnick et al. (eds.), *Resilience in Aging: Concepts, Research, and Outcomes*,
DOI 10.1007/978-1-4419-0232-0_6, © Springer Science+Business Media, LLC 2011

that will challenge their physiologic reserve. We have examined the recovery process from the relatively significant physiologic stressor of hip fracture.

Because hip fracture is an acute traumatic and disabling condition that affects older adults, it is a good model for the examination of the physiologic processes that might influence resilience.

Following a hip fracture, there is a sudden loss of physical function (as measured by ability to walk independently and walking speed) followed by a period of recovery that can continue for a year or more depending on the area of function examined (Magaziner et al. 1990, 2000). By the end of a year, half of those who were able to walk independently before their fracture are not able to walk independently (Magaziner et al. 1990, 2000), which translates into an excess loss of function of about 25% when compared to loss in similar persons who do not have a hip fracture (Magaziner et al. 2003). In elders post-hip-fracture, the average one-year mortality is 18–33 percent (Magaziner et al. 1997). The duration of recovery and the period of increased mortality risk extend beyond that required for fracture healing, implying that the hip fracture event may trigger other adverse physiologic consequences.

In the following sections, we outline some aspects of the physiologic responses to the trauma of hip fracture that may explain the propensity for the adverse consequences of physiologic stress is older adults. We then discuss how possible modifiers of this response might influence resilience in older adults.

Inflammatory Response in Older Adults

Inflammatory cytokines are intercellular signaling molecules that mediate various aspects of cell function. They are essential for the coordination of the inflammatory response and immune function. Aging is associated with increased levels of circulating inflammatory cytokines (Bruunsgaard et al. 1999; Wei et al. 1992). These chronic, low-grade increases are typically two to four times the normal level of young adults, which, although well below the levels seen during acute infections (Krabbe et al. 2004), may have adverse effects. In studies of older adults, higher serum levels of markers of chronic inflammation have been associated with sarcopenia, decreased strength, functional loss and the frailty syndrome (Cappola et al. 2003b; Cesari et al. 2004b; Cohen et al. 1997; Ferrucci et al. 1999; Payette et al. 2003; Reuben et al. 2002; Walston et al. 2002).

Frailty and Resilience

Elders who are frail have decreased resilience to physiologic stressors. The frailty syndrome has been defined as a biologic syndrome of decreased reserve and resistance to stressors, resulting from cumulative declines across multiple physiologic systems, and causing vulnerability to adverse outcomes in elders (Fried et al. 2001).

There is evidence to suggest that older adults, and in particular frail older adults, may respond differently to inflammatory stimuli compared to younger adults or non-frail older adults. Peripheral blood mononuclear cells (PBMC) taken from frail elderly subjects had a higher IL-6 production after lipopolysaccharide (LPS) stimulation than those from non-frail elders (Leng et al. 2004), and elders are believed to also have a prolonged response following an inflammatory stimulus with slower normalization of cytokine levels compared to younger adults (Bruunsgaard et al. 1999; Krabbe et al. 2001). Following abdominal surgery, older adults have been reported to have both an increased and delayed interleukin-6 (IL-6) response, compared to younger patients (Kudoh et al. 2001).

Older adults who suffer hip fractures are often frail, and following the trauma of hip fracture and subsequent surgical repair, inflammatory cytokines have been found to be elevated up to one year post-fracture (Miller et al. 2006). These levels are higher than published values in disabled older women who have not suffered a hip fracture (Cappola et al. 2003a).

An inflammatory reaction following an acute medical event or traumatic event such as hip fracture is a reflection of the normal physiologic response to the initial insult. However, in some older adults, for example frail older adults, this response may be prolonged and become detrimental to recovery. The inflammatory response may therefore be a physiologic factor that influences the resilience of older adults to these physiologic stressors, and may explain the decreased resilience to physiologic stressors that may be seen in frail elders.

Effect of Inflammation on Muscle

Remote inflammatory processes, such as cancer, congestive heart failure (CHF), arthritis, and chronic obstructive pulmonary disease (COPD), have been observed to be associated with muscle catabolism and loss of muscle function that have been attributed to circulating cytokines (Gosker et al. 2003; Reid and Li 2001; Vescovo et al. 2000). Inflammation can contribute to muscle weakness by two main mechanisms: accelerated protein loss and contractile dysfunction (Reid and Li 2001). Inflammatory cytokines have long been associated with catabolic states (Beutler et al. 1985). This effect is believed to result from nitrogen loss and catabolism of muscle protein, which is strongly linked to tumor necrosis factor alpha (TNF-α). In addition, the inflammatory response can also suppress trophic hormone production and activity, for example insulin-like growth factor 1 (IGF-1), which similarly results in decreased muscle mass (Barbieri et al. 2002; Cappola et al. 2003b; De Benedetti et al. 1997; Fernandez-Celemin et al. 2002; Fernandez-Celemin and Thissen 2001).

Muscle weakness, however, has also been found to occur without overt loss of muscle protein (Budgett 1998) suggesting that inflammation may result in changes intrinsic to the muscle itself. In fact, inflammatory cytokines have been associated with altered contractile protein composition and contractile dysfunction in laboratory animals and humans (Li et al. 2000; Vescovo et al. 2000). In addition to the catabolic effect of chronic inflammatory states (Beutler et al. 1985; Kotler 2000), TNF-α is believed to depress contractile force at the myofilament level, by a mechanism mediated by reactive oxygen species (ROS) and nitric oxide (NO) derivative generation (Reid et al. 2002).

In adults undergoing elective hip arthroplasty, peak IL-6 levels shortly after surgery were associated with time to recovery of walking (Hall et al. 2001). In hip fracture patients, serum levels of inflammatory markers were adversely associated with function, as individuals with higher serum inflammatory cytokine levels were observed to have worse performance on tests of lower extremity function in the year post-fracture than those with lower serum levels (Miller et al. 2006). If cytokine levels do in fact rise and remain high in some individuals following exposure to physiologic stressors, then this may result in similar consequences on muscle mass and function as seen in other chronic inflammatory conditions.

Oxidative Stress

Dating back to the 1950s, it has been suggested that oxidative damage, caused by free radicals, might be associated with the age-related functional decline and the development of frailty seen in older adults (De La Fuente 2002). Free radicals have been described as "any species capable of independent existence that contains one or more unpaired electrons" (Halliwell and Gutteridge 1999). Due to the unstable nature of these free radicals, biologic systems can be placed in a state of disequilibrium resulting in oxidative damage (Aust et al. 1985; Sevenian and Hochstein 1985). It has been theorized that oxidative damage may be, in large part, responsible for the sarcopenia (loss of muscle mass and strength) and resultant functional decline seen with typical aging (Fano et al. 2001). These sarcopenic changes are thought to be due to oxidative damage to DNA, proteins, and lipids that increases in human skeletal muscle (Semba et al. 2007b).

Early in the course of surgery an increase in ROS and a decrease in plasma antioxidant levels have been measured, suggesting that oxidative stress is one of the early responses to surgical stress (Clermont et al. 2002; Luyten et al. 2005). ROSs are important mediators and regulators of the inflammatory response, and are important to the intercellular messaging systems of nuclear factor Kappa B (NF-κB). Relatively low concentrations of hydrogen peroxide or a moderate oxidative shift in thiol-disulfide redox status have been shown to enhance NF-κB activation in various cell types. Expression of the inflammatory TNF-α is commonly induced by NF-κB and is accordingly increased under oxidative conditions (Dröge 2002). And NF-κB itself has been strongly implicated in pathological processes involved in muscle wasting (Cai et al. 2004).

In response to oxidative damage, the body has a natural antioxidant defense system that counters the rate of oxidation (Maxwell 1995; Clarkson and Thompson 2000). If the antioxidant system does not function properly in response to the oxidative damage caused by the proliferation of free radicals, then DNA damage and an acceleration of functional decline are likely consequences (Cesari et al. 2004a). Therefore, it is critically important that antioxidant levels are properly maintained among older adults to deal with the severe stressors that occur.

Potential Modifiers of Physiologic Resilience

Antioxidant Vitamins

Inflammation and oxidative stress are believed to play a significant role in many age-associated conditions such as sarcopenia, decreased strength, functional loss, and the frailty syndrome (Cappola et al. 2003b; Cesari et al. 2004b; Cohen et al. 1997; Ferrucci et al. 1999; Payette et al. 2003; Reuben et al. 2002; Semba et al. 2007a; Walston et al. 2002). Given the importance of ROS in the processes of inflammation and muscle wasting (Cai et al. 2004; Dröge 2002), there has been significant attention paid to the role of antioxidant vitamins in retarding these processes. Of these, vitamin E and the carotenoids are among the best studied. Vitamin E is a term that encompasses a group of potent, lipid-soluble, chain-breaking antioxidants that include four tocopherols and four tocotrienols (Brigelius-Flohe 1999). The carotenoids (α-carotene, β-carotene, β-cryptoxanthin, lutein, zeaxanthin, and lycopene) occur in a wide variety of fruits and vegetables. They are best known for their pro-vitamin A activity but in addition they are believed to be efficient scavengers of free radicals (Di Mascio et al. 1989). Selenium is an essential element and adequate selenium intake is required for optimal activity of key antioxidant enzymes, including glutathione peroxidases and thioredoxin reductases (Rayman 2000).

Because of their anti-oxidant effects, vitamin E, the carotenoids, and selenium have been extensively studied for their potentially preventive effects in chronic diseases believed to have an oxidative stress component such as cardiovascular diseases, atherosclerosis, and cancer (Navas-Acien et al. 2008; Rimm et al. 1993; Stampfer et al. 1993; Voutilainen et al. 2006). In studies of older adults, higher levels of both the tocopherols, carotenoids, and selenium have been associated with decreased frailty, increased muscle strength, and reduced disability (Bartali et al. 2008, 2006; Lauretani et al. 2007; Michelon et al. 2006; Semba et al. 2006; Semba et al. 2007b, 2007c).

In contrast to these observational studies, results from interventional studies with antioxidant vitamins have been less favorable. These studies have shown either no benefit or a risk of harm with the administration of supplemental antioxidant vitamins (Miller et al. 2005; Vivekananthan et al. 2003; Voutilainen et al. 2006). Many theories have been proposed for this disconnect between observational and interventional studies. One obvious explanation is that the serum markers of antioxidant vitamins may be markers of healthy lifestyle factors aside from diet that may result in the benefit seen in observational studies (Lichtenstein 2009). Another explanation is that the majority of intervention studies have relied on supplementation with single compounds, ignoring the complexity of whole food intake. For example, most carotenoid interventional studies have used high-dose β-carotene as the agent of supplementation, whereas intake of foods rich in carotenoids may also contain lycopene, α-carotene, lutein, zeaxanthin, and β-crytoxanthin (Voutilainen et al. 2006).

It is believed that in vivo the carotenoids exhibit their antioxidant properties in different locations in cellular structures, based upon their chemical composition. β-Carotene is a highly lipophilic structure and so would be located primarily deep within the interior of cell membranes, whereas zeaxanthin also has polar components and can span the cell membrane. Due to its lipophilicity, β-carotene would not be as effective a scavenger of water soluble peroxyl radicals, whereas zeaxanthin would (El-Agamey et al. 2004). It has been postulated that the carotenoids therefore act in concert to scavenge free radicals across cellular structures; again suggesting that supplementation cannot easily replicate the complexity of whole food intake.

Also, β-carotene is believed to have paradoxical pro-oxidant effects at high serum concentrations, and this pro-oxidant effect has been suggested as a potential explanation for the observed negative effects in intervention studies that have typically utilized high-dose β-carotene. The water soluble vitamin C is believed to inhibit the pro-oxidant effects of high concentrations of β-carotene. Because smoking generates a high burden of oxidizing radicals, and smokers are typically deficient in vitamin C, this has been suggested as one explanation for the observation that smokers have fared particularly poorly in studies on β-carotene supplementation (El-Agamey et al. 2004).

Similarly, interventional studies using vitamin E have primarily used α-tocopherol as the agent of supplementation. Here too this may ignore the complexity of whole-food intake. A recent study has suggested a mechanism by which that unbalanced intake of α-tocopherol may be harmful, as it can result in a depletion of two other forms of vitamin E, γ-tocopherol, and δ-tocopherol; both powerful antioxidants (Huang and Appel 2003).

In response to a more potent inflammatory stimulus, the role of inflammatory markers and free radicals is even more pronounced. Key to the pathogenesis of sepsis and the systemic inflammatory response syndrome (SIRS) is the production of free radicals and inflammatory cytokines (Berger and Chiolero 2007). In an effort to minimize the devastating effects of sepsis, numerous immunotherapeutic approaches have been attempted, with little success (Nasraway 2003). It has been suggested that the immune dysregulation and organ dysfunction that is seen in the sepsis syndrome may be too complex to be significantly modified by therapies directed at single molecules, such as the anti-TNF-α antibodies (Abraham 1999).

Plasma concentrations of antioxidant vitamins have been found to be depressed during critical illness and sepsis, and supplementation with selenium, vitamin E, and carotenoids appears to offer some protection from the effects of sepsis and SIRS in observational studies and in small human or animal intervention studies (Sakr et al. 2007; Berger and Chiolero 2007). The first randomized trial of enteral pharmaconutrition in sepsis has recently been published. This study demonstrated that the administration of nutritional supplementation, including vitamins C, E, β-carotene, and selenium, early in the course of sepsis, resulted in a significantly faster recovery of organ function compared to controls (Beale et al. 2008). Although it is premature to draw strong conclusions from a single study, it may be that this more holistic approach to nutritional therapy be of benefit. In contrast to sepsis, the levels of inflammatory cytokine elevations that have been observed following hip fracture or in post-operative patients are generally lower, and so may not require aggressive immunotherapy. For example, after cardiac surgery where serum levels of vitamin E have been observed to decrease shortly after surgery (Luyten et al. 2005), pre-operative supplementation was found to offer some protective effects in one small study (Yau et al. 1994).

Vitamin D

The importance of vitamin D in the maintenance of calcium homeostasis is well known. Vitamin D is now believed to also have important effects related to muscle strength and function, via both a direct influence and through its regulation of para-thyroid hormone (PTH) levels (Bischoff-Ferrari et al. 2004b; Visser et al. 2003). Vitamin D deficiency may result in decreased muscle strength from both an increase in muscle protein degradation as well as altered contractile properties of muscle (Rodman and Baker 1978; Wassner et al. 1983). The vitamin D receptor (VDR) is present on skeletal muscle (Simpson et al. 1985), and muscle protein synthesis is initiated by the binding of 1,25-dihydroxyvitamin D3 [1,25 $(OH)_2$ D3] to its nuclear receptor with subsequent gene transcription. The influence of 1,25 $(OH)_2$ D3 on calcium homeostasis in skeletal muscle is believed to influence the contractile properties of muscle cells via both a VDR-mediated genomic pathway and a non-genomic rapid mechanism involving membrane effects of 1,25 $(OH)_2$ D3 (Boland et al. 1995).

Vitamin D has also been studied for its immunomodulatory effects. The VDR, through which the majority of the biologic effects of vitamin D are mediated, has been identified in almost every tissue in the body including most cells of the immune system (Holick 2005; van Etten and Mathieu 2005). 1,25 $(OH)_2$D3 has been shown to inhibit the maturation of dendritic cells (DC) in vitro as well as the secretion by DCs and other antigen-presenting cells of the immuno-stimulatory cytokine IL-12. Since IL-12 stimulates the development of CD4+ T-helper 1 cells (Th-1) and inhibits the development of CD4+ T-helper 2 cells, this results in a shift away from a relatively pro-inflammatory Th1 profile (Ex: IL-1, TNF-α, IL-17, IL-18, IFN-γ) and toward a relatively anti-inflammatory Th2 type (Ex: IL-4, IL-10, IL-13) (van Etten and Mathieu 2005). In addition, the transcription of several key Th-1 cytokines such as IFN-γ and IL-2 is also inhibited by vitamin D (van Etten and Mathieu 2005). Vitamin D deficiency has been associated with an increased risk of Th-1 cytokine-mediated autoimmune diseases such as inflammatory bowel disease, rheumatoid arthritis, systemic lupus erythematosis, multiple sclerosis, and type 1 diabetes mellitus (Peterlik and Cross 2005). Furthermore, although vitamin D attenuates the antigen-presenting function of monocytes and macrophages, the chemotactic and phagocytic function of these cells is enhanced by exposure to 1,25 $(OH)_2$ D_3, suggesting an immune-modulating effect rather than merely an immunosuppressive one.

Unfortunately, vitamin D deficiency is common in older adults, especially among several groups of minority elders (Yetley 2008). We have found that the serum level of 25 (OH) D measured shortly after hip fracture is associated with IL-6 response post-fracture, with subjects deficient in vitamin D at the time of the fracture displaying higher serum levels of IL-6 at all follow-up time points in the year post-fracture. Vitamin D deficiency itself has also been associated with worse function post-hip fracture (LeBoff et al. 2008).

Vitamin D deficiency has been associated with functional decline, sarcopenia, and the frailty syndrome with studies indicating that vitamin D deficiency increases risk for decreased muscle strength, sarcopenia, falls, and frailty (Bischoff-Ferrari et al. 2004a; Puts et al. 2005; Visser et al. 2003), many of the same outcomes are associated with chronic inflammatory processes in elders. Whether the relative pro-inflammatory state that is conferred by vitamin D deficiency may explain, in part, the adverse effect of this deficiency is not known. Furthermore, if vitamin D deficiency is associated with frailty, then this deficiency may explain, in part, the increased cytokine response and the decreased functional resiliency to stressors in frail elders (Leng et al. 2004). If individuals who are deficient in vitamin D at the time of the fracture respond with a greater inflammatory response than those with sufficient levels following hip fracture surgery, then this would suggest that vitamin D may offer some protective effects from a detrimental inflammatory response following the inflammatory stimulus of hip fracture and surgical repair.

Exercise

Physical activity and exercise have also been associated with elevations in anti-inflammatory cytokines and cytokine inhibitors as well as lower levels of pro-inflammatory cytokines (Abramson and Vaccarino 2002; Colbert et al. 2004; Okita et al. 2004; Ostrowski et al. 1999, 2000; Wannamethee et al. 2002). In response to exercise, IL-6 is typically the first cytokine to appear, followed by interleukin-1 receptor antagonist (IL-1ra) and interleukin-10 (IL-10). The rise in IL-6 levels occurs shortly after initiation of exercise, peaking at approximately 3–4 hours after exercise termination, returning to baseline levels 24–48 hours post-exercise (Toft et al. 2002). Both IL-10 and IL-1ra have anti-inflammatory effects, while the effects of IL-6 are more complex, in this context it is believed to exert an inhibitory effect on TNF-α and IL-1β.

There is evidence that exercise may have prolonged anti-inflammatory effects and may result in blunting of the response to inflammatory stimuli. In healthy subjects, the performance of a cycling exercise at 75% of their VO_2 max had a blunted TNF-α response to an endotoxin bolus (Starkie et al. 2003). This suggests that exercise might also offer some protection against chronic systemic low-grade inflammation resulting from external stimuli. We have found that a low-intensity generalized exercise program can reduce levels of soluble TNF-α receptor 1 (sTNF-α R1) in the year after hip fracture.

The effect of exercise on resistance to oxidative stress is more complex, as exercise itself can generate oxygen-free radicals. Low levels of exercise-induced oxidative stress are believed to result in increased expression and synthesis of anti-oxidant enzymes, through a mechanism involving NF-κB as several important antioxidant enzymes contain NF-κB binding sites in their promoter region (Ji 2002; Gomez-Cabrera et al. 2008). In studies of older adults, physical activity has been found to be associated with an increased level of the intrinsic anti-oxidant enzyme glutathione peroxidase, but with a decreased level of carotenoids, perhaps as a result of consumption following the oxidative stress of exercise (Rousseau et al. 2006; Karolkiewicz et al. 2003).

In a randomized study, preoperative exercise was found to reduce the duration of stay at hospital and ICU stay in patients awaiting coronary artery bypass grafting surgery (Arthur et al. 2000). Cardio-pulmonary bypass results in the significant generation of free radicals and oxidative stress (Clermont et al. 2002). Whether the observed beneficial effects of pre-operative exercise may be due to a favorable attenuation of the oxidative stress and inflammatory responses following surgery is not known.

Statins

Key to the pathogenesis of sepsis and the SIRS is the production of free radicals and inflammatory cytokines (Berger and Chiolero 2007). 3-Hydroxy-methyl-glutaryl-COA reductase inhibitors (statins) are a class of medications that have been shown in observational studies to improve survival in sepsis (Almog et al. 2004). Statins have important anti-inflammatory effects; however statins do not target individual inflammatory mediators, but instead may reduce the overall magnitude of the systemic response (Ando et al. 2000; Terblanche et al. 2006, 2007). This broad action is believed to be an important distinguishing feature in the modulation of the host response to septic insults. A recent study estimated that between 1999 and 2004 over 24% of men over 50 and women over 60 had taken statins (Spatz et al. 2009), but whether these agents might favorably alter the inflammatory response in those who are exposed to acute stressors is unknown.

Conclusion

The physiologic response to stressors in older adults is complex, and tremendous variability exits in the ability of older adults to recover from physiologic stress. The oxidative stress and inflammatory response may suggest potential explanations for this variability. Early observational and experimental data suggest that modifiers of the inflammatory response and antioxidant vitamins may favorably impact resilience in older adults to physiologic stress. The disappointing results from antioxidant intervention trials, however, would argue for caution before advocating for the widespread use of these agents in older adults. Instead, diets rich in foods that contain anti-oxidants, the maintenance of adequate vitamin D levels, and physical activity are likely to be the most beneficial for the enhancement of physiologic resilience in elders.

References

Abraham, E. (1999) Why immunomodulatory therapies have not worked in sepsis. *Intensive Care Med, 25*, 556–566.

Abramson, J. L., & Vaccarino, V. (2002) Relationship between physical activity and inflammation among apparently healthy middle-aged and older US adults. *Arch Intern Med, 162*, 1286–1292.

Almog, Y., Shefer, A., Novack, V., Maimon, N., Barski, L., Eizinger, M., et al. (2004) Prior statin therapy is associated with a decreased rate of severe sepsis. *Circulation, 110*(7), 880–885.

Ando, H., Takamura, T., Ota, T., HNagai, Y., & Kobayashi, K. (2000) Cerivastatin improves survival of mice with lipopolysaccharide-induced sepsis. *J Pharmacol Exp Ther, 294*, 1043–1046.

Arthur, H. M., Daniels, C., McKelvie, R., Hirsh, J., & Rush, B. (2000) Effect of a preoperative intervention on preoperative and postoperative outcomes in low-risk patients awaiting elective coronary artery bypass graft surgery. A randomized, controlled trial. *Ann Intern Med, 133*(4), 253–262.

Aust, S. D., Morehouse, L. A., & Thomas, C. E. (1985) Role of metals in oxygen radical reactions. *Free Radic Biol Med, 1*, 3.

Barbieri, M., Ferrucci, L., Ragno, E., Corsi, A. M., Bandinelli, S., Bonafe, M., et al. (2002) Chronic inflammation and the effect of IGF-1 on muscle strength and power in older persons. *Am J Physiol Endocrinol Metab, 284*, E481–E487.

Bartali, B., Frongillo, E. A., Guralnik, J. M., Stipanuk, M. H., Allore, H. G., Cherubini, A., et al. (2008) Serum micronutrient concentrations and decline in physical function among older persons. *JAMA, 299*(3), 308–315.

Bartali, B., Semba, R. D., Frongillo, E. A., Varadhan, R., Ricks, M. O., Blaum, C. S., et al. (2006) Low micronutrient levels as a predictor of incident disability in older women. *Arch Intern Med, 166*(21), 2335–2340.

Beale, R. J., Sherry, T., Lei, K., Campbell-Stephen, L., McCook, J., Smith, J., et al. (2008) Early enteral supplementation with key pharmaconutrients improves Sequential Organ Failure Assessment score in critically ill patients with sepsis: outcome of a randomized, controlled, double-blind trial. *Crit Care Med, 36*(1), 131–144.

Berger, M. M., & Chiolero, R. L. (2007) Antioxidant supplementation in sepsis and systemic inflammatory response syndrome. *Crit Care Med, 35*(Suppl. 9), S584–590.

Beutler, B., Mahoney, J., Le Trang, N., Pekala, P., & Cerami, A. (1985) Purification of cachectin, a lipoprotein lipase-suppressing hormone secreted by endotoxin induced raw 264.7 cells. *J Exp Med, 161*, 984–995.

Bischoff-Ferrari, H. A., Dawson-Hughes, B., Willett, W. C., Staehelin, H. B., Bazemore, M. G., Zee, R. Y., et al. (2004a) Effect of Vitamin D on falls: a meta-analysis. *JAMA, 291* (16), 1999–2006.

Bischoff-Ferrari, H. A., Dietrich, T., Orav, E. J., Hu, F. B., Zhang, Y., Karlson, E. W., et al. (2004b) Higher 25-hydroxyvitamin D concentrations are associated with better lower-extremity function in both active and inactive persons aged 60 y. *Am J Clin Nutr, 80*, 752–758.

Boland, R., De Boland, A. R., Marinissen, M., Santillian, G., Vazquez, G., & Zanello, S. (1995) Avian muscle cells as targets for the secosteroid 1,25-dihyroxyvitamin D3. *Mol Cell Endocrinol, 114*, 1–8.

Brigelius-Flohe, R. T. M. (1999) Vitamin E: function and metabolism. *FASEB J,13*(10), 1145–1155.

Bruunsgaard, H., Skinhoj, P., Qvist, J., & Pedersen, B. K. (1999) Elderly humans show prolonged in vivo inflammatory activity during pneumococcal infections. *J Infect Dis,180*, 551–554.

Budgett, R. (1998) Fatigue and underperformance in athletes: the overtraining syndrome. *Br J Sports Med, 32*, 107–110.

Cai, D., Frantz, J. D., Tawa, N. E. J., Melendez, P. A., Oh, B. C., Lidov, H. G., et al. (2004) IKKbeta/NF-kappaB activation causes severe muscle wasting in mice. *Cell, 119*(2), 285–298.

Cappola, A., Xue, Q., Ferrucci, L., Guralnik, J., Volpato, S., & Fried, L. (2003a) Insulin-like growth factor I and interleukin-6 contribute synergistically to disability and mortality in older women. *J Clin Endocrinol Metab, 88*(5), 2019–2025.

Cappola, A. R., Xue, Q. L., Ferrucci, L., Guralnik, J. M., Volpato, S., & Fried, L. P. (2003b) Insulin-like growth factor I and interleukin-6 contribute synergistically to disability and mortality in older women. *J Clin Endocrinol Metab, 88*(5), 2019–2025.

Cesari, M., Pahor, M., Bartali, B., Cherubini, A., Penninx, B. W., Williams, G. R., et al. (2004a) Antioxidants and physical performance in elderly persons: the Invecchiare in Chianti (InCHIANTI) study. *Am J Clin Nutr, 79*, 289–294.

Cesari, M., Penninx, B. W. J. H., Pahor, M., Lauretani, F., Corsi, A. M., Williams, G. R., et al. (2004b) Inflammatory markers and physical performance in older persons: The InCHIANTI study. *J Gerontol A Biol Sci Med Sci, 59A*(3), 242–248.

Clarkson, P. M., & Thompson, S. (2000) Antioxidants: what role do they play in physical activity and health?, *Am J Clin Nutr, 72*, 637S–646S.

Clermont, G., Vergely, C., Jazayeri, S., Lahet, J. J., Goudeau, J. J., Lecour, S., et al. (2002) Systemic free radical activation is a major event involved in myocardial oxidative stress related to cardiopulmonary bypass. *Anesthesiology, 96*(1), 80–87.

Cohen, H. J., Pieper, C. F., Harris, T., Rao, K. M., & Currie, M. S. (1997) The association of plasma IL-6 levels with functional disability in community-dwelling elderly. *J Gerontol A Biol Sci Med Sci, 52*(4), M201–M208.

Colbert, L. H., Visser, M., Simonsick, E. M., Tracy, R. P., Newman, A. B., Kritchevsky, S. B., et al. (2004) Physical activity, exercise, and inflammatory markers in older adults: findings from The Health, Aging and Body Composition Study. *J Am Geriatr Soc, 52*, 1098–1104.

De Benedetti, F., Alonzi, T., Moretta, A., Lazzaro, D., Costa, P., Poli, V., et al. (1997) Interleukin 6 causes growth impairment in transgenic mice through a decrease in insulin-like growth factor-1. *J Clin Invest, 99*, 643–650.

De La Fuente, M. (2002) Effects of antioxidants on immune system ageing. *Eur J Clin Nutr, 56*, S5–S8.

Di Mascio, P., Kaiser, S., & Sies, H. (1989) Lycopene as the most efficient biological carotenoid singlet oxygen quencher. *Arch Biochem Biophys, 274*, 532–538.

Dröge, W. (2002) Free radicals in the physiological control of cell function. *Physiol Rev, 82*, 47–95.

El-Agamey, A., Lowe, G. M., McGarvey, D. J., Mortensen, A., Phillip, D. M., Truscott, T. G., et al. (2004) Carotenoid radical chemistry and antioxidant/pro-oxidant properties. *Arch Biochem Biophys, 430*(1), 37–48.

Fano, G., Mecocci, P., Vecchiet, J., Belia, S., Fulle, S., Polidori, M. C., et al. (2001) Age and sex influence on oxidative damage and functional status in human skeletal muscle. *J Muscle Res Cell Motil, 22*(4), 345–351.

Fernandez-Celemin, L., Pasko, N., Blomart, V., & Thissen, J. P. (2002) Inhibition of muscle insulin-like growth factor I expression by tumor necrosis factor-alpha. *Am J Physiol Endocrinol Metab, 283*, E1279–E1290.

Fernandez-Celemin, L., & Thissen, J. P. (2001) Interleukin-6 stimulates hepatic insulin-like growth factor binding protein-4 messenger ribonucleic acid and protein. *Endocrinology, 142*, 241–248.

Ferrucci, L., Harris, T. B., Guralnik, J. M., Tracy, R. P., Corti, M. C., Cohen, H. J., et al. (1999) Serum IL-6 level and the development of disability in older persons. *J Am Geriatr Soc, 47*(6), 639–646.

Fried, L. P., Tangen, C. M., Walston, J., Newman, A. B., Hirsch, C., Gottdiener, J., et al. (2001) Frailty in older adults: evidence for a phenotype.*J Gerontol A Biol Sci Med Sci, 56A*, M146–M156.

Gomez-Cabrera, M. C., Domenech, E., & Viña, J. (2008) Moderate exercise is an antioxidant: upregulation of antioxidant genes by training.*Free Radic Biol Med, 44*(2), 126–131.

Gosker, H. R., Kubat, B., Schaart, G., van der Vusse, G. J., Wouters, E. F., & Schols, A. M. (2003) Myopathological features in skeletal muscle of patients with chronic obstructive pulmonary disease.*Eur Respir J, 22*(2), 280–285.

Hall, G. M., Peerbhoy, D., Shenkin, A., Parker, C. J. R., & Salmon, P. (2001) Relationship of the functional recovery after hip arthroplasty to the neuroendocrine and inflammatory responses. *Br J Anaesth, 87*, 537–542.

Halliwell, B., & Gutteridge, J. M. C. (1999),*Free Radicals in Biology and Medicine.* (3rd ed.). Oxford, UK: Oxford University Press.

Holick, M. F. (2005) The vitamin D epidemic and its health consequences. *J Nutr, 135*, 2739S–2748S.

Huang, H. Y., & Appel, L. J. (2003) Supplementation of diets with alpha-tocopherol reduces serum concentrations of gamma- and delta-tocopherol in humans. *J Nutr, 133*(10), 3137–3140.

Ji, L. L. (2002) Exercise-induced modulation of antioxidant defense. *Ann N Y Acad Sci, 959*, 82–92.

Karolkiewicz, J., Szczesniak, L., Deskur-Smielecka, E., Nowak, A., Stemplewski, R., & Szeklicki, R. (2003) Oxidative stress and antioxidant defense system in healthy, elderly men: relationship to physical activity. *Aging Male, 6*(2), 100–105.

Kotler, D. P. (2000) Cachexia.,*Ann Intern Med, 133*(8), 622–634.

Krabbe, K. S., Bruunsgaard, H., Hansen, C. M., Moller, K., Fonsmark, L., Qvist, J., et al. (2001) Ageing is associated with a prolonged fever response in human endotoxemia. *Clin Diagn Lab Immunol, 8*, 333–338.

Krabbe, K. S., Pedersen, M., & Bruunsgaard, H. (2004) Inflammatory mediators in the elderly. *Exp Gerontol, 39*, 687–699.

Kudoh, A., Katagai, H., Takazawa, T., & Matsuki, A. (2001) Plasma proinflammatory cytokine response to surgical stress in elderly patients. *Cytokine, 15*, 270–273.

Lauretani, F., Semba, R. D., Bandinelli, S., Ray, A. L., Guralnik, J. M., & Ferrucci, L. (2007) Association of low plasma selenium concentrations with poor muscle strength in older community-dwelling adults: the InCHIANTI Study. *Am J Clin Nutr, 86*(2), 347–352.

LeBoff, M. S., Hawkes, W. G., Glowacki, J., Yu-Yahiro, J., Hurwitz, S., & Magaziner, J. (2008) Vitamin D-deficiency and post-fracture changes in lower extremity function and falls in women with hip fractures. *Osteoporos Int, 19*, 1283–1290.

Leng, S. X., Yang, H., & Walston, J. D. (2004) Decreased cell proliferation and altered cytokine production in frail older adults. *Aging Clin Exp Res, 16*, 249–252.

Li, X., Moody, M. R., Engel, D., Walker, S., Clubb, F. J. J., Sivasubramanian, N., et al. (2000) Cardiac-specific overexpression of tumor necrosis factor-alpha causes oxidative stress and contractile dysfunction in mouse diaphragm. *Circulation, 102*(14), 1690–1696.

Lichtenstein, A. H. (2009) Nutrient supplements and cardiovascular disease: a heartbreaking story.*J Lipid Res, 50*, S429–S433.

Luyten, C. R., van Overveld, F. J., De Backer, L. A., Sadowska, A. M., Rodrigus, I. E., De Hert, S. G., et al. (2005) Antioxidant defence during cardiopulmonary bypass surgery. *Eur J Cardiothorac Surg, 27*(4), 611–616.

Magaziner, J., Fredman, L., Hawkes, W., Hebel, J. R., Zimmerman, S., Orwig, D. L., et al. (2003) Changes in functional status attributable to hip fracture: a comparison of hip fracture patients to community-dwelling aged. *Am J Epidemiol, 157*(11), 1023–1031.

Magaziner, J., Hawkes, W., Hebel, J. R., Zimmerman, S. I., Fox, K. M., Dolan, M., et al. (2000) Recovery from hip fracture in eight areas of function. *J Gerontol Med Sci, 55A*(9), M498–M507.

Magaziner, J., Lydick, E., Hawkes, W., Zimmerman, S. I., Fox, K. M., Epstein, R. S., et al. (1997) Excess mortality attributable to hip fracture in white women aged 70 years and older. *Am J Public Health, 87*(10), 1630–1636.

Magaziner, J., Simonsick, E. M., Kashner, T. M., Hebel, J. R., & Kenzora, J. E. (1990) Predictors of functional recovery one year following hospital discharge for hip fracture: a prospective study. *J Gerontol Med Sci, 45*(3), M101–M107.

Maxwell, S. R. J. (1995) Prospects for the use of antioxidant therapies.*Drugs,349*(3), 345–361.

Michelon, E., Blaum, C., Semba, R. D., Xue, Q. L., Ricks, M. O., & Fried, L. P. (2006) Vitamin and carotenoid status in older women: associations with the frailty syndrome. *J Gerontol A Biol Sci Med Sci, 61*(6), 600–607.

Miller, E. R. R., Pastor-Barriuso, R., Dalal, D., Riemersma, R. A., Appel, L. J., & Guallar, E. (2005) Meta-analysis: high-dosage vitamin E supplementation may increase all-cause mortality. [see comment]. *Ann Intern Med, 142*(1), 37–46.

Miller, R. R., Cappola, A. R., Shardell, M. D., Hawkes, W., Hebel, J. R., Yu-Yahiro, J., et al. (2006) Persistent changes in interleukin-6 and lower extremity function following hip fracture. *J Gerontol A Biol Sci Med Sci, 61*, 1053–1058.

Nasraway, S. A. (2003) The problems and challenges of immunotherapy in sepsis. [Review] [65 refs].*Chest, 123*(Suppl. 5), 451S–459S.

Navas-Acien, A., Bleys, J., & Guallar, E. (2008) Selenium intake and cardiovascular risk: what is new? *Curr Opin Lipidol, 19*(1), 43–49.

Okita, K., Nishijima, H., Murakami, T., Nagai, T., Morita, N., Yonezawa, K., et al. (2004) Can exercise training with weight loss lower serum C-reactive protein levels? *Arterioscler Thromb Vasc Biol, 24*, 1868–1873.

Ostrowski, K., Rohde, T., Asp, S., Schjerling, P., & Pedersen, B. K. (1999) Pro- and anti-inflammatory cytokine balance in strenuous exercise in humans. *J Physiol, 515*, 287–291.

Ostrowski, K., Schjerling, P., & Pedersen, B. K. (2000) Physical activity and plasma interleukin-6 in humans - effect of intensity of exercise. *Eur J Appl Physiol, 83*, 512–515.

Payette, H., Roubenoff, R., Jacques, P. F., Dinarello, C. A., Wilson, P. W. F., Abad, L. W., et al. (2003) Insulin-like growth factor-1 and interleukin-6 predict sarcopenia in very old community-living men and women: the Framingham Study. *J Am Geriatr Soc, 51*, 1237–1243.

Peterlik, M., & Cross, H. S. (2005) Vitamin D and calcium deficits predispose for multiple chronic diseases. *Eur J Clin Invest, 35*(5), 290–304.

Puts, M. T. E., Visser, M., Twisk, J. W. R., Deeg, D. J. H., & Lips, P. (2005) Endocrine and inflammatory markers as predictive of frailty. *Clin Endocrinol, 63*, 403–411.

Rayman, M. P. (2000) The importance of selenium to human health., *Lancet, 356*(9225), 233–241.

Reid, M. B., Lannergren, J., & Westerblad, H. (2002) Respiratory and limb muscle weakness induced by tumor necrosis factor-alpha. *Am J Respir Crit Care Med, 166*, 479–484.

Reid, M. B., & Li, Y. P. (2001) Cytokines and oxidative signalling in skeletal muscle. *Acta Physiol Scand, 171*, 225–232.

Reuben, D. B., Cheh, A. I., Harris, T. B., Ferrucci, L., Rowe, J. W., Tracy, R. P., et al. (2002) Peripheral blood markers of inflammation predict mortality and functional decline in high-functioning community-dwelling older persons. *J Am Geriatr Soc, 50*(4), 638–644.

Rimm, E. R., Stampfer, M. J., Ascherio, A., Giovannucci, E., Colditz, G. A., & Willett, W. C. (1993) Vitamin E consumption and the risk of coronary heart disease in men. *N Eng J Med, 328*, 1450–1456.

Rodman, J. S., & Baker, T. (1978) Changes in the kinetics of muscle contration in vitamin D-depleted rats.*Kidney Int, 13*, 189–193.

Rousseau, A. S., Margaritis, I., Arnaud, J., Faure, H., & Roussel, A. M. (2006) Physical activity alters antioxidant status in exercising elderly subjects. *J Nutr Biochem, 17*(7), 463–470.

Sakr, Y., Reinhart, K., Bloos, F., Marx, G., Russwurm, S., Bauer, M., et al. (2007) Time course and relationship between plasma selenium concentrations, systemic inflammatory response, sepsis, and multiorgan failure. *Br J Anaesth, 98*(6), 775–784.

Semba, R. D., Bartali, B., Zhou, J., Blaum, C., Ko, C. W., & Fried, L. P. (2006) Low serum micronutrient concentrations predict frailty among older women living in the community. *J Gerontol A Biol Sci Med Sci, 61*(6), 594–599.

Semba, R. D., Ferrucci, L., Sun, K., Walston, J., Varadhan, R., Guralnik, J. M., et al. (2007a) Oxidative stress and severe walking disability among older women. *Am J Med,120*(12), 1084–1089.

Semba, R. D., Lauretani, F., & Ferrucci, L. (2007b) Carotenoids as protection against sarcopenia in older adults. *Arch Biochem Biophys, 458*(2), 141–145.

Semba, R. D., Varadhan, R., Bartali, B., Ferrucci, L., Ricks, M. O., Blaum, C., et al. (2007c) Low serum carotenoids and development of severe walking disability among older women living in the community: the women's health and aging study I. *Age Ageing,36*(1), 62–67.

Sevenian, A., & Hochstein, P. (1985) Mechanisms and consequences of lipid peroxidation in biological systems. *Annu Rev Nutr, 5*, 365–375.

Simpson, R. U., Thomas, G. A., & Arnold, A. J. (1985) Identification of 1,25-dihydroxyvitamin D3 receptors and activities in muscle. *J Biol Chem, 260*, 8882–8891.

Spatz, E. S., Canavan, M. E., & Desai, M. M. (2009) From here to JUPITER identifying new patients for statin therapy using data from the 1999–2004 National Health and Nutrition Examination Survey. *Circ Cardiovasc Qual Outcomes, 2*, 41–48.

Stampfer, M., Hennekens, C., Manson, J., Colditz, G., Rosner, B., & Willett, W. C. (1993) Vitamin E consumption and the risk of coronary disease in women. *N Eng J Med, 328*, 1444–1449.

Starkie, R., Ostrowski, S. R., Jauffred, S., Febbraio, M., & Pedersen, B. K. (2003) Exercise and IL-6 infusion inhibit endotoxin-induced TNF-alpha production in humans. *FASEB J, 17*, 884–886.

Terblanche, M., Almog, Y., Rosenson, R. S., Smith, T. S., & Hackam, D. G. (2006) Statins: panacea for sepsis? *Lancet Infect Dis, 6*(4), 242–248.

Terblanche, M., Almog, Y., Rosenson, R. S., Smith, T. S., & Hackam, D. G. (2007) Statins and sepsis: multiple modifications at multiple levels. *Lancet Infect Dis, 7*(5), 358–368.

Toft, A. D., Jensen, L. B., Bruunsgaard, H., Ibfelt, T., Halkjaer-Kristensen, J., Febbraio, M., et al. (2002) Cytokine response to eccentric exercise in young and elderly humans. *Am J Physiol Cell Physiol, 283*, C289–C295.

van Etten, E., & Mathieu, C. (2005) Immunoregulation by 1,25-dihydroxyvitamin D3: basic concepts. *J Steroid Biochem Mol Biol, 97*, 93–101.

Vescovo, G., Volterrani, M., Zennaro, R., Sandri, M., Ceconi, C., Lorusso, R., et al. (2000) Apoptosis in the skeletal muscle of patients with heart failure: investigation of clinical and biochemical changes. *Heart, 84*(4), 431–437.

Visser, M., Deeg, D. J. H., & Lips, P. (2003) Low vitamin D and high parathyroid hormone levels as determinants of loss of muscle strength and muscle mass (sarcopenia): the Longitudinal Aging Study Amsterdam. *J Clin Endocrinol Metab, 88*, 5766–5772.

Vivekananthan, D. P., Penn, M. S., Sapp, S. K., Hsu, A., & Topol, E. J. (2003) Use of antioxidant vitamins for the prevention of cardiovascular disease: meta-analysis of randomised trials. *Lancet, 361*, 2017–2023.

Voutilainen, S., Nurmi, T., Mursu, J., & Rissanen, T. H. (2006) Carotenoids and cardiovascular health. *Am J Clin Nutr, 83*(6), 1265–1271.

Walston, J., McBurnie, M. A., Newman, A., Tracy, R. P., Kop, W. J., Hirsch, C. H., et al. (2002) Frailty and activation of inflammation and coagulation systems with and without clinical comorbidities. *Arch Intern Med, 162*, 2333–2341.

Wannamethee, S. G., Lowe, G. D. O., Whincup, P. H., Rumley, A., Walker, M., & Lennon, L. (2002) Physical activity and hemostatic and inflammatory variables in elderly men. *Circulation, 105*, 1785–1790.

Wassner, S. J., Li, J. B., Sperduto, A., & Norman, M. E. (1983) Vitamin D deficiency, hypocalcemia, and increased skeletal muscle degradation in rats. *J Clin Invest, 72*, 102–112.

Wei, J., Xu, H., Davies, J. L., & Hemmings, G. P. (1992) Increase of plasma IL-6 concentrations with age in healthy subjects. *Life Sci, 51*, 1953–1956.

Yau, T. M., Weisel, R. D., Mickle, D. A., Burton, G. W., Ingold, K. U., Ivanov, J., et al. (1994) Vitamin E for coronary bypass operations. A prospective, double-blind, randomized trial.*J Thorac Cardiovasc Surg, 108*(2), 302–310.

Yetley, E. A. (2008) Assessing the vitamin D status of the US population. *Am J Clin Nutr, 88*(2), 558S–564S.

Chapter 7
Using the Arts to Promote Resiliency Among Persons with Dementia and Their Caregivers

Robert E. Roush, Michelle Braun, Anne Davis Basting, Jerald Winakur, Francesca Rosenberg, and Susan H. McFadden

Over 5 million persons aged 71 and older (22.2%) have some form of cognitive impairment without dementia that can adversely affect memory and other executive functional capacities (Plassman 2008). This prevalence level and the additional 5 million with Alzheimer's disease, coupled with the burgeoning older population that will double in another 10 years, call for more creative approaches to helping these persons and their caregivers become more resilient in coping with the marked changes in their lives. The arts may be a helpful adjunct to traditional health care practices for those persons who now and will have dementia. This chapter follows from the Humanities and Arts Symposium presented at the Gerontological Society of America's 62nd Annual Scientific Meeting in Atlanta, GA in November 2009. The authors explore how using various art forms help persons with dementia and their caregivers cope with those circumstances.

Neuropsychologist Michelle Braun begins with an explication of how the plasticity of the brain and the arts complement neurobiology, allowing persons with dementia to have a better quality of life. Anne Basting follows with *a first-person* account of her experience using creative engagement to work with older persons with dementia and to teach her students what this means for them and their future patients. This leads to geriatrician Jerald Winakur, who uses the literary device of narrative medicine with his patients, telling the reader how his father's art and the course of his father's dementia of the Alzheimer's type influenced his life. Francesca Rosenberg describes how the "Meet Me at MoMA" program uses great works of art to evoke emotional memory among persons with Alzheimer's disease. And Susan McFadden concludes with the interesting cases of Leo and Mrs. G. who are persons with dementia whose engagement in the arts has helped them become more resilient. In the discussion, the range of artistic expression is tied to ideas for clinical practice to improve the quality of lives of persons with dementia and of those who care for them.

R.E. Roush (✉)
Bastor College of Medicine, Houston, TX, USA
e-mail: rroush@bcm.tmc.edu

B. Resnick et al. (eds.), *Resilience in Aging: Concepts, Research, and Outcomes*,
DOI 10.1007/978-1-4419-0232-0_7, © Springer Science+Business Media, LLC 2011

Michelle Braun's "The Science of Artistic Engagement"

As with many scientific advances, our understanding of the value of artistic engagement for individuals with dementia began with poignant clinical observations. For many years, clinicians and caregivers reported that individuals with Alzheimer's disease seemed to respond positively to artistic engagement, as evidenced by behavioral changes including increased smiling and interaction, improved moods, and decreased agitation (Hanneman 2006; Stewart 2004). Over the past several years, a growing body of converging research has supported these observations, suggesting that artistic engagement is an important tool for improving quality of life, diminishing problem behaviors, and even improving some aspects of cognitive functioning in individuals with dementia. Interestingly, the benefits of artistic engagement do not appear to be isolated to certain types of artistic activities, and presently include varied techniques such as drawing, music, and dance. Although there are many other art forms yet to be studied and much more to learn about those that have been studied, this fresh field of scientific inquiry has started to provide important clues for guiding the care and maximizing the quality of life for individuals with dementia. To date, most research has focused on groups of individuals with dementia or case studies of individuals with dementia (usually artists), with findings suggesting important links between symptomatic improvement and artistic engagement, and providing rich hypotheses about underlying neurobiological mechanisms.

Artistic Engagement Helps Manage Symptoms

Clinicians and caregivers have long been interested in minimizing the agitation and depression that can accompany dementia and have been encouraged by recent evidence that these symptoms can be minimized with artistic engagement. The impact of music is perhaps the best studied art form in this regard, as it has been consistently linked with reductions in agitation. For example, in a study comparing normal controls to patients with dementia, Cho et al. (2009) showed that patients assigned to a music-intervention group versus care-as-usual group exhibited a significant decrease in depression and agitation. Another study showed significantly reduced agitation in patients with dementia who were exposed to music of their preference and to simulated family presence with average reductions in problem behaviors to 50% of the baseline rate (Garland et al. 2007). In an innovative study combining the use of endocrinological measurements, behavioral evaluations, and functional assessments, dementia patients receiving 16 sessions of music therapy demonstrated significantly decreased irritability, significant improvement on the "language" subscale of the Mini-Mental Status Examination, and a significant decrease in salivary chormogranin A (CgA) levels, a measure of stress and sympathetic nervous system activity (Suzuki et al. 2004). Such multi-modal assessment of outcome variables provides fruitful considerations for future studies that seek to expand upon traditional methods of behavioral assessment and examine links between physiological, cognitive, and behavioral variables.

Other studies have evaluated the impact of dance and wall art. In one study examining the outcome from nine weekly sessions of "Dance and Movement Therapy," dementia patients exhibited slight improvement in self-care abilities and improved performance on a cognitive measure of global planning and visuospatial ability (Clock Drawing), although no difference in memory or behavioral symptoms between the groups was evident (Hokkamen et al. 2008). Another study examined door testing behavior on a nursing home unit (a frequent source of agitation and distress for patients), and found significant reductions in door testing behaviors when the doors were disguised with a wall mural (Kincaid and Peacock 2003). In sum, findings from these studies and several others indicate that exposure to various forms of art results in improvement of behavioral symptoms and, in some cases, mild improvement in non-memory aspects of cognitive functioning (e.g. global planning, language).

Neurobiological Underpinnings of Artistic Engagement

By examining changes in artwork as a function of dementia subtype and/or stage, hypotheses about neurobiological changes have been developed. Most studies show an increase in abstraction in the artwork of patients with advancing Alzheimer's disease (Lev-Wiesel and Hirshenzon-Segev 2003), and decreased precision and color scheme (Crutch and Rossor 2006), all of which have been attributed to increased neuronal degeneration due to disease progression. Although few studies have examined how the artwork of patients with different subtypes of dementia might differ, a recent case-controlled study provides some evidence of a link between subtypes of dementia and different artistic changes (Rankin et al. 2007). In examining 49 patients with different subtypes of dementia [Alzheimer's disease (AD), semantic dementia (SD), frontotemporal dementia (FTD)] and normal controls, an interesting dissociation between subtypes of dementia and artistic style was noted: individuals with FTD created more bizarre art (presumably due to greater degeneration of frontal lobe areas), as did individuals with SD (the temporal lobe variant of FTD), while individuals with AD used a more muted color palette (attributed to potential deficits in visual association and decreased ability to recognize common objects). This study reflects a growing attempt to link dementia subtypes to specific features of artwork, and may help us to better understand the pathology of dementia and how we might compensate for it.

In addition to group studies, case studies have been utilized to drive speculation about the connections between artwork and neurobiological mechanisms. In contrast to the results of group studies discussed above, several case studies have depicted artists with *preserved* creativity into the later stages of dementia. For example, the artwork of well-known artist William de Kooning, as analyzed by

Espinel (2007), was judged to be generally consistent over the course of his dementia, even in the later stages of the disease. Espinel postulated a framework to explain this phenomenon – "Creating in the Midst of Dementia" – suggesting that the well-known deficit in semantic memory that characterizes AD may be offset by preserved functioning in three other memory systems (working, procedural, episodic), allowing continued consistency in the creation of artwork. Preserved drawing and creativity into the late stages of dementia was also demonstrated in the work of artist Danae Chambers (Fornazzari 2005). Although it is unclear why some studies show reduced artistic abilities in advancing AD and other studies show little to no change, some of this may be explained by the artist's prior experience (i.e. the well-learned abilities of experienced artists may be more resistant to neurodegeneration than the artwork of individuals with dementia who were not prior artists). Another important consideration in evaluating these findings is the lack of standardized criteria in judging the abstract nature of artwork (Crutch and Rossor 2006) which may complicate comparison of findings across studies.

It is also interesting to note an association between de novo artistic behavior and neurological conditions including FTD, epilepsy, subarachnoid brain hemorrhage, and Parkinson's disease (Pollak and Lythgoe 2007). Such research provides converging support that brain mechanisms are involved in artistic production. In comparison to the wealth of studies examining drawing in dementia, there are no known studies analyzing the neurobiological mechanisms of musical appreciation. In individuals without neurological compromise, activation in the emotional processing areas of the brain (limbic system structures) and right-hemisphere cortical areas is noted, although it is unclear if this association holds true in individuals with dementia. It is hoped that future studies will examine musical appreciation in individuals with dementia in order to elucidate specific neurobiological underpinnings and help inform future compensatory strategies and perhaps even therapies.

Becoming Artists Ourselves: Creating Research to Answer a Growing Need

While the work reviewed here provides us with empirically based hypotheses about why individuals with dementia appear to benefit from artistic engagement, and suggests underlying neurobiological mechanisms, we are only beginning to understand the scientific relationship between artistic engagement and dementia. Given that the number of individuals with AD in the United States is expected to increase by more than 50% by 2030 (from 5.1 million to 7.7 million; Alzheimer's Association 2009), and given that there are few if any other treatments available that can improve quality of life and behavioral symptoms as consistently as artistic engagement, continued creative research into the link between art and dementia is more important than ever.

Anne Davis Basting's Reflections on "Creative Resilience: Using the Arts to Strengthen Response to Aging and Stress"

I have been working in the applied arts with people in the mid-to-late stages of dementia for 15 years. Opening emotional and symbolic communication to people whom rational language has failed is a powerful experience, one that has given me great appreciation for the resiliency of people for whom much of the world is considered beyond growth and learning. At the moment, the core challenge in demonstrating the resilience of older adults with disabilities is the attitudes of their care providers. The assumption that growth, expression, skill building, even learning is not possible among older adults with physical and cognitive disabilities stultifies efforts to research and explore the benefits of arts and community development programs.

I approach this work as an artist and scholar of the humanities teaching students of all ages and abilities to develop and hone their skills in creative expression and shaping the world around them. In my case, "students" include my traditionally aged college students enrolled in my service-learning courses, people with memory loss living in congregate care settings, and the staff/family who partner in their care.

Research shows us that creative engagement can improve the quality of life of elders. There is another body of research on the environmental impact of art, like walking by art in the hallways or piping age-appropriate music into facility speaker systems. But my interest is in engagement-creativity that is used to simultaneously build a sense of self and community, not just in a given facility, but bridging that facility with the larger, outside world.

I recently organized and held a Think Tank at the Center on Age & Community in which we wrestled with the question of how to "radically transform activities" in long-term care to more fully reflect what we know from research – that the power of activities comes from creative expression, social interaction, and both skill and community building.

Several ideas emerged from the Think Tank. Activities need to morph into creative engagement projects that have meaning and purpose for a variety of participants connected to the older adult, including grandchildren, children, friends, paid care partners, and the general public. They need to allow for individual expression. They need to approach and depict the elder as a person, not a disease (or an accumulation of conditions). They need to build toward a product or event that can be invested in and shared with pride.

The Think Tank we held in May 2009 featured cutting edge media makers and artists, artists and writers working in community-building, leaders in long-term care, older adults, caregivers, and even a high school student who worked in a nursing home. We broke into small groups that blended artists with those working in long-term care in the hopes that the innovative thinking in each group would spur out-of-the-box ideas. In one exercise, I presented the small groups with a list of 10 activities suggested for people with dementia. The list included things such as "toss a ball," "collect baseball cards," and "make lemonade." I asked the groups to "enchant" the activity – to add a layer of mystery and meaning. The results were consistently inventive and playful, enabling us to see a model for projects that open opportunities for one-on-one engagement, intra-facility groups, and extra-facility groups.

An example of such a creative project is "The Communal Table" (Fig. 7.1). Building off an activity suggestion to "sort silverware," the Think Tank group designed a series of activities around a larger project – to share in a meal that reflects the unique character of a given group. They suggested that the group:

1. choose a reason to celebrate together with a meal;
2. design the menu;
3. perhaps grow some food for the meal;
4. make some of the food for the meal;
5. design and make invitations for the meal;
6. create a guest list;
7. set the table;
8. create decorations;
9. create a "welcoming" ritual for the guests;
10. figure out what to ask guests to bring;
11. discuss celebrations they might have had in their family, or wish they would have had;
12. hold the meal;
13. document the meal with photos, video;
14. possibly live webcast the meal to another care facility as a way to "share" the meal more broadly;
15. clear the table;
16. work together to put away decorations and silverware (sort silverware);
17. write and share stories about "fantasy" meals you would like to have (fantasy dinner guests).

The model for the Communal Table project looked like this:

Engagement inside the group
Can include families, residents, and staff

Design invites — Plan menu — Prepare table — Plan invite list — Prepare/share meal

PROJECT:Communal Table

Share stories of special menus — Share stories of special meals in the past — Share list of fantasy dinner party guests — Web cam the meal and watch others

Engagement with the larger world
Can include families, general public, sister facility or school groups

Fig. 7.1 The model for the Communal Table project

Research on the impact of creative engagement and its contribution to and support of resilience in older adults is limited. Studies tend to be small, not use control groups, and test only one side of the engagement – the older adults. The crucial component of these programs is that they build relationships and community. They increase the social connectivity of people whom the medical framework of institutional care sees not as people, but as an accumulation of diseases and losses.

A recent study on the TimeSlips storytelling method expanded the inquiry to look at the quality and quantity of engagement between staff and residents in nursing homes, as well as attitude changes among staff. Another research study (forthcoming) looked at the impact of the Storycorps Memory Loss Initiative on people with dementia and the family/friend who interviews them. These relational (dyad or triad) studies can start to capture the effect of creative engagement on the resiliency of older adults with physical and cognitive disabilities.

Jerald Winakur's Reflections on "His Father and the Impact of Art"

When I was a child I remember crawling into my father's lap, a pencil and a notebook in my hands. "Draw a dog, Daddy," I might say. Or a bird, or a tree. And he did. A few deft strokes and there it was. I thought it was magic, those figures coming to life on the paper through my father's hand. I have never been able to do this. Whatever the magic is, it is not in me.

My father spent his life working 6-day weeks in a dreary shop opened by his own father who then had the bad luck to die when my dad was only seven. His mother, an illiterate immigrant caught with her family of six children in the desperate circumstances of the Depression, had no choice but to take each child in turn out of school and put them to work in the store. At age 16, and 6 months shy of high school graduation, my father's turn came. And, aside from 5 years spent in the Army Air Corps photographing ground damage after the bombers made their runs, the shop became his life.

An old wooden easel gathered dust in a corner of our basement. During the years I grew up in that house, I never saw him put brush to canvas.

When I was a teenager, I worked with him after school and on Saturdays. We were driving home together one night after a long, busy day. He said, "You know, when I was in junior high – about your age – I had an art teacher who took an interest in me. He sent me home with a note for my mother. She beat me before I could read it to her. I guess she must have thought I'd gotten into some kind of trouble. She didn't need any more trouble. Anyway, when she finally let me read her the note, it said that this teacher wanted me to go to the Maryland Institute of Art. He'd make sure I got in and that it wouldn't cost anything…" I was moved in some way I didn't understand then. My voice caught. "So what did Granny say?" "Nothing," he said. "She tore up the note and walked away."

My father died of Alzheimer's disease 3 years ago. He was 87 years old. He had been going downhill for 7 years; I, his son the geriatrician, helped to keep him at home until the end. One might think I had some special insight into his disease, that somehow I could make it better, slow it down, figure out something. Who else, if not someone like me? But I muddled through like the rest of us do.

In a twist of fate, my father began painting again. His business was destroyed in one night during the civil unrest that occurred in Baltimore in the aftermath of the assassination of Dr. Martin Luther King. That left my father, with no other skills or education, unemployed at the age of 50. He careened into a deep depression, worked a series of dead-end jobs. My mother began a new career as a receptionist in a doctor's office – my office to be specific – where she worked for the next 30 years.

One day, the old easel appeared in a clearing in the garage. My father set up a series of bright lights, a table on which to place his study objects. He started going to the library almost every day and taught himself art history, coming home and talking to my mother about the lives of Renoir and Monet, Picasso, and Rousseau.

Paintings began to flow from his studio: the roses and irises from his garden, portraits of his family members done from memory and with the help of old photographs. His work encompassed every phase of modern art from the Impressionists through the Cubists and Abstract Expressionists. He would spend hours in the museum, studying how each artist applied the paint to the canvas. He experimented with sand and straw, watercolors, and pastels.

I began to hang his works in my medical office, which gave him immense pleasure. My patients would exclaim over them, offer to buy them. My father occasionally gave one away, but he could not bring himself to sell any. "I'm just a piker," he said. "I don't know what I'm doing."

Once I entered one of his oils in a local contest without his knowledge and took him to the gallery where all the works were to be hung after judging. There was his painting, "Wild Wren," a white and gold ribbon hanging from the frame. He had won the competition and I never saw him more ebullient than on that day.

This went on for over 20 years. His health began to fail. He had a couple of heart attacks and then prostate cancer. His production slowed but he kept painting. I began to notice that the works were changing, the perspective dimming, the faces on the portraits less realistic.

And then he painted no more. I would talk to him about it, trying to cajole him back into his studio. He would shrug his shoulders and say, "I just don't know what to paint anymore." Not long after, I realized he could no longer sign his name.

At age 80, during a hospitalization for heart failure, he developed delerium. He was never the same after that, and although I took him home and my family cared for him over the next 7 years, his decline was inexorable. When I visited, even during the worst times of his paranoia and belligerency, if I pulled out one of his old art books, sat down next to him, the book opened across our laps, and began to turn the pages, he would become engrossed. "Oh, I've always loved that one!" he would say.

My father is gone now. I have spent the last few years thinking about his life. He had all the risk factors for developing a dementing illness: a harsh childhood, the lack of educational achievement, severe blows to his self-esteem, bouts of depression, vascular disease, etc. His father died young, his mother by a series of strokes, his brother while still in his 50s and his sisters with cancer.

I cursed the disease that stole my father's selfhood; I was brought to my knees on the day he could no longer remember my name. But he was in his mid-80s by then, and with all nature and nurture arrayed against him, I have to conclude that he was, in the end, saved by his art. The magic served him well.

Francesca Rosenberg's "Creative Resilience: Using the Art at MoMA to Strengthen Response to Aging and Stress"

Alzheimer's disease is a progressive illness that impacts not only memory, thinking, and behavior but also affects work, lifelong hobbies, and/or one's social life. Alzheimer's disease also adversely affects caregivers who often experience depression, increased anxiety, stress, and have less time to tend to their own lives. Since there is no available cure in sight, people with dementia and caregivers are looking for a way to help manage the disease. The Museum of Modern Art has found that looking at all kinds of visual art – paintings, sculpture, drawings, photographs, and prints – can positively impact both caregivers and care recipients.

Being one of the first museums in the country to offer programs to make its collection and special exhibitions accessible to people with Alzheimer's disease and their caregivers, in 2006 the Museum of Modern Art launched *Meet Me at MoMA*. This monthly program features interactive tours of the Museum's renowned collection of modern art and its special exhibitions for individuals in the early and middle stages of the disease, along with their family members and caregivers. *Meet Me at MoMA* gives those living with the degenerative disease an expressive outlet and forum for dialogue through guided tours and discussion in the Museum's galleries during non-public hours. Specially trained Museum educators engage participants during a tour of four or five artworks, including works by such modern masters as Henri Matisse, Pablo Picasso, Jackson Pollock, and Andy Warhol, related to a theme and presented in a predetermined sequence. Each tour lasts roughly one and a half hours, with about 15–20min spent at each artwork. Several discussion questions are posed to engage participants in observing, describing, interpreting, and connecting to the works and to each other. Historical points about the artworks are conveyed throughout the tour, and smaller group discussions are also often used to spark further interaction among participants.

Why Art?

While no one has attempted to scientifically prove why art is an effective tool, MoMA's ideas include these:

- Art looking as well as art making provides mental stimulation and learning possibilities as well as an outlet to spark expression and creative interpretation.

Preliminary research suggests that these kinds of activities might offer benefits to people with dementia.

- Art can tap into one's long-term and emotional memories – feelings he or she have had before relating to events and people in their lives.
- Looking at art puts patient and caregiver on level playing field – both can engage with the work at various levels and feel validated and empowered.
- Art can be a tool for communication thereby enabling human and social connection and understanding between patient and caregiver, and between patients and other patients and caregivers and other caregivers.
- Art offers the means to make connections between individual experience and the world at large.

NYU Center of Excellence for Brain Aging and Dementia Evaluation Study of *Meet Me at MoMA*

This initiative was funded through a generous grant from MetLife Foundation, enabling the Museum to produce resources, including a publication and a website, designed to equip museum professionals, care organizations, and individual families with methods for making art accessible to people living with early and middle-stage Alzheimer's disease.

Although anecdotal evidence exists, very little research has been conducted on the effects of the visual arts on brain function and mood. Thus, the NYU Center of Excellence for Brain Aging and Dementia (CEBAD) conducted a formal evaluative study that (1) assessed whether programs such as *Meet Me at MoMA* positively impact people with early-stage Alzheimer's, and (2) examined benefits for caregivers. The study was carried out over the course of 9 months by (1) Mary Mittelman, Dr.P.H., Director of the Psychosocial Research and Support Program of the CEBA&D and Research Professor in the Department of Psychiatry at the NYU School of Medicine and (2) Cynthia Epstein, LCSW, Social Worker and CEBA&D Clinical Investigator. The overall aim of this research project was to evaluate the impact of the Meet Me at MoMA program on quality-of-life outcomes for persons with dementia and their family caregivers. It was hypothesized that people with early stage dementia and their family caregiver would report: (1) decreased social isolation; (2) enhanced self-esteem; (3) fewer symptoms of depression; (4) improved mood; and (5) enhanced quality of life.

Thirty-seven dyads (74 individuals) in total were enrolled as study participants. To be eligible for inclusion in the study, one member of the dyad had to have a diagnosis of early-stage Alzheimer's disease or related dementia, have been accompanied by a family member, and have been attending the Meet Me at MoMA program for the first time.

The format of the study was as follows: prior to the start of a regularly scheduled monthly session of ,*Meet Me at MoMA*, participants completed an intake questionnaire, had lunch, and rated their mood before and after the session using a visual assessment scale. During the session, trained MoMA and NYU staff observed previously identified participants with Alzheimer's noting mood, level of engagement, and other behavior using a form tested for inter-rater reliability. After the session, members of the study were provided with a take-home questionnaire to be returned by mail. Study participants returned to MoMA 1 week later to complete a follow-up questionnaire (identical to the intake questionnaire), had lunch, and talked with MoMA educators informally about art.

Study Results in Brief

Findings were these:

- *The importance of the educator.* Beyond doubt, it is the style and approach of the educators – which is never overtly didactic or condescending, but rather warm and interactive – and the interaction with them that participants single out as being of exceptional importance to them. The way in which they involve the participants with dementia and elicit their comments, which are then met with genuine interest and appreciation, rekindles feelings of self-worth.
- *Intellectual stimulation.* Having the opportunity to learn, to be intellectually stimulated, to experience great art together was felt to be a "blessing."
- *Shared experiences.* The family members that participated in the project expressed profound gratitude that the person they care about had the opportunity to have this special experience and, just as important, that they shared it with their care recipient. For married couples, the opportunity to share an activity that was of interest to both partners validated their identity as a couple. Sons and daughters also expressed their pleasure in taking part in an activity with their parent in which both could be relaxed and engaged.
- *Social interaction.* For so many couples in which one has dementia, what were once "normal" social interactions become events fraught with strain and shame. While they did remark that the program was inherently a socializing activity, many participants expressed the wish that the program could be extended to include more social interaction after the gallery tour.
- *Accepting environment.* The educators, together with the entire MoMA staff, create a sense of safety and convey feelings of regard for the participants. The value placed on the person at least temporarily removes the stigma of Alzheimer's disease so that participants can enjoy the MoMA experience. It is possible that the extraordinary attention that was lavished on study participants may have heightened their feelings of being welcome and important, but this also serves to point out how much people with dementia feel the loss of status and nurture

in the community and how much they appreciate the efforts made on their behalf. The wish to continue to attend as a couple, where the limitations of the ill spouse would not affect the experience for the well, makes this kind of program particularly valuable.

- *Emotional carryover.* For both the persons with dementia and their caregivers there were positive changes to mood both directly after the program and in the days following the Museum visit. Caregivers reported fewer emotional problems, and all but one person with dementia reported elevated mood.
- *Program extension.* Almost all caregivers planned to return to the Museum for future programs, which is a testament to their positive experiences. The Meet Me at MoMA program also served as a catalyst, inciting new conversation in the days to follow.

Conclusion

Participants were very grateful for the *Meet Me at MoMA* program. As they began to know each other from repeated visits, the desire for more socializing became clear. The setting itself sends the message to the person with dementia that he or she continues to be a person of value, and those participants for whom it was a familiar place can now return with their self-esteem safe and even nurtured. Considering the small sample of participants, findings from this study were suggestive of the potential of the *Meet Me at MoMA* program to improve the lives of people with dementia and their caregivers. The investigators recommend a longer term study with larger numbers of participants to corroborate initial findings. For more information about the study or making art accessible to people with Alzheimer's and other dementias, visit http://www.moma.org/learn/programs/alzheimers or send an e-mail to alzheimersproject@moma.org.

Susan McFadden's *"Resilience and Creative Engagement: The Role of Relationships"* [1]

Psychologists and other social scientists borrowed the idea of "resilience" from the physical sciences. Resilient materials revert to their original forms after being stretched, bent, or twisted. Resilient people can "bounce back" when life circumstances stretch, bend, and twist them; resilient older adults are often described as aging successfully.

---

[1]This section is adapted from the following paper: McFadden, S. H., & Basting, A. D. (2010). Healthy aging persons and their brains: promoting resilience through creative engagement. *Clinics in Geriatric Medicine, 26, 149–162.* doi:10.1016/j.cger.2009.11.004.

Although much research currently examines predictors of individuals' resilience, health outcomes of resilience, and interventions to support and improve resilient responses to life challenges, we rarely hear about persons living with dementia as having a "bounce back" capacity. Because gerontology's focus on "successful aging" seems to exclude these persons, Harris (2008) has argued that we need to start paying attention to resilience among elders with dementia. They "bounce back" by employing various coping strategies, showing positive emotions, accepting change, and acting in ways that reveal a sense of life meaning (McFadden et al. 2001).

Creative engagement, through story-telling, painting, song-writing, dance, and other art forms, enables people with dementia to communicate their resilience to others. According to a leading researcher on resilience, creative activities reveal the "capacity for positive emotions and generative activities" (Bonnano 2005, p. 136) following loss or trauma.

Individuals living with dementia know plenty about loss and the trauma of forgetfulness, and yet if they live within a supportive community designed to meet their needs appropriately, they can thrive and flourish. When given the opportunity to create something, they get the satisfaction of working toward a goal and feeling a sense of purpose and pride in their achievement. These are characteristics of persons who are creative (Lindauer 2003) and resilient (Connor and Davidson 2003) – persons like Leo and Mrs. G. Leo lives with advanced dementia and Mrs. G. is in the early stages of memory loss. They show us how to draw lines of connection among research and scholarship on late life resilience, creativity, and the significance of social acceptance and support for persons living with dementia.

The Interesting Cases of Leo and Mrs. G

Leo has lived in a county-run nursing home for several years. His dementia has progressed to the point where he utters very few words. Nevertheless, Leo was selected to participate in an artist-led program that enabled a group of about ten residents to make and paint clay pots, take photographs using Polaroid cameras, paint on canvas, draw with colored pencils, assemble a mosaic, and do the preparatory work that resulted in brightly colored fused glass objects. Each time the group met, someone pushed Leo's wheelchair into the room and up to the table holding the art. Leo soon showed his capacity for concentration and meticulous attention to detail. For example, when working with mosaics, he used a small paintbrush to swab on the glue, and then turned it around so he could use the other end to push the mosaic piece into position. Occasionally, he looked up from his work and smiled at the group. About halfway through the 10-week program, the person in charge of activities at the facility commented that Leo was starting to look forward to the arts group. She inferred this from his facial expressions when she said things such as "tomorrow the arts group meets." Also around this time, Leo's wife died. He missed a couple of arts group gatherings and the staff respected his wishes not to participate. He returned on the day of the glass fusing project, and again showed intense concentration, carefully working with his pieces of glass.

Is Leo resilient? We can only know by observing him, for he is not capable of completing a survey or responding to interview question such as the ones Harris posed in her research on resilience in persons with dementia. Harris's (2008) assertion that the notion of "successful aging" needs to be replaced with a focus on resilience was based on interviews with persons living with the early stages of memory loss, people who could answer her questions like Mrs. G. did:

> I'm very productive at the moment, so I am going with it. I do [silk] flower floral arrange-ments for weddings. I am very creative. With silk flowers, I can always have them on hand and keep a prototype. I keep it so I can refer to it because I won't be able to remember how I did that. These things come from my mind. It's my creation. (p. 56)

Leo and Mrs. G. exercised control through their creative activities – activities that also strengthened their connections to others. Leo knew just where he wanted to place the mosaic and glass pieces; Mrs. G. had control over the silk flower arrange-ments. Leo's creativity occurred in a group setting, and required the support and guidance of an artist, volunteers, and staff members. At the end of each session, each person showed what had been made and received applause and cheers from the others. Mrs. G. made her flower arrangements for the happy occasions of wed-dings and presumably she got satisfaction from their appreciation of her work.

Like any person who lives to old age, Leo and Mrs. G. have known their share of loss and trauma. Both have been diagnosed with dementia, and it is likely that their brains and vascular systems show the cumulative effects of meeting the chal-lenges of human life. Does this mean they failed at aging, that instead of "aging well" they are "aging ill"? After all, Leo needs considerable assistance from others for most activities of daily life. As reported by, Mrs. G. has "very bad asthma and emphysema and a few years earlier had cancer surgery" (p. 3). She was forced to retire early because of the dementia diagnosis and she gets little help from her sons and 12 siblings. On the other hand, Leo lives in a progressive facility dedicated to supporting personhood in all residents and Mrs. G. has a loving husband, a support network in her community, and an understanding physician. Within the constraints of their lives, both show resilience. One might even say that within these con-straints, they are flourishing and their creative expressions are but one example of the lived-experience of the "paradox of well-being" (Mroczek and Kolarz 1998) we see in so many older persons.

Discussion

What this writer (RER) took away from his co-authors' pieces was this: each of them has a body of experience in how persons with dementia respond to heightened senses evoked by seeing the graceful dancer's leap in *Swan Lake*, hearing the next Pavarotti hit Puccini's high note in *Madama Butterfly*, the pure joy of sitting before Renoir's *Luncheon of the Boating Party* at The Phillips Collection wondering what all those people were saying to each other on that sunny afternoon down the Seine, or being enraptured by a Richard Burton alone on a stage standing behind a lectern reciting line after line of Shakespeare's prose to a hushed, mesmerized audience. These and other artistic experiences like an Ansel Adams exhibit of his timeless and wonderful photographs of the beauty of nature are meaningful and important in that his photographic art reminds us of the need to preserve the splendor of wilderness. And when one gazes upon an exhibit of exquisite quilt art designed and hand-made by little known creative persons from rural areas, we are also reminded that art is everywhere and that the old adage, "beauty is in the eye of the beholder," is true.

If only we were able to capture and repeat those visual, auditory, and emotional stimuli to effect the outcomes across all persons with dementia that we see in some. Can the present day technology of fMRI or some future imaging process help us do that by "enjoying" the "art" of seeing one's own the brain light up that, in turn, lessens anxiety and depression and slows the rate of cognitive decline? It is to the neurobiologists and biogerontologists that we leave that question.

Like everything else in the clinician's array of treatment choices, more research needs to be targeted on how one chooses an art form as the independent variable and measures the hypothesized change on the dependent one (Roush et al. 2001). Until that happens, we should continue to expose persons with and without dementia to the wonderful world of the creative arts for their own and our enjoyment. Perhaps other "Sarah's," like the frail elderly lady about whom Hart (1992) wrote will have better times in their latter days. When taught about art and philosophy at the nursing home where she lived in Washington, DC, Sarah, a retired nurse thought to have dementia, "came out of her foggy tunnel." She loved Matisse and attended an exhibition of his works, exclaiming upon having seen the 11-foot high *Large Composition with Masks*, "This has been one of the best days of my life." She died peacefully in her sleep that night. In an interesting sidebar, Matisse painted that magnificent piece in the last year of his 85-year-long life.

This chapter is for the caregivers of all the Mr. Winakur's, Leo's, Mrs. G's, and Sarah's of the world. When we work with them and their countless counterparts across the land, we should document what we do via the arts, always asking questions about what seemed to work and why. And as we all are marching inexorably toward our own old ages, keep in mind Goethe's maxim: "Science and Art belong to the whole World and the barriers of nationality vanish before them."

References

Alzheimer's Association (2009) 2009 Alzheimer's disease facts and figures. http://www.alzheimersassociation.org/national/documents/report_alzfactsfigures2009.pdf

Alzheimer's Foundation of America Web address http://www.alz.org/national/documents/report_alzfactsfigures2009.pdf accessed 10.01.09

Bonnano, G. A. (2005) Resilience in the face of potential trauma. *Current Directions in Psychological Science, 14,* 135–138.

Cho, A., Lee, M.S., Cheong, K., & Lee, J. (2009) Effects of group music intervention on behavioral and psychological symptoms in patients with dementia: a pilot-controlled trial. *International Journal of Neuroscience, 119,* 471–481.

Cohen, G. (2006) The mature mind: the positive power of the aging brain. Basic Books, New York

Connor, K. M., & Davidson, J. R. T. (2003) Development of a new resilience scale: the Connor–Davidson Resilience Scale (CD-RISC). *Depression and Anxiety, 18*, 76–82.

Crutch, S. J. & Rossor, M. N. (2006) Artistic changes in Alzheimer's disease. *International Review of Neurobiology, 74*, 147–161.

Espinel, C. H. (2007) Memory and the creation of art: the syndrome, as in de Kooning, of 'creating in the midst of dementia' – an 'ArtScience' study of creation its 'brain methods' and results. In J. Bogousslavsky & M. G. Hennerici (Eds.), *Neurological disorders in famous artists* (pp. 75–88). Basel, Switzerland: Karger.

Fornazarri, L. R. (2005) Preserved painting creativity in an artist with Alzheimer's disease. *European Journal of Neurology*, 12, 419–424.

Garland, K., Beer, E., Eppingstall, B., & O'Connor, D. W. (2007) A comparison of two treatments of agitated behavior in nursing home residents with dementia: simulated family presence and preferred music. *American Journal of Geriatric Psychiatry, 15*, 514–521.

Hanneman, B. T. (2006) Creativity with dementia patients. Can creativity and art stimulate dementia patients positively? *Gerontology, 52*, 59–65.

Harris, P. B. (2008) Another wrinkle in the debate about successful aging: the undervalued concept of resilience and the lived experience of dementia. *International Journal of Aging and Human Development, 67*, 43–61.

Hart, J. (1992) Beyond the tunnel: the arts and aging in America. Museum One Publications, Washington, DC

Hokkamen, L., Rantala, L., Remes, A. M., Harkonen, B., Viramo, P., & Winblad, I. (2008) Dance and movement therapeutic methods in management of dementia: a randomized, controlled study. *Journal of the American Geriatric Society, 56*, 771–772.

Kincaid, C. & Peacock, J. R. (2003) The effect of a wall mural on decreasing four types of door-testing behaviors. *Journal of Applied Gerontology* 22(1): 76–88.

Lev-Wiesel, R. & Hirshenzon-Segev, E. (2003) Alzheimer's disease as reflected in self-figure drawings of diagnosed patients. *The Arts in Psychotherapy, 30*, 83–89.

Lindauer, M. S. (2003) *Aging, creativity, and art: a positive perspective on late-life development.* New York: Kluwer Academic/Plenum Publishers.

McFadden, S. H., Baldauf, C., & Ingram, M. (2001) Actions, feelings, and values: foundations of meaning and personhood in dementia. *Journal of Religious Gerontology 11*, 67–86.

Mroczek, D. K., & Kolarz, C. M. (1998) The effect of age on positive and negative affect: a developmental perspective on happiness. *Journal of Personality and Social Psychology, 75*, 1333–1349.

Plassman, BL et al (2008) Prevalence of cognitive impairment without dementia in the United States. *Annals of Internal Medicine* 148(6): 427–434

Pollak, T. A. & Lythgoe, M. F. (2007) De novo artistic behavior following brain injury. In Bogousslavsky J. and Hennerici, M. G.'s *Neurological disorders in famous artists*, 75–88. Basel, Switzerland: Karger.

Rankin, K. P., Liu, A. A., Howard, S., Slama, H., Hou, C. E., Shuster, K., et al. (2007) A case-controlled study of altered visual art production in Alzheimer's and FTLD. *Cognitive Behavioral Neurology, 20*, 48–61.

Roush, R.E., White, P.L., and Denis, K.B. (2001) Art for pleasure, art for therapy. *The Gerontologist* 41(1):156.

Stewart, E. G. (2004) Art therapy and neuroscience blend: working with patients who have dementia. *Art Therapy: Journal of the American Art Therapy Association, 21*, 148–155.

Suzuki, M., Kanamori, M., Watanable, M., Nagasawa, S., Kojima, E., & Nakahara, D. (2004) Behavioral and endocrinological evaluation of music therapy for elderly patients with dementia. *Nursing and Health Sciences, 6*, 11–18.

Chapter 8
Promoting Worker Resilience Over the Lifecourse

Christopher McLoughlin, Philip Taylor, and Philip Bohle

Introduction

In Australia, as in most other industrialized economies, there is growing concern about the work capacity of older workers and their retention in the workforce against a background of population aging and efforts to prolong working lives. It is widely recognized that working later will be promoted by equipping industry and workers with instruments that can gauge working potential. Although policy makers in most industrialized nations now consider an extension of working lives as the basis of sustaining welfare systems and offsetting decline in the number of young labor market entrants, globalization and the competition this fosters present as a strong countervailing force for both government and employers. Certain groups, including older workers with few or outdated skills, and those with declining health may be particularly affected by job insecurity and long-term unemployment. Reconciling these seemingly countervailing tensions is a problem now facing a number of industrialized economies. A resilient older worker whose skills and capabilities can easily adjust as the requirements of the market shift would help maintain labor productivity growth even as populations age (Hagemann and Nicoletti 1989).

A potentially useful concept when considering the fit between personal capabilities and changing job demands is Work Ability, which originated in Finland and is now widely used in Europe (Ilmarinen and Rantanen 1999). Work ability concerns how well an individual's capabilities, health, and well-being match job demands. However, the degree to which individual workers will rate their work ability level as high or low will depend upon their employment context. This includes the wider social culture, industrial and labor market situation, workplace conditions, employer practices, and, of course, their occupation and other personal characteristics. Figure 8.1 demonstrates the various elements of work ability. In considering the status of older workers, it is apparent from the research literature that many interrelated factors determine their relationship with the labor market (Taylor et al. 2000). The emerging

C. McLoughlin (✉)
Monash University, Churchill, VIC, Australia
e-mail: cmcloughlin@me.com

B. Resnick et al. (eds.), *Resilience in Aging: Concepts, Research, and Outcomes*, DOI 10.1007/978-1-4419-0232-0_8, © Springer Science+Business Media, LLC 2011

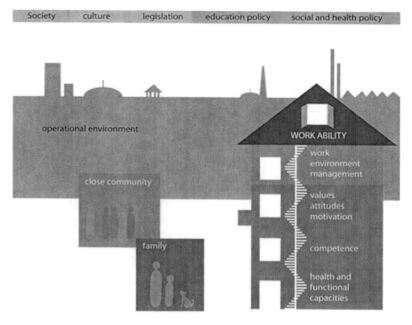

Fig. 8.1 The Work Ability House (Source: Finnish Institute of Occupational Health)

consensus is that tackling the issue of the ongoing employment of older workers requires multifaceted and integrated workplace strategies (Walker 1999).

Finnish studies indicate that at an individual level, the factors that predict work ability include health, functional capacities, competences, and attitudes. Work and workplace also influence work ability through factors including the physical, technological, mental, and social demands of work, work community and management, organizational culture, and work environment. A third level of factors consists of aspects or characteristics of the wider society such as employment, education and exit policies, social and health services, and other preventive measures such as prevention of age discrimination (Ilmarinen 2001). Tuomi et al. (2001) found that the main predictors of work ability were work demands and the environment, followed by work organization and the work community. Professional competence and lifestyle factors have been found to be weaker predictors. Good predictors of high work ability are the use of knowledge and work experience. Strong predictors of low work ability are poor work postures, work climate, an increase in mental workload, uninspiring work, and a lack of satisfaction with working time arrangements. Good perceived work ability is associated with high self-assessments in terms of work quality and productivity.

The concept of work ability promotion is based on four different actions: (1) adjustments to the physical work environment, (2) adjustments to the psychosocial work environment, (3) health and lifestyle promotion, and (4) updating skills. The first two activities are focused on work content and work environment, and the latter two on individuals. Research has indicated that (1) reducing repetitive movements, (2) increased satisfaction with supervisors, and (3) an increase in vigorous physicalexercise during leisure time are predictors of improved work ability among men and women aged 51–62 years in physical, mixed, and mentally demanding work (Ilmarinen and Rantanen 1999; Ilmarinen 2001).

The promotion of work ability has been found to reduce the incidence of work disability and the likelihood of premature retirement and absenteeism; increase productivity and competence among the workforce; improve the public image of a company; and improve quality of life and well-being among workers themselves, effects which appear to carry over into retirement (Ilmarinen and Rantanen 1999; Tuomi et al. 2001).

The *"Redesigning Work for an Ageing Society"* (RWAS) project, supported by an Australian Research Council grant, examined the utility of the work ability construct in Australia. Drawing on this study, this chapter explores the measurement of work ability based on a new diverse sample, and examines how work ability may moderate the influence of job demands on critical outcome measures: job satisfaction, personally meaningful work, and job insecurity. Furthermore, the potential value of work ability promotion in terms of facilitating resilience of older workers and the sustainability of labor supply over the long term as populations age is demonstrated.

Project Description

The participants in this project were from across Australia, with a majority working in various locations in the state of Victoria. Sampling was undertaken in four case study organizations: a small national university, two international freight terminals of an international airline, a national manufacturing company, and the roadside assistance division of a motoring organization. Within these organizations, respondents were drawn from different levels, from entry level to management levels. Although response rates varied across case organizations, the survey had an approximate overall response rate of 40%, yielding a total sample of 1,687 respondents. The manufacturing company and the national university made up the vast majority of the sample, representing 53 and 39%, respectively. Males were slightly overrepresented (males, $n = 919$; females, $n = 713$; unanswered, $n = 55$). The average age of respondents was 45 years, with a range of 21–75 years. Occupational group was categorized according to the ANZCO (Australian Bureau of Statistics 2006) coding guidelines. In a very general amalgamation of this coding, 72% of the sample reported their job as white collar and 27% reported their occupation to involve manual work.

It is important to note some details of the configuration of the sample, particularly the gender specificity of certain organizations. As shown in Table 8.1, most of the females in the sample are from the university. It is possible that these female workers are different from the smaller groups in the manufacturing firm or freight terminals. Also shown in Table 8.1 are similarities in the average age of respondents from the different organizations.

Questions have been raised regarding the validity of the Work Ability Index (WAI) as a measure of work ability based on prior work when used with Australian respondents (Healy et al. 2007; Oakman 2007; Parker et al. 2006; Palermo et al. 2009). This motivated the development of a new measure labeled the Work Ability Survey (WAS). The Work Ability Survey (WAS) was developed to be used in this

project. This measure is based on the most recently developed conceptual model of
work ability from the Finnish Institute of Occupational Health, presented graphi-
cally in Fig. 8.1. Included in this measure are two overall scales reflecting personal
and organizational components of work ability, which are the combination of
subscales capturing the following factors:

Work ability	
Organizational capacity	Personal capacity
Control of work methods	Intrinsic work benefits
Control of work time	Extrinsic work benefits
Learning opportunities	Work schedule
Trust	Home–work balance
Respect	Work–home balance
Career development support	Physical health
Supervisor consultation	Mental health
Everyday discrimination	Job insecurity
Training	

The relationship between individuals' level of work ability, the demands of their
work, and their resilience in working life has an easily grasped, intuitive link. The
core of the work ability concept captures how the individuals' resources, the design
of their work, and the physical and psychosocial environment at work are matched

Table 8.1 Firm- and gender-specific sample sizes

Organization	Sample size	Average age of respondent		Gendered sample size	Work type	Percentage
Manufacturing firm	896	42.89	Male	619	White collar	55
					Manual work	42
			Female	253	White collar	91
					Manual work	9
Roadside assistance	59	49.88	Male	59	White collar	–
					Manual work	100
			Female	0	White collar	–
					Manual work	–
National university	656	48.11	Male	187	White collar	84
					Manual work	15
			Female	440	White collar	92
					Manual work	8
Air freight terminals	76	44.84	Male	54	White collar	51
					Manual work	48
			Female	20	White collar	91
					Manual work	8

to job demands. The notion of providing tools, resources, and supportive frameworks which assist a worker to respond to and meet changing environmental demands, be they in their place of work or external, may be viewed as engendering resilience. In this case, the different types of demands encountered in one's working life represent stressors. The personal and organizational capacity components of the present conceptualization of work ability define areas where protective measures against the stressors or risk factors presented in the demands of working life may be initiated. Supporting individual work ability can be viewed as providing protection from the potential negative effect of demands that exceed personal capacity, for instance the potentially adverse effects of changing production methods may be countered by adequate training in new skills while adequate health and safety policies may reduce the incidence of absence due to sickness or injury. The extent of resilience to stressors or adversity can be determined through the extent of positive outcomes or the absence of negative outcomes despite the adversity present. In order to explore this, work-related psychosocial factors were used to determine: (1) the influence of different types of stressors (work demands) on job satisfaction, job insecurity, and level of personal meaning of work and (2) how different levels of work ability (protective factor) affect the influence of work demands (stressor) in terms of job satisfaction, job insecurity, and level of personally meaningful work (positive and negative outcomes related to stressor).

In addition to the WAS and measurement of work demands, three measures of work-related psychosocial factors were used to demonstrate the potential for improving the resilience of a workforce through improving work ability. These were job satisfaction, personally meaningful work, and job insecurity. The factor structure of these measures and the measures of work demands are presented in Appendix 8.1. The measure of job satisfaction used was a single item scored on a five-point Likert-type response scale. Personally meaningful work and job satisfaction were measured using the existing subscales adapted from the Copenhagen Psychosocial Questionnaire (Kristensen and Borg 2003). The measure of job insecurity was developed and piloted for use in the case study organizations. The items that make up these subscales were scored on a five-point Likert-type response scale. The personally meaningful work measure consisted of five items, while that of job insecurity consisted of four items, and larger scores on all these scales indicated greater job satisfaction, job insecurity, and meaningfulness of individuals' work. Statistical analysis indicates that WAS scores decrease as the demands of an individual's work increase, except in the case of cognitive demands, where an increase in WAS scores by 1.5 points is predicted for every one-point increase in the cognitive demands while controlling for the other variables in the equation. There was also a significant relationship between WAS scores and the outcome measures as presented in Table 8.2. Specifically, WAS scores explained 6% of the variance in job insecurity, 29% of job satisfaction, and 16% of personally meaningful work. The predictive regression models based on measures of work demands explained 7, 10, and 18% of the variance in job insecurity, job satisfaction, and personally meaningful work, respectively, and when WAS scores were introduced, the variance explained became 11, 31, and 19%, respectively.

Table 8.2 Linear regression showing the relationship between WAS scores and the outcome measures

		B	Std error	Beta	t	Sig.
Job satisfaction	(Constant)	4.752	0.123		38.622	0
	WAS	0.023	0.001	0.539	23.422	0
Meaningful work	(Constant)	7.178	0.728		9.857	0
	WAS	0.092	0.006	0.397	15.844	0
Job insecurity	(Constant)	12.492	0.518		24.139	0
	Organizational capacity	−0.045	0.005	−0.257	−9.734	0

Taking each of these work-related psychosocial factors individually, their relationship with work demands and work ability is elucidated. Notably higher scores on the job design, task demand, and emotional demand scales predicted higher levels of job insecurity. Countercurrent to this, higher levels of work pace and cognitive demands predicted lower levels of job insecurity. When respondents' WAS scores were introduced into the model, the job design and the task demand measures showed partial mediation. The work pace measure remained unchanged, and the emotional demand and cognitive demand measures showed full mediation. These results suggest that a high pace of work buffers against job insecurity at any level of work ability. Also, work ability level influences the relationship between problems with the design of a job or the work environment and the difficulty of the tasks in respondents' work and job insecurity. Interestingly, WAS score mediated fully the increase in job insecurity observed with higher emotional and cognitive demands.

The predictive regression model of job satisfaction included four measures of work demands as significant contributors to the model. Notably, higher scores on the job design, and excess workload scales predicted higher levels of job satisfaction. Countercurrent to this, higher levels of emotional demands and cognitive demands predicted lower levels of job satisfaction. When respondents' WAS score was introduced into the model, the job design measure showed partial mediation. The emotional demand, excess workload, and cognitive demand measures showed full mediation. Work ability level influences the relationship between problems with the design of a job or the work environment in respondents' work and job satisfaction. Interestingly, WAS score mediated fully the increase in job satisfaction associated with increased excess workload scale scores and the reduced job satisfaction associated with increased emotional and cognitive demands.

The predictive regression model of personally meaningful work included six measures of work demands as significant contributors to the model. Notably, higher scores on the cognitive demand, work pace, and emotional demand scales predicted higher levels of personally meaningful work. Countercurrent to this, higher levels of job design, excess workload, and task demands predicted lower levels of personally meaningful work. When respondents' WAS score was introduced into the model, the emotional demand, job design, cognitive demand, and work pace measures showed partial mediation. The job design and the task demand measures showed full mediation. These results suggest that work ability level influences the relationship between problems with the design of a job or the work environment, the cognitive demands, emotional demands and the work pace in respondents' work, and the level of personal meaning in work perceived by respondents. Interestingly, WAS score mediated fully the increase in personally meaningful work associated with reduced excess workload and task demand scale scores. The full tabulated output from these analyses is presented in Appendix 8.2.

Concluding Remarks

Taking the above results as a whole, interesting inferences can be drawn regarding the influence of the demands of individuals' work, their level of work ability, and work-related psychosocial factors. The first interesting facet of the project is the nuanced relationship between different types of work demands and job satisfaction, job insecurity, and personally meaningful work. It was evident in each of the predictive models based on work demand variables that increases in some types of work demands were related to increases in job satisfaction and personally meaningful work and reductions in job insecurity, while increases in other types of work demands showed the inverse relationship. It is suggested that this is a critical aspect of this analysis. The configuration of the types of work demands that showed a differentiated influence on the various outcome measures demonstrates that some work demands may actually promote greater job satisfaction, more meaning in individual's work and less job insecurity. If the conceptual content of the outcome measures and the work demand measures is considered, it appears logical that the analysis demonstrated the particular directionality of the relationship between these measures of work demands and psychosocial factors related to work.

The next notable aspect of this analysis is the manner in which work ability offsets the influence of work demand measures on the outcome variables, demonstrating the potential gains offered through the promotion of work ability. It was evident that work ability offsets both the positive and negative influence of various types of work demands on work-related psychosocial factors. If organizational and personal capacities are of sufficient magnitude, the importance of job demands is mitigated, partially or completely, in terms of job satisfaction, personally meaningful work, and job insecurity. This is of particular practical significance. In the pursuit of greater productivity, workplace interventions can usefully focus on enabling and improving personal and organizational capacities, as work ability is conceptualized here, that promote worker resilience and potentially moderate the demands of a given job.

The results of the analysis reported in this chapter are in line with previous work ability research. A large body of work in Europe has shown that long-term and multifaceted interventions have improved and sustained employee work ability. If work ability is considered as a protective factor against the influence of the stressors of work demands, its promotion offers a potentially useful approach to maintaining resilience as workers age. Through collaboration between government, management, and employee groups, work ability promotion can be used to improve both individual and organizational components of work ability. The complex interrelation of protective and risk factors that are key to resilience and which may prohibit the clear planning and implementation of workplace interventions aimed at supporting older workers may be circumvented through the application of the work ability concept and the body of work relating to its promotion. With debate increasing about the steps that will be necessary to respond adequately to the vast array of issues that will manifest as the populations of the industrialized nations age, in particular that of maintaining a sustainable supply of labor, issues of maintaining resilience over a working life will inevitably come to the fore. Work ability provides a lens through which to view the responses that will be required.

Appendix 8.1 Items and factor structure of measures used in the linear regression analysis

	Job design
To what extent does your job involve repetitive movements?	0.417
To what extent does your job involve awkward positions?	0.812
To what extent does your job involve working beyond physical capacity?	0.548
To what extent does your job involve poor work stations?	0.493

	Work pace	Excess workload
Is your workload unevenly distributed so it piles up?		−0.773
Do you work at a high pace throughout the day?	0.763	
Do you have enough time for your work tasks?		0.672
Do you have to work very fast?	0.794	
Do you get behind with your work?		−0.794
Is it necessary to keep working at a high pace?	0.854	

	Cognitive demands	Task demands
Do you have to keep your eyes on lots of things while you work?		0.547
Does your work demand that you come up with new ideas?	0.734	
Does your work require you to make difficult decisions?	0.802	
Do you need to meet precise quality standards?		0.512
Do you carry out monotonous tasks?		0.516
Do you carry out complex tasks?	0.714	
Does your work require you to shuffle priorities?	0.598	

	Emotional demands
Does your work put you in emotionally disturbing situations?	0.725
Do you have to relate to other people's personal problems in your work?	0.74
Do you get emotionally engaged in your work?	0.626

	Meaningful work
Do you feel that the work you do is important?	0.781
Is your work meaningful to you?	0.908
Do you feel motivated and involved in your work?	0.868
Do you feel that the problems at your place of work are yours too?	0.506
Do you feel that your place of work is of great personal importance?	0.731

	Job insecurity
Becoming unemployed?	0.739
New technology making you redundant?	0.73
Finding it difficult to find another job if you became unemployed?	0.681
Being transferred to another job against your will?	0.609

Appendix 8.2 Tabulated output showing the statistical evidence of work ability moderating the influence of work demands on work-related psychosocial factors

Linear regression for a work demands predictive model of WAS scores

	Unstandardized coefficients		Standardized coefficients		
	B	Std error	Beta	t	Sig.
(Constant)	157.52	3.47		45.396	0
Job design	−1.595	0.171	−0.273	−9.303	0
Excess workload	−0.965	0.348	−0.077	−2.772	0.006
Work pace	−1.025	0.231	−0.135	−4.438	0
Cognitive demands	1.502	0.185	0.255	8.132	0
Task demands	−0.953	0.218	−0.128	−4.369	0
Emotional demands	−1.21	0.206	−0.175	−5.863	0

Predictive regression model for job insecurity based on work demand variables

Job insecurity	Unstandardized coefficients		Standardized coefficients			
	B	Std error	Beta	t	Sig.	Raw correlation
(Constant)	5.344	0.571		9.353	0	
Job design	0.178	0.035	0.153	5.129	0	0.22
Work pace	−0.11	0.045	−0.073	−2.414	0.016	0.002
Cognitive demands	−0.124	0.037	−0.106	−3.338	0.001	−0.06
Task demands	0.192	0.045	0.128	4.269	0	0.203
Emotional demands	0.127	0.042	0.092	3.02	0.003	0.07

Predictive regression model for job insecurity based on work demands and WAS score

Job insecurity	Unstandardized coefficients		Standardized coefficients			Partial correlations
	B	Std error	Beta	t	Sig.	
(Constant)	9.225	1.017		9.075	0	
Job design	0.117	0.037	0.103	3.13	0.002	0.088
Work pace	−0.154	0.049	−0.104	−3.13	0.002	−0.088
Cognitive demands	−0.07	0.041	−0.061	−1.716	0.086	−0.048
Task demands	0.16	0.047	0.11	3.438	0.001	0.097
Emotional demands	0.086	0.044	0.064	1.955	0.051	0.055
Organizational capacity	−0.032	0.005	−0.179	−5.892	0	−0.164

Predictive regression model for job satisfaction based on work demand variables

Job satisfaction	Unstandardized coefficients		Standardized coefficients			Raw correlation
	B	Std error	Beta	t	Sig.	
(Constant)	0.979	0.13		7.536	0	
Job design	0.069	0.006	0.276	11.079	0	0.307
Excess workload	0.041	0.014	0.077	2.918	0.004	0.134
Cognitive demands	−0.022	0.007	−0.09	−3.068	0.002	0.016
Emotional demands	0.032	0.009	0.108	3.711	0	0.141

Predictive regression model for job satisfaction based on work demands and WAS score

Job satisfaction	Unstandardized coefficients		Standardized coefficients			Partial correlation
	B	Std error	Beta	t	Sig.	
(Constant)	4.161	0.208		20.038	0	
Job design	0.03	0.006	0.121	4.717	0	0.13
Excess workload	0.018	0.014	0.034	1.339	0.181	0.037
Cognitive demands	−0.002	0.007	−0.009	−0.305	0.761	−0.008
Emotional demands	−0.003	0.008	−0.011	−0.375	0.708	−0.01
WAS	−0.021	0.001	−0.495	−19.009	0	−0.468

Predictive regression model for personally meaningful work based on work demands

Meaningful work	Unstandardized coefficients		Standardized coefficients			Raw correlation
	B	Std error	Beta	t	Sig.	
(Constant)	15.592	0.748		20.851	0	
Job design	−0.334	0.038	−0.251	−8.886	0	−0.212
Excess workload	−0.227	0.075	−0.08	−3.009	0.003	0.039
Cognitive demands	0.414	0.04	0.31	10.228	0	0.339
Emotional demands	0.158	0.046	0.099	3.45	0.001	0.205
Work pace	0.16	0.05	0.092	3.174	0.002	0.14
Task demands	−0.149	0.049	−0.087	−3.056	0.002	−0.088

Predictive regression model for personally meaningful work based on work demands and WAS score

Meaningful work	Unstandardized coefficients		Standardized coefficients			Partial correlation
	B	Std error	Beta	t	Sig.	
(Constant)	1.195	1.24	·	0.964	0.335	
Job design	−0.202	0.039	−0.149	−5.171	0	−0.145
Excess workload	−0.116	0.077	−0.04	−1.517	0.13	−0.043
Cognitive demands	0.3	0.042	0.22	7.177	0	0.199
Emotional demands	0.268	0.046	0.167	5.808	0	0.162
Work pace	0.249	0.051	0.142	4.858	0	0.136
Task demands	−0.066	0.048	−0.038	−1.367	0.172	−0.039
WAS	0.09	0.006	0.391	14.548	0	0.381

References

Australian Bureau of Statistics. (2006). *Australian and New Zealand Standard Classification of Occupations*. Available at: http://www.abs.gov.au

Hagemann, R. P., & Nicoletti, G. (1989). *Ageing Populations: Economic Effects and Implications for Public Finance*, OECD Working Papers, No. 61.

Healy, P., Taylor, P., Brooke, L., Bohle, P., & Ilmarinen, J. (2007). Adapting the Work Ability Index (WAI) for use in Australia. *Third International Symposium on Work Ability*. Unpublished Conference Paper.

Ilmarinen, J. (2001). Aging workers. *Occupational and Environmental Medicine*, 58, 8, 546–552.

Ilmarinen, J., & Rantanen, J. (1999). Promotion of work ability during ageing. *American Journal of Industrial Medicine Supplement*, 1, 21–23.

Kristensen, T. S., & Borg, V. (2003). *Copenhagen Psychosocial Questionnaire (COPSOQ): A Questionnaire on Psychosocial Working Conditions, Health and Well-being in Three Versions*. Psychosocial Department, National Institute of Occupational Health, Copenhagen, Denmark. Available at: http://www.arbejdsmiljoforskning.dk/upload/english_copsoq_2_ed_2003-pdf.pdf

Oakman, J. (2007). Does work ability influence employees intention to retire? *Third International Symposium on Work Ability*. Unpublished Conference Paper.

Palermo, J., Webber, L., Smith, K., & Khor, A. (2009). Factors that predict work ability: Incorporating a measure of organizational values towards ageing. In Kumashire, M. (Eds.) *Promotion of Work Ability towards Productive Ageing*. Taylor & Francis, London.

Parker, T., Worringham, C. J., Greig, K., & Woods, S. D. (2006). *Age-Related Changes in Work Ability and Injury Risk in Underground and Open-Cut Coal Miners*. Available at: http://eprints.qut.edu.au

Taylor, P., Steinberg, M., & Walley, L. (2000). Mature age employment: Recent developments in public policy in Australia and the UK. *Australasian Journal on Ageing*, 19, 125–129.

Tuomi, K., Huuhtanen, P., Nykyri, E., & Ilmarinen, J. (2001). Promotion of workability, the quality of work and retirement. *Occupational Medicine*, 51, 5, 318–324.

Walker, A. (1999). *Managing an Ageing Workforce: A Guide to Good Practice*. European Foundation for the Improvement of Living and Working Conditions. Official Publications of the European Communities, Luxembourg.

Chapter 9
Resilience in Aging: Cultural and Ethnic Perspectives

Darlene Yee-Melichar

This chapter shows that comprehensive research on resilience and aging would benefit from an examination and inclusion of cultural and ethnic perspectives relevant to older people. It shows the heterogeneity in resilience of older people as well as the cultural and ethnic perspectives in what older people will need addressed to be resilient in their lives. It also reveals that the older individual within a cultural or ethnic group is not a common stereotype, but still much their own person. Health and human service providers who interact with an older person must adjust their responses to that individual by taking into consideration the person's level of resilience, culture and ethnicity. More research in cultural and ethno-gerontology is required in order to better understand the diverse aging population and their current resilience and future needs. Forthcoming research on resilience and aging would benefit from a comprehensive and systematic approach by navigating the multi-dimensional perspectives of resilience at the individual, community, and cultural levels for intervention.

Resilience and Aging

The scientific community has begun to recognize resilience as a central component of success in later life. Although there is no consensus definition, resilience or the ability to recover from adversity and stress in life is a key factor of aging successfully. While resilience is often differentiated from coping and adaptation, how and why it is realized by some people and not others is still unclear. Resilience and aging has received inadequate attention; while some information is presented here, more research is required on the multidimensional perspectives of resilience in older people.

It is possible for older people to prevent or recover from physical decline. In a group of 213 people aged 72 and above who were living independently but needed

D. Yee-Melichar (✉)
San Francisco State University, San Francisco, CA, USA
e-mail: dyee@sfsu.edu

B. Resnick et al. (eds.), *Resilience in Aging: Concepts, Research, and Outcomes*,
DOI 10.1007/978-1-4419-0232-0_9, © Springer Science+Business Media, LLC 2011

assistance with at least one activity of daily living (such as bathing, dressing or going to the bathroom), it was noted that 28% of the participants 85 or younger had regained their ability to care for themselves (Gilbert 1999). This suggests that older adults have the power to help prevent or forestall the loss of independence with regular training and support. This type of behavior further suggests that resilience of individuals in later life is possible, but is often related to the individual and his/her willingness to recover.

A comprehensive review of the literature on resilience summarized key concepts and definitions as well as biological and psychosocial factors (Lavretsky and Irwin 2007). Treatment approaches to promote resilience, and implications for future research and interventions were discussed. The authors (Lavretsky and Irwin 2007, p. 309) indicated that "Successful aging is associated with a positive psychological outlook in later years, general well-being, and happiness... With global aging on the rise, many nations are developing and implementing healthy aging policies to promote quality and years of healthy life."

The processes and circumstances that create vulnerability among older people residing in Europe were examined by Grundy (2006). Vulnerability occurs when the balance between reserve capacity and environmental challenge falls below a level that ensures a reasonable quality and quantity of life. Vulnerable older people were defined as those whose reserve capacity falls below the threshold needed to cope successfully with the challenges that they face in life. The most vulnerable elderly are those who are lacking in autonomy, income, and social relationships. Preventive and compensatory interventions have been shown to be effective in preserving and/ or restoring the reserve capacity and reducing the vulnerability of older people.

Grundy (2006) proposed various interventions to minimize vulnerability and increase resiliency; these interventions included promotion of healthy lifestyles and coping skills, strong family and social relationships, savings and assets; environmental improvements to reduce the risk of falls, social and policing programs to reduce street crime, influenza immunization programs; access to good acute care and rehabilitation, psychological and social work services, long-term assistance, and income support.

Although most interventions in Europe have evolved randomly and have not been thoroughly evaluated; some interventions have been shown to be effective in preserving or restoring the reserve capacity and reducing the vulnerability of older people. Grundy (2006) was careful to point out that more research is needed to learn about what is most effective in reducing vulnerability in different subsets of elderly individuals. Despite heterogeneity in age, there may be cultural and other differences in what each age cohort might need. In Europe, there are such diverse populations that understanding these differences are crucial. The same is certainly true here in the United States.

For example, in a recent study involving data from over 1,000 women related to the Women's Health Initiative, researchers aimed to understand how resilience might change over the lifespan. Research results indicated that resilience appeared to relate to other healthy aging determinants, and the way one ages (within a cultural and/or other context) may change the way that resilience is expressed (Vahia 2008).

Bauman et al. (2001) examined resilience in the oldest-old. The authors reviewed three separate studies. One was a qualitative study of resilience in 18 women aged

72–98 years conducted by Neary (1997) who identified common strategies the older participants used to get through difficult times. These strategies were similar to the processes in the selective optimization with compensation model discussed by Baltes and Baltes (1990). Personal traits common to the resilient older women in this study included flexibility, tolerance, independence, determination, and pragmatism (Neary 1997). These traits are similar to those identified in the LaFerriere and Hamel-Bissell (1994) study.

The second study was conducted by Felten (2000) who examined seven women, representing a variety of ethnic groups, who had had serious physical impairments from which they had recovered. These older women displayed the traits of determination, previous experience with hardship, knowledge of available services, strong cultural and religious values, family support, self-care activities, and care giving for others.

The third study was conducted by Talsma (1995) who studied 5,279 people from the Netherlands with a mean age of 69.6 years. Three dimensions of resilience were identified including physical functioning, psychological functioning, and well-being. The conclusion was that resilient older people have high levels of physical functioning, are willing to take initiative and to develop behaviors, believe they have control over their current life and are generally satisfied with their lives. The Netherlands is a more homogenous society than the United States; hence, the applicability of this latter study to the diverse elderly residing in the United States has not yet been established.

Hawkley et al. (2005) summarized that resiliency is impacted partly by genetics but is also influenced by individual responses to stress. These differences include frequency of exposure to stress, nature and intensity of psychological and physiological reactions to stress, and the efficacy of restorative and preventative measures to stress. The authors explained the net impact of human frailties and strengths on physiological resilience and health during the aging process. They summarized how people might be genetically influenced by physiology, but that people have astonishing capacities to minimize or contain the long-term costs of stress, thereby maintaining a resilient physiology and helping them ensure a long and healthy life. This capacity comes from choices that limit exposure to stress, adapting coping strategies, and sleep and exercise patterns. Aging is inevitable, but limiting stress can considerably slow down the degradation of the body limiting even one's need to be resilient.

Fry (1997, p. 150) concluded that "Older people are people... Older people are people who have been here longer than others." In summary, it is apparent that resilient older people have shared and will hopefully continue to share similar circumstances and experiences that promote their security and/or decrease their vulnerability as they age.

Cultural Perspectives on Aging

Five issues have been noted, from a cultural perspective, to promote security or delineate increased vulnerability for older people. These include: (1) material factors, (2) health factors, (3) social linkages, (4) cultural values, especially those of independence, and (5) cultural change (Fry 1997). Resilience is not examined specifically, but cross-cultural perspectives that impact an individual and how each may confront aging have been explored. Specifically, it was noted that growing older is not a uniformly "good" or "bad" practice; rather studies must look at culture, life experience, and local circumstance to demonstrate people's responses to aging.

Older people's experience and relationship to aging must not be separated from their earlier life stages. Younger life cannot be "divorced" from the stages of later life because that stage in life impacts later stages in life. The author explained that to understand someone's reaction to later life the overall picture of their individual experience must be examined.

Fry (1997, pp. 146–150) reflected that "Culture gives meaning to life. Values define what is good and what is bad. Aging has its valences… Independence is a dominant value orientation in American culture." However, the differences we see in other cultures are major differences in productive organization, family structures, political centralization, stratification, and worldviews.

Gunnestad (2006) examined resilience in a cross-cultural perspective with a study about: (1) protective factors, (2) different ways of creating resilience, (3) resilience and vulnerability from culture, and (4) minority and majority cultures, biculturalism and resilience. Although this discussion is not specific to older people, it examines cultural, familial, and social issues which both aid and hinder the development of resilience in children. The author outlined protective factors and processes which help to create resilience. These protective factors include: (1) Network factors (external support), (2) Abilities and Skills (internal support), and (3) Meaning, Values, and Faith (existential support).

According to Gunnestad (2006, pp. 2–3), "Network factors" include external support from family, friends, neighbors, teachers, etc. "Abilities" include internal support such as physical and mental strength, temperament and emotional stability, intellect and appearance. "Skills" include communication skills, social and emotional skills. "Meaning, Values, and Faith" include existential support such as perception of values and attitudes. The author pointed out that culture is contained in all three protective factors, and that these protective factors are interrelated. Culture affects the way we form external support and network systems. Culture decides what abilities and skills are appreciated. And, culture is an integral part of meaning, values and faith.

Gunnestad (2006, p. 3) described the need to create resilience. Resilience is created when the protective factors initiate certain processes in the individual. Identified different ways of creating resilience: (1) building a positive self-image; (2) reducing the effect of risk factors and (3) breaking a negative cycle and opening up new opportunities.

The author examined resilience and vulnerability in different cultures: (1) Latino youth; (2) North American Indian First Nation; and (3) South African youth. The author illustrates how the culture over a long period of time has developed ways of behavior that generate resilience within that setting. Culture can be said to be a way of living facing the challenges in a certain environment with both extrinsic and intrinsic factors (Gunnestad 2006, p. 10).

Gunnestad (2006, p. 17) studied minority and majority cultures, biculturalism, and resilience. Culture relates to the meaning of life of a group of people, it relates to how they live and work (skills), what they hold as right and important for them (values) and it also goes with faith and religion. Culture is a vital part of the identity. Identity is a central part of our personality; it may be seen as the core.

From the perspective of resilience, it can be seen that if you take the culture from a people, you take their identity, and hence their strength – the resilience factors. If people are stripped of what gives them strength, they become vulnerable, because they do not automatically gain those cultural strengths that the majority culture has acquired over generations.

Stutman et al. (2002) report on resilience among immigrants and people from minority cultures. Immigrants and people from minority cultures who master the rules and norms of their new culture without abandoning their own language, values and social support seem more resilient than those who just keep their own culture and cannot acclimate to their new culture or those who become highly acculturated.

Cultural Differences in the Expression of Resilience

Katzko et al. (1998) examined the self-concept of the elderly in a cross-cultural comparison. A sample of elderly Spanish participants ($n = 83$) and elderly Dutch participants ($n = 74$) were compared to gain an idea of the cross-cultural content of self-concept. The research required participants to provide information through the use of the SELE-Instrument. The SELE Instrument is a sentence completion test with a set number of stem questions. The test determines whether the statements made by participants are either motivational or dispositional statements. Motivational statements are beliefs or perceptions while the dispositional statements are self-evaluations of the physical and mental self. The SELE-Instrument maintains specific procedures and coding methods to examine the differences and similarities of the responses between the elderly Dutch and Spanish participants.

Katzko et al. (1998) analyzed and discussed the research results; they acknowledged that the most striking differences were questions related to the "Family" and "Activities" categories. It appears that the elderly participants are looking for new ways to continue to lead meaningful lives after previous goals related to family, marriage, and career are met. In terms of Planning, it appeared that the elderly Spanish participants were more concerned about "Family" while the elderly Dutch participants were more concerned about "Activities." In terms of Possible, it appeared that the elderly Spanish participants were more concerned about "Family, Habitation and Helping" while the elderly Dutch participants were more concerned about "Autonomy and Activities."

Questions related to "future possibilities" (personal expectations and goals of the participants) also exposed differences in personal desires between the two cultures. Additional responses to various questions exposed the differing goals, plans, and desires of the two cultures. Overall, the results of the study indicated that in both cultures, the elderly participants maintain a "still-healthy" image of themselves and often look for opportunities with which to fill their day-to-day existence with meaningful activities.

Katzko et al. (1998) examined the self-concept of the elderly Dutch participants to elderly Spanish participants. They looked at what made these groups age well. They found that each cultural group chose to fill their time differently; the elderly Spanish participants spent more time with family while the elderly Dutch participants spent more time on activities. However, either way, finding fulfillment in their choice was crucial in being content and satisfied as they aged.

Lewis (2008) defined "culture as a shared, learned, symbolic system of values, belief, and attitudes that shapes and influences perception and behavior – an abstract 'mental blueprint' or 'mental code'." Defined "resilience as the strengths that people and systems demonstrate that enable them to rise above adversity" and described ways to build resilience. According to, "cultural resilience refers to a culture's capacity to maintain and develop cultural identify and critical cultural knowledge and practices." Defined "community resilience as the ability of a community to establish, maintain, or regain an expected or satisfactory level of community capacity in the face of adversity and positive challenge." Lewis (2008) summarizes the role of Alaskan elders in the cultural resilience of Native communities.

Cultural Resilience

Lewis (2008) comments on cultural resilience, examining the obstacles that specific societies face in establishing and maintaining their various traditions and social norms. He explores resilience and cultural resilience within the elderly community and defines the typical roles of elders (i.e., grandfather, mentor). "Cultural Identity" is an important topic since the elderly relies upon it to maintain status within their community. It is a social support system that allows them to share their culture with younger generations.

Lewis focuses upon maintaining a community's level of resiliency, highlighting the peoples of Native Alaska to provide examples of how a specific culture maintains its identity. Examples he includes are the Alaskan natives' effort to speak and teach their native language and share traditional stories. Lewis also points out issues such as Alaska's reliance on imported goods and out-migration of youth, as variables which decrease that community's resiliency. Lewis turns to issues of the elder community within the Alaskan Native people and remarks upon the challenges they face such as: younger generations moving away and leaving elders to support themselves. Tensions between personal and communal resilience address the elders' desire to maintain independence while maintaining a valuable and useful identity within their culture. Lewis concludes his presentation by emphasizing that the issue of resilience sparks innovative efforts within a specific culture to maintain its identity.

Culture and Aging

Moody (1998) cites the differences among cultures in regards to aging. He describes how different cultures view, and tend to, elders in geriatric medical care. His article features a case study of a family who is taking care of their aged Chinese family member who is still currently a citizen of China, but is residing in the United States. The family is tending to their elder family member and making medical decisions on her behalf. The scenario is the Chinese elder complains of increasing pain and the family takes her to the hospital. The family learns that the elder family member in fact has cancer. The family asks the doctor not to tell the Chinese elder that she has cancer and opts for herbal remedies instead of traditional remedies such as radiation. The family is adamant about their decision citing their cultural values, but this leaves the healthcare team shocked about the family's decision and in disagreement with their choices.

Moody (1998) portrays the increasing complexity of "ethnic ethics" in the medical community in relationship to the aging population. The idea of "ethnic ethics" rests on the idea that as elders of different cultures age, there are different practices that varying cultures abide by. Moody depicts some of the most common arguments that arise when discussing differences in cultural medical care. First, there is the argument that rights and values are relative to the culture in which are expressing them. Some cultures value familial solidarity in later age; whereas other cultures, like the United States, value individualism and independence. Others believe that certain rights are universal and should not be questioned among cultures. Some believe that the argument of the "right thing to do" must be looked at on an individual basis and not in larger context. These viewpoints set the stage for the complexity of different cultures within the American healthcare system.

Moody (1998) also describes a study by the Fan Fox and Samuels Foundation. This study brought together different elders of different ethnicities and surveyed them about their views on aging. Although many of the predicted different responses occurred, there were also many similar statements across different cultures. Some ideas that were similar among cultures included: shared belief of fatalism, reluctance to communicate with healthcare professionals, and the belief that healthcare professionals did not want their opinion in relationship to care. The study predicted they would find differences among cultures, but were not prepared for the similarities they found.

It is clear that there are cultural differences that medical professional should be aware of and consider when having to provide care. In fact, future medical care might include the need to "negotiate differences" or to understand differences of cultures and look for ways to incorporate compromises between cultures. Despite a family's wish to use an alternative or less scientific intervention, doctors should still work hard to try and educate the family about the benefits of tested medicine. In summary, no matter the ethnic group, they all share "a concern for the dignity of elders."

Resilience Across Ethnic Groups

Consedine et al. (2004) explain that there are a variety of ways that older adults employ in adapting to the changes that aging brings. The authors explain that as individual's age, they come to resemble each other less, rather than more. What is known is that older adults engage in a diverse range of self-care efforts and different attempts to anticipate future difficulties related to aging.

Consedine et al. (2004) considered socioemotional adaptation among individuals from six ethnic groups: African Americans, Jamaicans, Trinidadians, Bajians, US-born Whites, and Immigrant Europeans, predominantly Russians and Ukrainians from the former Soviet Union. The study examined a sample of 1,118 community-dwelling older adults from Brooklyn, New York based on data from the Household Income and Race Summary Tape File 3A of the 1990 Census files. The mean age of the sample was 73.8 years. Data were collected during face-to-face interviews that lasted about one and a half hours in the respondent's home or in a location of their choice such as a church or senior center.

Consedine et al. (2004) used the following measures to look at ethnic constraints on later life adaptation: Demographics, Resiliency, Quality of Social Networks, Stress, Trait Emotions (Negative vs. Positive), Emotion inhibition, Religiosity, and Interpersonal conflict. For the purposes of the study, resiliency was defined as functionality relative to health impairment. Data were analyzed and results were reported. Consedine et al. (2004, pp. 124–125) concluded that "later life is associated with both gains and losses; aging brings with it a variety of challenges in coping with losses in physical, social, and economic realm."

The data also suggested that resilient members of African descent (African Americans, Jamaicans, Trinidadians, and Bajians) were more likely to manifest patterns of adaptation characterized by religious beliefs, while resilient US-born Europeans and immigrant Europeans were more likely to benefit as a result of a nonreligious social connectedness. Social networks, religion, emotions, and emotion regulation are among the key proximal components underlying ethnic difference in later life adaptation.

Aging and Culture

Holzberg (1982) described how little is written about the cultural factors that differentially affect the aging individual or social group. She explained that most contemporary literature focuses on the biological, psychological, and sociological factors of aging, but not on the cultural perspectives of aging. The author gave details on some of the anthropological perspectives to ethnicity and aging. First she explained that "cultural patterning of the human life cycle" is an effort to demonstrate how dominant societal values may structure, facilitate, or hinder individual and group adjustments to aging. Through understanding these patterns, one can better understand the diverse ways individual's age separate from the overall age group.

It is important not to place all "old" in group such as AARP or NCSC, but rather look at elders more closely. Holzberg (1982) criticized research as often placing minority elderly in the category of impoverished or attributing them with unemployment, low levels of education, and high dropout rates. She explained that it does impact the aging experience, but cannot be the only thing that is viewed as important. She gave specific examples of ethnicities including Asians, Native Americans, and Indians and how each group ages differently. Holzberg (1982) explained that understanding the nature of cultural experiences can aid us in our search for explanations of why certain people age differently from others.

Woehrer (1978) has said "The fact that people of different cultural backgrounds put their social worlds together differently means that their needs and resources as well as the ways in which they use the services available to them will vary." Holzberg (1982) concludes with a call for more research in cultural and ethnic gerontology in order to better understand the diverse elder populations and their current and future needs.

Nandan (2007) examined three "waves" of Asian Indian Elderly (AIE) immigrants. The author asserted policy makers and helping professionals have lumped the Asian Indian Elderly (AIE) immigrants with other Asian groups without considering the specific needs and unique perspectives of this population. The author detailed the time periods and numbers in which Asian Indian Elderly immigrated to the United States. Tracing the Asian Exclusion Acts of the early twentieth century, Nandan (2007) stated that the Asian Indian Elderly immigrants did not make much of an impact on the country's population demographics until well after the US repealed these laws. Therefore, the biggest immigration stages took place in the mid-1963s, during the economic boom in 1970s and mid-1980s, and during the 1990s after the "Family Reunification Act of 1990" was passed. Nandan noted that most of these Asian Indian Elderly are aged 55 and over, and therefore have specific needs based upon the circumstances surrounding their particular time of immigration.

Nandan (2007) described the differences in present experiences, legal status, reasons for marriage, adaption and challenges, and pre-immigration culture and values, of each wave of immigrants. The author noted that unlike the second and third wave immigrants, first wave immigrants may not as often visit family members in India because much of their family has already migrated to the US or other countries. Also, the support and community life in India is vastly different from the time they left, and therefore they do not recognize their native homeland. On the contrary, second wave immigrants do visit their native India to see family and friends, and seem to hold closer ties with their native culture as they are more often settled in rural areas in the USA (unlike the first wave immigrants who migrated to large cities for work). In addition, the second wave of Asian Indian Elderly seems to have retained specific cultural and religious customs of their native homeland, fueling their desire to make visits.

Nandan (2007) remarked upon the loneliness and alienation experienced by third wave immigrants, coupled with the financial and medical burden of caring for their elderly parents. These burdens are compounded by their parents' (immigrants as well) status as "permanent residents" rather than citizens, which makes them inapplicable from benefiting from most public services. In some situations, children may send their elderly parents back to India in order to give them better care.

The author discussed the proper approach a "helping professional" should take in regards to Asian Indian Elderly, stating that those "competent" persons will keep in mind the specific cultural change, age group, and migration experience during the past 50 years of Asian Indians, rather than grouping their research and goals within the larger Asian Immigrant group. Nandan (2007) has 11 propositions in which helping professionals should engage with Asian Indian immigrants based upon the different time in which each group came to America, including the age group in which they now belong.

For example, the first wave of AIE immigrants should be viewed very similarly to United States-born citizens. They are familiar with American values, and often have retired with substantial financial security. Second wave AIE immigrants are in their 50s with college/marriageable age children and, more often than first wave immigrants, come from a variety of countries: India, Kenya, South Africa, along with Guyanese cultures and might have adapted faster to American custom than those who directly migrated from India. Many of the third wave immigrants may not be legal citizens, coming after the reunification clause of the American immigration policy. Nandan (2007) concludes that helping professionals must receive ongoing training to adequately address the specific differences within the three waves of Asian Indian Elderly immigrants in addition to not grouping this specific culture within the larger group of Asian Immigrants.

Nandan (2007) described the increase of Asian Indian Elderly Americans since the mid-1960s. The author discussed the three distinct waves of immigration since 1960 and what services and or resources each may need as they age. Recently in the 2000 US Census, Asian Indians ranked fourth highest with regard to number of immigrants over the age of 55. The author explained that the country is experiencing a "browning" and "graying" of America. Since the needs and experiences of three waves of AIE immigrants are different because of the time, age, and stage in life of their migration to the U.S., their needs will be different.

Example of Impact of Culture on Resilience

Yin (2006) described how elderly white men are most afflicted by high suicide rates. Overall, in the U.S. population, there are 11 suicide deaths per 100,000; however, white males commit suicide three times the existing national average, and are eight times more likely to kill themselves than women of the same age group.

The author described the high suicide rates of elderly white males and why they seem to be at substantially greater risk for suicide than females. Some researchers claim that the lack of resilience in males is from weak coping abilities. For example, men are accustomed to asserting their will and taking charge; however, later in life, as they age, men have unrealistic expectations and are less likely to ask help from others, making aging more isolating. Also, the author explained how much of the research around male suicide explains an elderly person's act of suicide as "tragic but rational," making it seem normal and acceptable.

The author explained that women have lower suicide rates because of their existing physical and role changes they experience through life making them more apt to accept change when it happens in later life. Further, women also tend to build more robust social networks with family and friends which is necessary for resilience. Suicide is found to be less common in those with strong social networks. In addition, race might affect resilience in males. Researchers noted that the lower suicide rates in male Hispanics and non-Hispanic whites might be because of "familism" or their increased emphasis on close relationship with extended kinship. The author indicates that lower suicide rates in older male African Americans might be due to more connectedness to social institutions such as family, church, and social-support systems. Researchers found in interviews that African American Pastors in the south viewed suicide as a "white thing," and furthered this by saying that their community had developed a culture of resilience in which suicide was counter to the black experience. The author explained that culture, tradition, and family connections seem to lower suicide rates because of increased resilience.

Yin (2006) described why there are such obstacles in detecting depression in the elderly. The author explains that in later life depression can manifest into fatigue and or other physical systems, making the diagnosis of depression much more difficult. The author also explains that there is the persisting public view that suicide in the elderly is less tragic and more acceptable than in youth, even viewed as part of the natural aging process. Finally, the author concludes with whatever the reasons are that treating depression in later life is treatable and should be treated as aggressively in later life as in youth. The elders are an important and critical part of society and need to be treated that way.

Yin (2006) included a graph that shows suicide by age and sex (which shows elderly white men having a significantly higher number of suicides). The next chart shows male death rates for suicide by race, Hispanic origin and age. It shows how White males have the highest number of suicides per 100,000 later in old age. Some researchers argue that elderly white males lack the resilience and coping mechanisms that make white women and older black people less prone to suicide. Researchers show that Hispanic males might have a significantly smaller percentage of suicides because of the cultural emphasis on close relationships with extended kinship. The author concluded that social institutions such as family, church, and social support systems might serve to protect against things that may influence suicide. The author showed how resilience is probably stronger in culturally rich minorities.

Next Steps in the Area of Cultural Impact on Resilience

This chapter shows that comprehensive research on resilience and aging would benefit from an examination and inclusion of cultural perspectives and ethnic variations relevant to the sample population of older people. Information on resilience and aging indicate that the elderly have the power to help prevent or forestall the loss of independence with regular training and support; successful aging is associated with a positive psychological outlook; some interventions have been shown to be effective in preserving or restoring the reserve capacity and reducing the vulnerability of older people; and the way one ages may change the way that resilience is expressed.

Research on resilience in aging and cultural perspectives reveal that studies must look at culture, life experience, and local circumstance to demonstrate people's responses to aging; culture affects the way we form external support and network systems, decides what abilities and skills are appreciated, and is an integral part of meaning, values and faith; culture over time has developed ways of behavior that generate resilience within that setting; immigrants and people from minority cultures seem more resilient than those who cannot acclimate to their new culture or those who become highly acculturated; differences in goals exist between cultures yet cultures look for opportunities with which to fill their existence with meaningful activities; need for individual resilience as well as cultural resilience and community resilience and need for ethnic ethics in cultural medical care to address differences and similarities in cultural perspective.

Studies on resilience in aging and ethnic variations suggest that as individuals age, they come to resemble each other less; social networks, religion, emotions, and emotion regulation are among the key components underlying ethnic difference in later life adaptation; little is written about the cultural factors that differentially affect the aging individual or social group; understanding the nature of cultural experiences can aid us in our search for explanations for why certain people age differently from others; culture, tradition, and family connections seem to lower suicide rates because of increased resilience; and resilience is probably stronger in culturally rich minorities.

This review of the literature shows the heterogeneity in resilience of older people as well as the cultural and ethnic perspectives in what older people will need addressed to be resilient in their lives. It also reveals that the older individual within a cultural or ethnic group is not a common stereotype, but still much their own person.

A "strengths perspective for social work practice" indicates that "people have untapped, undetermined reservoirs of mental, physical, emotional, social and spiritual abilities that can be expressed. The presence of this capacity for continued growth and heightened well-being means that people must be accorded the respect that this power deserves. The capacity acknowledges both the being and the becoming aspects of life." (Weick et al. 1989, p. 352).

Health and human service providers who interact with an older person must adjust their responses to that individual by taking into consideration the person's level of resilience, culture and ethnicity. More research in cultural and ethnogerontology is needed in order to better understand the diverse aging population and their current resilience and future needs. Forthcoming research on resilience and aging would benefit from a comprehensive and systematic approach by navigating the multidimensional perspectives of resilience at the individual, community, and cultural levels for intervention.

References

Baltes, P.B., and Baltes, M.M. (1990). Psychological Perspectives on Successful Aging: The Model of Selective Optimization with Compensation. In P.B. Baltes and M.M. Baltes (Eds.), *Successful Aging: Perspectives from the Behavioral Sciences* (pp. 1–34). Cambridge: Cambridge University Press.

Bauman, S., Harrison, A., and Waldo, M. (2001). Resilience in the Oldest-Old. Retrieved March 19, 2009, from Health Care Industry, Website: http://findarticles.com/p/articles/mi_qa3934/is_200110/ ai_n8959937

Consedine, N., Magai, C., and Conway, F. (2004). Predicting Ethnic Variation in Adaption to Later Life: Styles of Socioemotional Functioning and Constrained Heterotypy. *Journal of Cross Cultural Gerontology*, 19(2), 97–131. Retrieved from http://search.ebscohost.com

Felten, B.S. (2000). Resilience in a Multicultural Sample of Community Dwelling Women Older than Age 85. *Clinical Nursing Research*, 9(2), 102–124.

Fry, C. (1997). Cross-Cultural Perspectives on Aging. In K. Ferraro (Ed.), *Gerontology: Perspectives and Issues* (pp. 138–152). New York, NY: Springer.

Gilbert, S. (1999). Study Upbeat on Resilience of Elderly. Retrieved March 28, 2009, from *New York Times: Women's Health*. Website: http://www.nytimes.com/specials/women/warchive/980203 _96.html

Grundy, E. (2006). Aging and Vulnerable Elderly People: European Perspectives. *Aging and Society*, 26, 105–129. Doi: 10.107/s0144686X05004484

Gunnestad, A. (2006). Resilience in a Cross-Cultural Perspective: How Resilience in Generated in Different Cultures. In A. Jens (Ed.) Retrieved from http://www.immi.se/intercultural/nr11/gunnestad.html

Hawkley S et al. (2005). Stress, Aging and Resilience: Can Accrued Wear and Tear be Slowed? *Canadian Psychology*, 46(3), 115–125. Retrieved from http://psychology.uchicago.edu/people/faculty/ cacioppo/jtcreprints/hbemmc05.pdf

Holzberg, C. (1982). Ethnicity and Aging: Anthropological Perspectives on More than Just the Minority Elderly. *The Gerontologist*, 22(3), 249–257. Retrieved from http://0-ejournals.ebsco.com. opac.sfsu.edu/Article.asp?ContributionID=19839628

Katzko, M., Steverink, N., Dittmann-Kohli, F., and Herrera, R. (1998). The Self-Concept of the Elderly: A Cross-Cultural Comparison. *International Journal of Aging & Human Development*, 46(3), 171–187. Retrieved from http://search.ebscohost.com

LaFerriere, R.H., and Hamel-Bissell, B.P. (1994). Successful Aging of Oldest Old Women in the Northeast Kingdom of Vermont. *IMAGE: Journal of Nursing Scholarship*, 26, 319–323.

Lavretsky, H., and Irwin, M. (2007). Resilience and Aging. *Aging Health*, 3(3), 309–323. Doi: 10.2217/1745509X.3.309

Lewis, J. (2008). Preserving our Future. The Role of Elders in the Cultural Resilience of Native Communities. Retrieved from http://elders.uaa.alaska.edu/powerpoints/elder-resilience_lewis.pdf

Moody, H. (1998). Cross-Cultural Geriatric Ethics: Negotiating Our Differences. *Generations*, 22(3), 32. Retrieved from http://search.ebscohost.com

Nandan, M. (2007). Waves of Asian Indian Elderly Immigrants: What Can Practitioners Learn? *Journal of Cross-Cultural Gerontology*, 22(4), 389–404. http://search.ebscohost.com

Neary, S.R. (1997). Room to Maneuver: Preserving Choice in Resilient Old Age, Doctoral Dissertation, Boston College. *Dissertation Abstracts International*, 58-12B, AAG9818636.

Stutman, S., Baruch, R., Grotberg, E., and Rathore, Z. (2002). *Resilience in Latino Youth*. Working Paper, Institute for Mental Health Initiatives. Washington, DC: The George Washington University.

Talsma, A.M. (1995). Evaluation of a Theoretical Model of Resilience and Select Predictors of Resilience in a Sample of Community-Based Elderly, Doctoral Dissertation, University of Michigan. *Dissertation Abstracts International*, 56-08B, AA19542967.

Vahia, I. (2008). Resilience in Aging. *Healthwise*, 26(8). Retrieved March 18, 2009, from Healthwise. Website: sira.ucsd.edu

Weick, A., Rapp, C., Sullivan, W., and Kisthardt, W. (1989). A Strengths Perspective for Social Work Practice. *Social Work*, 34(4), 350–354.

Woehrer, C.E. (1978). Cultural Pluralism in American Families: The Influence of Ethnicity on Social Aspects of Aging. *The Family Coordinator*, 27, 328–339.

Yin, S. (2006). *Elderly White Men Afflicted with High Suicide Rates*. Population Reference Bureau. Retrieved from http://www.stormfront.org/forum/showthread.php?t=492316

Chapter 10
Civic Engagement: Policies and Programs to Support a Resilient Aging Society

Nancy Morrow-Howell, Greg O'Neill, and Jennifer C. Greenfield

Introduction

Civic engagement among older adults is gaining attention in both the popular and academic press. As the health and education of aging Americans continue to increase, so does the opportunity to engage this growing population in civic activities aimed at improving communities. At the same time, this engagement has the potential to promote the health and resiliency of older adults. Evidence suggests that volunteering improves health, mental health, and socialization, and is protective in the face of loss and other challenges of later life. Thus, it has a place in the discussion of resilience as defined in this book, the *ability to achieve, retain, or regain a level of physical or emotional health after illness or loss*. In this chapter, we review the current status of volunteering among older adults in the United States, and we highlight over two decades of research demonstrating the positive association between volunteering and wellbeing of older adults. We then consider the relationship of volunteering to resilience. We review current policies and programs that promote volunteering, and finally, we address challenges to wider participation among the older population.

Definitions and Current Status of Volunteering Among Older Adults

There is no standard definition of "civic engagement" in the literature, although many have been offered (see Definitions of Civic Engagement, GSA, http://www. civicengagement.org). Definitions include varying activities undertaken by individuals, but a common theme is that these activities have public consequence for communities and the polity (Christiano 1996). Two spheres of activity often are

N. Morrow-Howell (✉)
Washington University, St. Louis, MO, USA
e-mail: morrow-howell@wustl.edu

B. Resnick et al. (eds.), *Resilience in Aging: Concepts, Research, and Outcomes*,
DOI 10.1007/978-1-4419-0232-0_10, © Springer Science+Business Media, LLC 2011

included: political and social. "Political engagement" refers to those behaviors that influence governmental processes at the local, state, and national levels. "Social engagement" refers to actions that connect individuals to others and that relate to care or development (Wuthnow 1991). In both spheres, actions are usually voluntary and include mutual aid, volunteerism, and civic service. In this chapter, we focus on formal volunteering, given the vast potential of the aging population to serve communities in these roles. We define volunteering as an activity undertaken by an individual that is uncoerced, unpaid (or minimal compensation to offset costs), structured by an agency or organization, and directed toward a community concern (Cnaan et al. 1996). We include a wide range of volunteer activities, from episodic, such as serving a Thanksgiving meal at a homeless shelter, to high commitment, like participating in the Foster Grandparent or Senior Companion programs where older adults serve their communities for at least 15 h a week.

Prevalence of Volunteer Engagement

Older Americans have a strong history of volunteering. Many adults engage in service well into their retirement years, and volunteer rates do not decline significantly until later life when health concerns make volunteer engagement more difficult. In 2008, 61.3 million people volunteered in the United States, representing an overall volunteer rate of 27% (Corporation for National and Community Service [CNCS] 2009). The volunteer rate among older adults is slightly lower (23.5%), but this rate has increased steadily since 1974, in contrast with declining rates of volunteer engagement among younger adults in the same time period (CNCS 2009; Foster-Bey et al. 2007).

There are several explanations for the lower rates of volunteering among older adults. Younger and middle-aged adults take on volunteer roles related to their children's activities as well as their work roles. Older adults are generally more separated from educational and work institutions and are thus less likely to be presented with volunteer opportunities (Morrow-Howell 2007). Health issues are related to declining rates of volunteering for those over the age of 75 (AARP 2003). Further, research demonstrates that older adults are less likely than younger and middle-aged adults to be asked to volunteer, but if asked, older adults are more likely to agree (Independent Sector 2000). Also, once in volunteer roles, older adults commit more time, reporting a median of 96 h a year, while the 45–54 age group reports 50 h a year, and those 55–64 years report 56 h (U.S. Bureau of Labor Statistics 2005). These numbers increase when definitions of "service" are expanded to include informal help to others. According to AARP, as many as 68% of older Americans report having performed some type of service – formal or informal – in 2008 (Koppen 2009). Another estimate comes from the Health and Retirement Survey where about 33% of respondents aged 55 years and over reported engagement in formal volunteerism, while 52% reported engagement in informal volunteerism (Zedlewski and Schaner 2005). Indeed, a full accounting of the helping activity of older adults must extend beyond the boundaries of formal voluntary activities (Rozario 2007).

Older adults with more resources – those with more education, income, health, and social resources – are more likely to volunteer (Musick and Wilson 2008; Tang et al. 2009). Although findings are inconsistent, researchers often document that females, whites, and married older adults are more likely to volunteer than their male, non-white, and unmarried counterparts (Choi 2003; Peters-Davis et al. 2001). Non-Hispanic whites have higher representation among formal volunteers than do African Americans: 30.4% compared to 22.1% (U.S. Bureau of Labor Statistics 2005). Differential rates in volunteering can be attributed to disparities in economic and health resources, and competing demands of caregiving and working (Center for Health Communication, Harvard School of Public Health 2004; McBride 2007).

Great hope is placed in the rising cohort of older Americans. Baby Boomers tend to volunteer in greater numbers than previous generations. This is explained by higher levels of education as well as the propensity to have children later in life (which keeps them involved in volunteering at educational institutions and child-related activities into later ages) (Corporation for National and Community Service [CNCS] 2007). Baby Boomers may work longer, but there is evidence that employment, especially part-time employment, is related to volunteering (Morrow-Howell 2007). In addition, up to two-thirds of older adults not currently engaged in volunteer service express a desire to become engaged (National Governors Association [NGA] 2008). Clearly, there is tremendous potential for increasing the civic engagement of older adults in the future.

Outcomes of Volunteering

Volunteering has been associated with many positive outcomes for older adults (CNCS 2007), including reduced mortality (Musick et al. 1999), increased physical function (Lum and Lightfoot 2005; Moen et al. 1992), increased levels of self-rated health (Morrow-Howell et al. 2003), reduced depressive symptomatology (Musick et al. 1999; Musick and Wilson 2003), reduced pain (Arnstein et al. 2002), higher self-esteem (Omoto et al. 2000), and greater life satisfaction (Van Willigen 2000). The above findings generally were derived from longitudinal surveys, where well-being outcomes at a subsequent observation period are associated with volunteer activities in previous observation periods, controlling for as many confounding variables as possible.

More recently, experimental and quasi-experimental studies are emerging. Fried et al. (2004) at Johns Hopkins University completed a randomized trial to evaluate the effects of participating in the Experience Corps (EC) program, a high commitment volunteer program in which older adults perform service in elementary schools. In the study, 149 new recruits to the program were assigned to EC or to a waitlist. Compared to the waitlist controls, EC volunteers reported increased physical strength and an increase in the number of people they could turn to for help. They also showed less decline in walking speed (Fried et al. 2004) and a trend toward improved cognitive function (Carlson et al. 2008). EC participants also reported being more physically active (Tan et al. 2006). In another study of the health effects of participation in the EC program, EC participants were matched with a comparison group from the Health and Retirement Study sample. The two groups were equal on health status at baseline and volunteer history; 2 years later, EC participants reported fewer depressive symptoms and fewer functional limitations, and the effect sizes were substantial (Morrow-Howell et al. 2009b).

Role theory has often been used to explain the beneficial effects of volunteering. By assuming the role of volunteer, individuals may gain access to resources, social contacts, status, and recognition (Moen et al. 1992). Researchers have pointed out that, compared to other productive activities (like work or caregiving), volunteering is usually more discretionary. The choice involved in volunteering (picking the type of volunteer activity, for example) may increase its potential to produce feelings of usefulness or personal satisfaction (Musick and Wilson 2003). A study of volunteering in Israel suggested that volunteering has positive effects above and beyond activities such as physical exercise and hobbies (Shmotkin et al. 2003).

Volunteering may provide unique opportunities for older adults, who report more gains in life satisfaction and self-esteem, and more improvement in depressive symptoms than do younger volunteers (Omoto et al. 2000; Van Willigen 2000). These age differences may be due to the fact that the volunteer experience assumes a different meaning among the specific role sets that vary across the life course. Midlarsky (1991) suggested that volunteering may substitute for paid work; Moen (1995) suggested that it may contribute to social connections that may otherwise diminish after retirement. Musick and Wilson (2003, p. 268) suggest that different motivations to volunteer between young and older adults might lead to the "elevated" significance of this activity among older population; older adults are more intrinsically motivated while younger adults are more motivated by extrinsic rewards (i.e., gaining work experience, or making social connections).

Volunteering and Resiliency

The literature on the positive effects of volunteering for health, mental health, self-esteem, social connections, and life satisfaction of older adults suggests that volunteering is related to resiliency in several ways. Volunteering increases the potential for an adult to be resilient when faced with adversity, and may serve as a coping strategy in the recovery process. As summarized by Musick and Wilson (2003), volunteering increases the personal and social resources of an individual. It is these resources that are part of an *individual's capacity to make a "psycho-social comeback."*

Individuals with fewer personal and social resources may be at greater risk for difficulty in recovering from an adverse event. That is, they may be more vulnerable and less resilient. These same individuals are those that research suggests may benefit most from volunteering (Spring et al. 2007). For example, Musick et al. (1999) found that older adults with less social interaction experience a greater protective effect from volunteering than those with more social interaction. Morrow-Howell et al. (2003) found that older adults with functional limitations benefit more from volunteering than those who are more functional. Further, lesser educated and lower income older adults report more benefits from volunteering than their better educated and higher income counterparts, including better health, improved self-esteem, increased socialization, and greater generativity (Morrow-Howell et al. 2009a). In sum, it appears that volunteers who are more vulnerable to poorer quality of life outcomes, especially in the face of loss and other challenges, benefit the most from volunteering. Thus, volunteering can be seen as strategy to bolster resources to better prepare for loss or crisis.

It has long been suggested that volunteer work may substitute for the loss of other roles in later life (Chambre 1987), especially the productive and social roles of a workplace. An older adult who volunteers may be less disrupted by the loss of another role. Greenfield and Marks (2006) demonstrate that volunteering can protect older adults with role-identity absences (e.g., partner, employee, parent) with regard to purpose in life. In a study of Japanese older adults, volunteering attenuated the negative effect of losing a job for men; and for women, involvement in multiple roles, including volunteerism, was related to fewer depressive symptoms compared to women involved only in housework (Sugihara et al. 2008).

Finally, volunteering is a specific coping technique that an adult can utilize in response to adversity, or as a way to recover after a crisis or loss. Volunteering can provide a means to deal with emotional needs or feelings of uselessness, and individuals report that their volunteer work is therapeutic (Musick and Wilson 2008). Regarding the challenge of losing a spouse, Pillemer and Glasgow (2000) suggest that the volunteer role may provide meaningful social activity that can facilitate adaptation. Li and Ferraro (2007) found that widows who adopted a volunteer role after spousal loss were protected against depressive symptoms; those who increased volunteer hours after widowhood experienced gains in self-efficacy. Brown et al. (2008) studied the effects of helping behavior on recovery from spousal loss and found that bereaved individuals who engaged in helping others experienced a more rapid decline in depression than those who did not, even after controlling for social support and health.

Given the potential of volunteering to increase the health and resiliency of the aging population, policymakers and program leaders increasingly are interested in strategies to maximize the involvement of older adults in volunteer activities. In the next section of this chapter, we review policy and program initiatives aimed at volunteering and older adults.

Maximizing Participation Through Programs and Policies

Government Programs

The federal government currently supports a variety of volunteer programs targeting older adults. Most prominent are the three national Senior Corps programs: the Foster Grandparent Program, the Senior Companion Program, and the Retired and Senior

Volunteer Program (RSVP). Together, these programs engage over half a million older Americans in service to their communities each year (Eisner et al. 2009).

The Foster Grandparent Program is Senior Corps' oldest program, dating back to the War on Poverty initiatives of Lyndon Johnson's administration in the mid-1960s (Freedman 1999). The program provides a small stipend to low-income adults age 60 and over who serve as mentors, tutors, and caregivers for disadvantaged or disabled youth. The Senior Companion program pays a small stipend to low-income adults age 60 and over who provide support to frail persons – most of them elderly – who require assistance to live independently in their homes or communities. RSVP, the youngest, largest, and most flexible of the three programs, promotes the engagement of adults age 55 and over in a diverse range of service activities, including organizing neighborhood watch programs, tutoring children, building houses, and assisting victims of natural disasters.

Although Senior Corps programs operate through the Corporation for National and Community Service (CNCS) – an independent federal agency established in 1993 to coordinate federal and state volunteer efforts – additional programs that support service and volunteering opportunities for older adults operate through other federal agencies. Among these programs are the Senior Community Service Employment Program (SCSEP), Service Corps of Retired Executives (SCORE), Troops to Teachers, the Senior Environmental Employment Program, and Experience Corps.

SCSEP – established by Congress in Title V of the Older Americans Act of 1965 and operated through the U.S. Department of Labor – offers low-income adults age 55 and over paid volunteer positions through public and non-profit agencies, such as senior centers, governmental agencies, schools, hospitals, and libraries. Although SCSEP began as an anti-poverty program rooted in community service, its mission has expanded to include work-based training and job placement. The U.S. Small Business Administration also provides volunteer opportunities for older adults through SCORE – a non-profit organization that encourages working and retired executives and business owners to provide free counseling and training to aspiring entrepreneurs and small business owners. Like SCORE, Troops to Teachers – a program administered by the U.S. Department of Education and Department of Defense – is not specifically targeted to older adults, although it often enlists the service efforts of older individuals. This program helps eligible military personnel begin new careers as teachers in public schools. Through financial incentives, the program encourages participants to seek placement in high poverty area schools. The Senior Environmental Employment Program, administered by the Environmental Protection Agency (EPA), provides an opportunity for retired and unemployed Americans age 55 and over to remain active using their skills in meaningful tasks that support a wide variety of EPA's environmental programs. Experience Corps, which began as a national demonstration project under the auspices of CNCS in 1995, supports adults age 55 and older who work in teams for at least 15 h per week to tutor and mentor elementary school students, help teachers in the classroom, and lead after-school enrichment activities. Today, the program operates in 23 cities with funding from AmeriCorps (the national service program administered by CNCS), state and local public and private funds, private foundations, and in-kind donations.

Non-profit Sector Initiatives

Over approximately the last decade, a number of non-profit organizations have spearheaded innovative efforts to advance opportunities for volunteering, employment, lifelong learning, advocacy, and public service in later life (see "The Civic Enterprise" at http://www.civicengagement.org). Although too numerous to list here, they include: national networks of retired health care professionals working in free clinics (e.g., Volunteers in Medicine); networks of pro bono business consultants for non-profits, schools, and government agencies (e.g., The Taproot Foundation); faith-based initiatives to engage older adults in civic work (e.g., Shepherd's Centers, Faith in Action); national campaigns to advance federal and state policies to promote older adult civic engagement (e.g., Experience Wave); social innovation awards for individuals age 60 or older who have demonstrated vision and entrepreneurialism in addressing community and national problems (e.g., Civic Ventures' Purpose Prize); awards for employers and organizations creating pathways to social impact work in the second half of life (e.g., Civic Ventures' Encore Opportunity Award); clearinghouse-type organizations that facilitate the link between older adults and volunteer opportunities (e.g., VolunteerMatch); as well as several initiatives to help working or retired adults transition into new careers in the public sector (e.g., Partnership for Public Service), non-profit sector (e.g., ReServe, The Transition Network, Bridgestar, Executive Service Corps), or international service (e.g., Encore! Service Corps International, International Senior Lawyers Project). In addition, all three of the major non-profit national professional associations in aging – the American Society on Aging (ASA), The Gerontological Society of America (GSA) and the National Council on Aging (NCOA) – recently have made civic engagement a focus of their programmatic, research, and policy efforts.

Political Momentum

Over the past 5 years, political interest in the civic engagement of older Americans has increased considerably. Prompted by the research evidence that volunteering is good for older adults and that the country could benefit from tapping this pool of human capital, politicians have stepped up their efforts to mobilize older adults for volunteer work.

In 2005, civic engagement was a focus of the fifth White House Conference on Aging (WHCoA). Among the 50 policy recommendations that the delegates voted to bring forward to the President and Congress, two were related to civic engagement: the first was a resolution calling for a national strategy to promote meaningful volunteer activities for older Americans; and the second was a resolution calling for renewal of the laws that authorize national service programs (O'Neill 2007). With regard to civic engagement, one of the delegates' major policy goals was achieved in late 2006 when President Bush signed into law the 5-year reauthorization of the Older Americans Act (H.R. 6197). The law included several areas of expansion, building upon ideas and language developed in the WHCoA policy recommendations. The law included a definition of civic engagement, required that the Assistant Secretary for Aging develop a comprehensive strategic plan for engaging older adults in meeting critical community needs, and authorized a new program of demonstration, support, and research grants for projects that engage older adults in multigenerational and civic engagement activities.

At the state level, new efforts to engage older adults in volunteer work have emerged. In 2007, California Governor Schwarzenegger launched the "EnCorps Teachers" program, an initiative that recruits skilled soon-to-be-retired employees to serve as math and science teachers in public secondary schools. In 2008, California and New York were the first two states to create cabinet-level positions for service and volunteering, giving volunteers a voice at the highest levels of state government. Facing tight budgets, states are experimenting with various incentives to increase volunteering by older adults. In 2008, Illinois granted free public transportation to all senior citizens with the expectation that it would facilitate greater access to community volunteer opportunities. In several other states, local districts offer residents over age 60 the opportunity to volunteer in schools and earn a modest tax credit against their property taxes (see, for example, Senior Tax Exchange Program, http://www.brf.org/partnership/programs/step/geninfo.htm).

The 110th (2008) session of Congress also saw the introduction of several bills to expand service opportunities for baby boomers and older adults. In three separate bills – the GIVE (Generations Invigorating Volunteerism and Education Act, H.R. 5366), the Encore Service Act (S. 3480), and the Serve America Act (S. 3487) – members of the U.S. House and Senate laid out their visions for service by Americans of all ages. And, at a summit on national service held 2 months prior to the November 2008 election, both presidential candidates John McCain and Barack Obama committed to signing into law major expansions for the nation's service programs if they were elected (Stengel 2008).

The Edward M. Kennedy Serve America Act

In his first 100 days in the White House, President Barack Obama signed into law the Edward M. Kennedy Serve America Act of 2009; the largest expansion of national service programs since the Depression-era Civilian Conservation Corps (Public Law 111-13 [H.R. 1388] 2009). The Act includes several provisions that specifically benefit midlife and older adults. The law – in effect as of October 2009 – establishes an Encore Fellowship program for individuals age 55 or older to serve in leadership or management positions in public and private non-profit organizations for 1 year; it targets 10% of AmeriCorps funds for organizations that enroll adults age 55 and older; and it creates Silver Scholarships that provide a $1,000 higher education award – transferable to children, foster children, and grandchildren – to older volunteers who contribute at least 350 h of service per year. The new law also requires that the nation's 50 State Commissions on National and Community Service complete detailed plans to recruit and leverage the resources of the baby boomer generation. It also expands service options for older Americans by lowering the age requirement for the Foster Grandparent and Senior Companion programs from 60 to 55, and increasing hourly stipend eligibility for the programs from 125% of the federal poverty level to 200%.

Evaluation of Program Effectiveness

Another important innovation introduced in the Serve America Act is the establishment of an ongoing, uniform evaluation process for all service programs. Until this point, evaluation of effectiveness and outcomes has been relatively inconsistent, with periodic studies of program accomplishments but no comprehensive effort to evaluate program outcomes longitudinally (see http://www.seniorcorps.gov/about/role_impact/research.asp for a list of past research on program impacts). In contrast, in addition to the ongoing reporting required by Congress, the Serve America Act requires regular program evaluations of all national service programs under the umbrella of the CNCS, and increases competition in the funding of the Senior Corps programs.

Performance measures for use across the various Senior Corps programs will help facilitate comparative analysis of program implementation strategies and may provide opportunities to further investigate the comparative effects of different types of volunteer engagement. Also, the transition to a more evidence-based implementation style will enhance the availability and consistency of data about the impacts of volunteer engagement on volunteers, service recipients, and communities. Lastly, the shift to competitive funding, supported by uniform performance measures, has the potential to enhance the quality and consistency of these national programs that engage older adults in service. Similar means of evaluating the impacts of volunteer programs outside of those administered by the CNCS would significantly advance efforts to improve program effectiveness while enhancing research on how volunteering supports the wellbeing and resilience of individuals and communities.

Challenges and Future Directions

Policy Directions

Although the landmark Edward M. Kennedy Serve America Act offers an historic opportunity to leverage the experience of older Americans on behalf of their communities' needs, federal programs represent only a small minority of senior volunteering. The federal government can encourage more volunteering by helping to remove barriers that older adults face, such as transportation costs, competing caregiving demands, and limitations from chronic conditions. Volunteers provide critical driving services to those who cannot otherwise conduct personal errands or get to and from medical appointments or other activities, yet individuals and non-profit organizations carry the cost of liability insurance. Driving services could be expanded if the Good Samaritan laws were broadened to include volunteer drivers. In addition, raising the charitable mileage deduction from 14 cents per mile to the 58.5 cents per mile that is deductible for business driving likely would have a major impact on allowing volunteers to serve those who live in places that require driving (Bridgeland et al. 2008). Expanding home- and technology-based volunteer opportunities (via telephone or computer) could increase access to volunteer roles for older adults with disabilities, transportation limitations, or remote residences (O'Neill 2007).

Policymakers also can make use of rewards and incentives to encourage activities that benefit the public. Research suggests that small incentives – such as education credits, access to group health insurance, or a modest monthly stipend – might reap large benefits by attracting more adults into community service (Bridgeland et al. 2008). Going forward, policy experts have recommended that the President charge a national commission to develop a "blueprint" for tapping the time, energy, and talents of millions of older adults to strengthen America's communities. The commission might be tasked to explore how tax, pension, education and retraining, and health-care policies could be reformed to maximize the involvement of older adults and baby boomers in their communities (Gomperts 2007). The commission also might highlight existing individual and organizational role models and develop strategies for translating the most promising ideas into policy and practice (Freedman 1999).

The corporate sector also can play an important role. Almost 70% of America's volunteers are in the labor force (U.S. Bureau of Labor Statistics 2009). Volunteering peaks in mid-life, not retirement. Therefore, the workplace is an ideal location to connect with and engage potential volunteers, including retirees. Companies can implement or expand corporate volunteer programs for their employees, and offer programs for their retirees to stay involved in community service. For example, through its Transition to Teaching program, IBM trains some of its most experienced employees to become fully accredited teachers in their local communities upon leaving the company. Policymakers might offer subsidies, tax credits, and other incentives to encourage businesses to create volunteer time policies, such as paid and unpaid leave for volunteering (Gerontological Society of America [GSA] 2005).

Recruitment and Outreach

Non-profit and public agencies need volunteer labor at the same time that many older adults state they currently are not engaged because they have not been asked (Rozario 2007). Clearly, one challenge is bringing together older adults and non-profit agencies in need of volunteers. Unless older adults are recruited actively, they will not likely come forward in large numbers to serve. Currently, organizations make contact with potential volunteers through a variety of channels: electronic and written media, local fairs and festivals, and presentations at community events and civic organizations (Civic Ventures 2004). Additionally, websites are being developed that may prove more effective over time as more older adults become comfortable with using the Internet to connect with resources (see, for example, http://www.volunteermatch.com and http://www.allforgood.org). Leaders in the public and non-profit sectors could reach out to older adults with national social marketing campaigns that would stimulate a new spirit of volunteerism and convey the positive outcomes of volunteering for older adults. The Obama administration's launch of the Serve.gov initiative to engage Americans of all ages in addressing community needs in education, health, energy and the environment, community renewal, and safety and security is a promising step in this direction. AARP also is moving in this direction with the launch of their Create the Good Facebook page (http://www.facebook.com/createthegood), which promotes volunteer opportunities around the country by posting announcements, pictures, and profiles of middle-aged and older adult volunteers.

Yet the recruitment method that seems most effective is the "personal ask." Older adults who are asked to volunteer do so at rates five times higher than those who are not asked, and yet, certain subpopulations, like African Americans, are less likely than Caucasians to be asked to volunteer (Independent Sector 2000). These findings have clear implications for identifying effective methods for recruiting volunteers, especially those who may benefit most from engagement but are least likely to be recruited. Targeting recruitment to more isolated, lower socioeconomic status (SES), and ethnic minority older adults may depend on effective messages and messengers who can connect with these adults more personally. Focus group studies indicated that key messages to convey to older adults include: sharing experience, leaving a legacy, having a sense of purpose, and developing meaningful relationships; and that African Americans respond more than other populations to the urgency of a need to help others in the community (Mark and Waldman 2002). Identifying individuals to engage in personal communications and recruitment may be difficult, but if health and social service providers, family members, and informal community leaders understand the potential benefits of volunteering and know about volunteer opportunities in the area, targeted outreach may be feasible.

Inclusion

Concern has been expressed that the current movement toward increasing volunteer involvement among older adults is elitist and fails to capture the diversity of the older population in terms of ethnicity and SES (Estes and Mahakian 2001; Martinson and Minkler 2006). Further, it is possible that the widening gaps in health and wealth among boomers may further marginalize certain subgroups of older adults (McBride 2007). Common structural barriers to participation include lack of knowledge about volunteering opportunity, associated costs of meals, transportation, and supplies; insufficient transportation options, and inadequate volunteer management (Caro and Bass 1995; Center for Health Communication, Harvard School of Public Health 2004). These barriers exert unequal influence on older adults, and those with fewer social and economic resources may not overcome them. McBride (2007) points out that volunteering can be inaccessible to older adults who need to earn income, provide caregiving, or have certain disabilities – all circumstances that are more common among older adults of lower SES.

The lack of inclusion of certain subgroups of older adults is a disservice to communities and to older adults themselves, and could potentially lead to increased disparities in health and well-being (Martinez et al. 2006). Thus, inclusion of diverse populations in formal volunteering is a priority. Policymakers, program leaders, and researchers should consider diversity widely to include ethnicity, education, skill levels, and functional ability. As an example, Project Shine (Temple University, http://www.projectshine.org/materials/cea) focused on immigrant elders, their engagement in civic roles, and how best to maximize their involvement in communities. This work emphasized the importance of language and pointed out that "volunteering" and "community service" may need to be replaced with more culturally appropriate language. Further, policymakers, program leaders, and researchers must recognize roles as informal volunteers and caregivers. The report concludes that trusted ethnic-based organizations, religious institutions, and informal social groups can serve as access points for more formal opportunities. Recent research on the effects of stipends demonstrates that a minimal amount of compensation (about $290/month for Americorps stipends) facilitates inclusion (McBride et al. 2009). Compared to non-stipended volunteers in the Experience Corps program, stipended volunteers are more likely to belong to ethnic minority groups and to have lower incomes. Also, stipended volunteers report higher perceived benefits of participation than non-stipended volunteers. The expansion of stipend programs, as discussed above, is a step in the right direction toward increasing inclusion.

Research Needs

This area requires more research to inform program and policy development in civic engagement. We have accumulated evidence that volunteering is good for older adults, but we lack research to determine what programs and policy initiatives will maximize the engagement of older adults in volunteer roles. We still need research that seeks to identify: (1) the volunteer behaviors and motivations of the baby boomer generation, (2) effective strategies to mobilize baby boomers and older adults, (3) best practices for volunteer program structures and design to attract and support older volunteers, and (4) extent of inclusion of diverse older adults, not only in terms of ethnicity, but also all ranges of education, income, functional abilities. At the same time, outcomes research that identifies the economic consequences of engaging older adults in civic engagement programs will be critical for building a constituency among policymakers and legislators. We also need to develop strategies to support capacity building by non-profit groups to attract and retain older adult volunteers. Researchers have observed that most non-profit groups are not prepared for the challenge of engaging large numbers of older adults in meaningful volunteer roles (Casner-Lotto 2007; Eisner et al. 2009). Older volunteers generally are seen in low-skill service positions rather than professional or leadership roles (National Council on the Aging [NCOA] 2006). In order to take full advantage of baby boomers' professional skills and experience, non-profit groups should be encouraged to invest more resources in volunteer management and recognition, and to create more opportunities for highly skilled volunteers to play a role in non-profit operations.

Conclusion

Research suggests that volunteering is a component of resilience in older adults, because it supports both physical and mental health while assisting individuals in developing networks of social support. Efforts are underway to expand the availability and diversity of volunteer roles available to older adults, while policymakers at the national, state and local levels are seeking ways to facilitate further engagement through infrastructure supports and more effective outreach programs. Further research is needed on how civic engagement relates to resilience, how volunteer programs can improve inclusion of diverse populations, and how organizations can maximize the benefits of their programs for all stakeholders, including the volunteers, the organizations, and the larger community. The baby boomer generation holds vast potential to leverage their skills, education and experience to solve society's most challenging problems; policies and programs must continue to evolve in order to capitalize on this unique opportunity.

References

AARP. (2003). *A synthesis of member volunteer experience*. Washington, DC: AARP.

Arnstein, P., Vidal, M., Wells-Federman, C., Morgan, B., & Caudill, M. (2002). From chronic pain patient to peer: Benefits and risks of volunteering. *Pain Management Nursing, 3*(3), 94–103.

Bridgeland, J. M., Putnam, R. D., & Wofford, H. L. (2008). *More to give: Tapping the talents of the baby boomer, silent and greatest generations*. Washington, DC: AARP.

Brown, S. L., Brown, M., House, J. S., & Smith, D. M. (2008). Coping with spousal loss: Potential buffering effects of self-reported helping behavior. *Personality and Social Psychology Bulletin, 34*, 849–861.

Carlson, M. C., Saczynski, J. S., Rebok, G. W., Seeman, T., Glass, T. A., McGill, S., et al. (2008). Exploring the effects of an "everyday" activity program on executive function and memory in older adults: Experience Corps®. The Gerontologist, *48*, 793–801.

Caro, F. G., & Bass, S. A. (1995). Increasing volunteering among older people. In S. A. Bass (Ed.), *Older and active: How Americans over 55 are contributing to society* (pp. 71–96). New Haven, CT: Yale University.

Casner-Lotto, J. (2007). *Boomers are ready for nonprofits, but are nonprofits ready for them?* New York, NY: The Conference Board.

Center for Health Communication, Harvard School of Public Health. (2004). *Reinventing aging: Baby boomers and civic engagement.* Boston: Harvard School of Public Health.

Chambre, S. (1987). *Good deeds in old age.* Lexington, MA: D.C. Heath and Co.

Choi, L. H. (2003). Factors affecting volunteerism among older adults. *The Journal of Applied Gerontology, 22*(2), 179–196.

Christiano, T. (1996). *The rule of many.* Boulder, CO: Westview Press.

Civic Ventures. (2004). Experience after school: Engaging older adults in after-school program: An Experience Corps tool kit. San Francisco, CA: Civic Ventures.

Cnaan, R. A., Handy, F., & Wadsworth, M. (1996). Defining who is a volunteer: Conceptual and empirical considerations. *Nonprofit and Voluntary Quarterly, 25*(3), 364–383.

Corporation for National and Community Service. (2007). *The health benefits of volunteering: A Review of recent research.* Washington, DC: Author. Retrieved July 28, 2009, from http://www.nationalservice.gov/pdf/07_0506_hbr.pdf.

Corporation for National and Community Service. (2009). *Volunteering in America: 2009.* Retrieved July 28, 2009, from http://www.volunteeringinamerica.gov/national.

Eisner, D., Grimm, R. T., Maynard, S., & Washburn, S. (2009). The new volunteer workforce. *Stanford Social Innovation Review, Winter,* 32–37.

Estes, C. L., & Mahakian, J. (2001). The political economy of productive aging. In N. Morrow-Howell, J. E. Hinterlong, & M. N. Sherraden (Eds.), *Productive aging: Concepts and challenges.* Baltimore: Johns Hopkins University Press, 197–213.

Foster-Bey, J., Grimm, R., & Dietz, N. (2007). *Keeping baby boomers volunteering: A research brief on volunteer retention and turnover.* Washington, DC: Corporation for National and Community Service.

Freedman, M. (1999). *Prime time: How baby boomers will revolutionize retirement and transform America.* New York: Public Affairs.

Fried, L., Carlson, M., Freedman, M., Frick, K., Glass, T., Hill, J., et al. (2004). A social model for health promotion for an aging population: Initial evidence on the Experience Corps Model. *Journal of Urban Health, 81,* 64–78.

Gerontological Society of America. (2005). *Civic engagement in an older America.* Washington, DC: Gerontological Society of America. Retrieved July 25, 2009, from http://www.civicengagement.org/agingsociety/2005WHCOArec.pdf.

Gomperts, J. S. (2007). Toward a bold new policy agenda: Five ideas to advance civic engagement opportunities for older Americans. *Generations, 30*(4), 85–89.

Greenfield, E. A., & Marks, N. F. (2006). Formal volunteering as a protective factor for older adults' psychological well-being. *Journal of Gerontology: Social Sciences, 59,* S258–S264.

Independent Sector. (2000). *American Senior Volunteers 2000.* Retrieved February 24, 2005, from http://www.indepsec.org/programs/research/senior_volunteers_in_america.html.

Koppen, J. (2009). *Volunteering perceptions and realities: A national survey of adults aged 18+.* Washington, DC: AARP.

Li, Y., & Ferraro, K. F. (2007). Recovering from spousal bereavement in later life: Does volunteer participation play a role? *Journal of Gerontology: Social Sciences, 62,* S257–S266.

Lum, T. Y., & Lightfoot, E. (2005). The effects of volunteering on the physical and mental health of older people. *Research on Aging, 27,* 31–55.

Mark, M., & Waldman, M. (2002). *Recasting retirement: New perspectives on aging and civic engagement.* San Francisco, CA: Civic Ventures.

Martinez, I., Frick, K., Glass, T., Carlson, M., Tanner, E., Ricks, M., et al. (2006). Engaging older adults in high impact volunteering that enhances health: Recruitment and retention in the Experience Corps Baltimore. *Journal of Urban Health: Bulletin of the New York Academy of Medicine, 83*(5), 941–953.

Martinson, M., & Minkler, M. (2006). Civic engagement and older adults: A critical perspective. *The Gerontologist, 46*(3), 318–324.

McBride, A. M. (2007). Civic engagement, older adults, and inclusion. *Generations, 30*(4), 66–71.

McBride, A., Gonzales, E., Morrow-Howell, N., & McCrary, S. (2009). A case for stipends. Working paper. St. Louis, MO: Center for Social Development, Washington University.

Midlarsky, E. (1991). Helping as coping. In M. Clark (Ed.), *Prosocial behavior* (pp. 238–264). Newbury Park, CA: Sage.

Moen, P. (1995). A life course approach to post-retirement roles and well-being. In L. Bond, S. Cutler, & A. Grams (Eds.), *Promoting successful and productive aging.* (pp. 239–256). Thousand Oaks, CA: Sage.

Moen, P., Dempster-McClain, D., & Williams, R. (1992). Successful aging. *American Journal of Sociology, 97,* 1612–1638.

Morrow-Howell, N. (2007). A longer worklife: The new road to volunteering. *Generations, Spring,* 63–67.

Morrow-Howell, N., Hinterlong, J., Rozario, P. A., & Tang, F. (2003). Effects of volunteering on the well-being of older adults. *Journal of Gerontology: Social Sciences, 58B*(3), S137–S145.

Morrow-Howell, N., Hong, S., & Tang, F. (2009a). Who benefits from volunteering? Variations in perceived benefits. *The Gerontologist, 49*(1), 91–102.

Morrow-Howell, N., Hong, S.-I., McCrary, S., & Blinne, W. (2009b). *Experience Corps: Health outcomes of participation* (CSD Research Brief 09-09). St. Louis, MO: Center for Social Development, Washington University.

Musick, M. A., & Wilson, J. (2003). Volunteering and depression: The role of psychological and social resources in different age groups. *Social Science & Medicine, 56*(2), 259–269.

Musick, M. A., & Wilson, J. (2008). *Volunteers.* Bloomington: Indiana University Press.

Musick, M. A., Herzog, A. R., & House, J. S. (1999). Volunteering and mortality among older adults: Findings from a national sample. *Journal of Gerontology: Social Science, 54B*(3), S173–S180.

National Council on the Aging. (2006). *Respect ability in America: Promising practices in civic engagement among adults 55+.* National Council on the Aging. Retrieved July 25, 2009, from http://www.ncoa.org/Downloads/PromisingPracticesReport.pdf.

National Governors Association. (2008). *Increasing volunteerism among older adults: Benefits and strategies for states.* Washington, DC: Author.

O'Neill, G. (2007). Civic engagement on the agenda at the 2005 White House Conference on Aging. *Generations, 30*(4), 101–108.

Omoto, A., Synder, M., & Martino, S. (2000). Volunteerism and the life course. *Basic and Applied Social Psychology, 22*(3), 181–197.

Peters-Davis, N. D., Burant, C. J., & Braunschweig, H. M. (2001). Factors associated with volunteer behavior among community dwelling older persons. *Activities, Adaptation, & Aging, 26*(2), 29–44.

Pillemer, K., & Glasgow, N. (2000). Social integration and aging. In K. Pillemer, P. Moen, E. Wethingon, & N. Glasgow (Eds.), *Social integration in the second half of life* (pp. 20–47). Baltimore: Johns Hopkins University Press.

Public Law 111-13. (2009). Retrieved May 30, 2009, from http://thomas.loc.gov/cgi-bin/bdquery/z?d111:H.R.1388.

Rozario, P. A. (2007). Volunteering among current cohorts of older adults and baby boomers. *Generations, 30*(4), 31–36.

Shmotkin, D., Blumstein, T., & Modan, B. (2003). Beyond keeping active: Concomitants of being a volunteer in old-old age. *Psychology and Aging, 18,* 602–607

Spring, K., Dietz, N., & Grimm, R. (2007). *Youth helping America: Leveling the path to participation: Volunteering and civic engagement among youth from disadvantaged circumstances.* Washington, D.C.: Corporation for National and Community Service.

Stengel, R. (2008, September 22). A sense of community. *Time, 172*(12), 48–64.

Sugihara, Y., Sugisawa, H., Shibata, H., & Harada, K. (2008). Productive roles, gender, and depressive symptoms: Evidence from a national longitudinal study of late-middle-aged Japanese. *Journal of Gerontology: Social Sciences, 63B,* 227–234.

Tan, E. J., Xue, Q.-L., Li, T., Carlson, M. C., & Fried, L. P. (2006). Volunteering: A physical activity intervention for older adults – The Experience Corps® Program in Baltimore. *Journal of Urban Health, 83*(5), 954–969.

Tang, F., Morrow-Howell, N., & Hong, S. (2009). Inclusion of diverse older populations in volunteering: The importance of institutional facilitation. *Nonprofit and Voluntary Sector Quarterly, 38*(5), 810–827.

U.S. Bureau of Labor Statistics. (2005). *Volunteering in the United States, 2005*. Washington, DC: U.S. Department of Labor.

U.S. Bureau of Labor Statistics. (2009). *Volunteering in the United States, 2008*. Washington, DC: United States Department of Labor. Retrieved July 27, 2009, from http://www.bls.gov/news.release/volun.nr0.htm.

Van Willigen, M. (2000). Differential benefits of volunteering across the life course. *Journal of Gerontology: Social Sciences, 55B*(5), S308–S318.

Wuthnow, R. (1991). *Act of compassion*. Princeton, NJ: Princeton University Press.

Zedlewski, S. R., & Schaner, S. G. (2005). Older adults' engagement should be recognized and encouraged. *The retirement project: Perspectives on productive aging*. Washington, DC: Urban Institute.

Chapter 11
Strengthened by the Spirit: Religion, Spirituality, and Resilience Through Adulthood and Aging

Carol Ann Faigin and Kenneth I. Pargament

Introduction

Human beings endure a multitude of life events, from daily frustrations to the terror of combat. What factors determine whether people flourish or flounder in the face of adversity? Traditional approaches to this question have investigated the biological, sociological, and psychological. These discoveries have led to a greater understanding of the framework of resilience. However, another growing body of research, generated by the field of psychology of religion and spirituality, may further inform our appreciation of resilience pathways.

In this chapter, we briefly review traditional understanding of resilience and how religious and spiritual approaches broaden that perspective. The sections are organized by life stage (adulthood and aging) and include an overview of how religious and spiritual coping can be both a positive source of resilience and potentially lead to detrimental outcomes. We provide a summary of these religious resilience pathways and offer suggestions for potential spiritual interventions that promote growth and elude religious pitfalls at these various stages of life.

Background on Traditional Perspectives of Resilience

There are multiple definitions of resilience (see Masten 1994; Egeland et al. 1993; Rutter 1987; Haimes 2009; Knight 2007); however, for this purpose, we describe it as the "ability to recover readily from illness, depression, adversity, or the like" (Webster's Dictionary 2003, p. 1638). Researchers in the fields of sociology, psychology, and biology have tried to understand and identify the mechanism that underlies this "ability" to overcome great odds. Specifically, social status, socioeconomic status (Schooler and Caplan 2009), social support (Florian et al. 1995; King et al. 1998),

C.A. Faigin (✉)
Togus VA Medical Center, 1 VA Center, Augusta, Maine 04330, USA
e-mail: caprini7@gmail.com

B. Resnick et al. (eds.), *Resilience in Aging: Concepts, Research, and Outcomes*,
DOI 10.1007/978-1-4419-0232-0_11, © Springer Science+Business Media, LLC 2011

perceived control over one's life (Schooler and Caplan 2009), high levels of self-esteem, problem-solving strategies (Dumont and Provost 1999), intelligence (Masten et al. 1999), hardiness (Kobasa 1979), physical health (Schooler and Caplan 2009), and positive emotions (Cohn et al. 2009) all can bolster recovery in response to adverse life events. However, some (Windle et al. 2008) have argued that the current models of resiliency do not provide a complete picture. The area of psychology of religion might offer additional, essential information for better understanding the mechanisms of resilience.

Religion and Spirituality[1] as a Unique Feature of Resilience

Historically, theorists in the field of psychology have viewed religion and spirituality through a reductionist lens. Specifically, it has been argued that beliefs in the divine serve more basic purposes, such as a defense mechanism for anxiety (Freud 1927), an attachment figure (Kirkpatrick 2005), an object representation (Rizzuto 1979), a physiological response (D'Aquili and Newberg 1998), or a source of identity and community (Durkheim 1915). However, others (Frankl 1984; James 1961; Pargament 2002; Miller and C'de Baca 2001) have argued that there is something unique to one's relationship with the sacred in religiousness and spirituality and thus to its role in resilience.

Religion and spirituality play a distinctive and important role for many individuals. National polls in the USA reveal that 93% of people believe in God (Gallop Poll, May 2008) and 83% of people acknowledge religion as important to them (Gallop Poll, September 2006). Why does religion draw so many to its shores, especially when under duress? This is perhaps due to the very nature of religion and spirituality. Pargament (1997) posited, "Religion offers a response to the problem of human insufficiency" and can complement nonreligious coping through offering solutions to "the limits of personal powers" (p. 310). People can look toward the ultimate for solace or unique solutions to life problems when pushed beyond their resources. Specifically, "The solutions may come in the form of spiritual support when other forms of social support are lacking, explanations when no other explanations seem convincing, a sense of ultimate control through the sacred when life seems out of control, or new objects of significance when old ones are no longer compelling" (Pargament 1997, p. 310). Thus, religion and spirituality are drawn upon in ways that positively impact the quality of life and resilience across the lifespan.

However, the realm of the sacred or divine may also cause unique distress in individuals and lead to negative outcomes throughout the lifespan. Given the central

---

[1]Although many regard the definition of "religion" to reference institutionalized doctrines and "spiritual" to mean a personal experience of the divine or sacred, there is debate about the overlapping meanings of these terms (see Zinnbauer et al. 1997; Zinnbauer and Pargament 2005) thus we will use the terms interchangeably in this review.

and distinctive place of religion and spirituality in the lives of many people in the USA, threats and challenges to this life domain may be particularly problematic. Those who wrestle with spiritual struggles may experience a unique form of distress due to the profound nature and core relevance of these questions, doubts, and tensions. For those who are disenfranchised or struggling with illness or distress, the perception of a divine force as punishing or abandoning may imply an ultimate unforgiveability or unacceptability of the individual (Pargament et al. 2005b). Doubting whether one is accepted or loved by a divine force may highlight existential questions that have no apparent answer, which may lead to disorientation or misinterpretation of religious tenets. Furthermore, believing that God is vengeful, angry, or has no power over evil can lead to disillusionment, fear, and distrust, which can shatter one's perspective of God, others, and the world (Pargament et al. 2005b). Thus, spiritual struggles can be a unique source of stress.

Powerful as spiritual struggles may be, more often than not people experience positive benefits from their faith. Empirical data underscore the notion that religion serves a distinct and compelling role in resilience. For instance, multiple studies have identified the positive impact of religious forms of coping, even after controlling for secular strategies and other demographic factors (Pargament et al. 2005a). One such study identified the unique, positive contribution of the domain of the transcendent. In the 1995 Detroit Area Study, Ellison and colleagues (2001) found that the relationship between religious involvement and psychological distress and well-being was not mediated by access to psychological or social resources (e.g., social support, self-esteem). They concluded that the salutary effects of religion could not be "explained away in terms of social or psychological resources" and "may foster distinctive sets of spiritual or psychosocial resources [...] that bolster or undermine health and well-being" (p. 243).

Another such study by Trenholm et al. (1998) highlights the unique role of spiritual struggles in people with panic disorder. Researchers investigated religious conflict, state-trait anxiety, rational behavior, illness attitude, and symptoms of panic disorder in 60 women who were classified into one of the three groups (panic disorder with therapy, panic disorder without therapy, and therapy clients without panic disorder). Data revealed that religious conflict (e.g., religious guilt) uniquely predicted panic disorder in both groups, even after controlling for irrational thinking, state anxiety, abnormal illness behavior, and hypochondriacal beliefs. The researchers conclude that the anxiety fueling the panic disorder "goes beyond the concept of an individual who becomes frightened by the catastrophizing of body sensations"; but instead encompasses perceptions of failing religious ideals, causing feelings of guilt and fears of moral transgressions. These two studies provide examples of both sides of the coin of religious coping and highlight their individual roles in building or breaking resilience.

As researchers acknowledge the domain of the sacred, some encourage incorporating spirituality on the road to resilience (Wolin and Wolin 1993; Park and Folkman 1997; Farley 2007). We argue that while integrating spiritual models of resiliency is an important next step for the field, it is *critical* to consider both sides of the religious experience. To better frame these methods of coping, we provide a background of positive religious coping and spiritual struggles.

Positive Religious Coping

In 1998, Pargament and colleagues introduced a framework for organizing the concept of positive and negative religious coping with major life stressors. They define positive religious coping as a way of interpreting and responding to life events that reflect a secure relationship with the divine, a sense of meaning and purpose in life, benevolent religious appraisals, a collaborative approach with the divine to solve problems, and searching for spiritual connectedness with others. This approach to coping with life's problems can help people conserve their beliefs in a higher power, help to surrender control, and to draw meaning from stressful circumstances (Pargament 2007). This profound trust in the divine is best exemplified by the following reflection from a woman who suffered paralysis from a terrible car accident. "I know God doesn't screw up. He doesn't make mistakes. Something very beautiful is going to come out of this" (Baker and Gorgas 1990, p. 5A). This quote demonstrates a flexible and open style of religious coping, which proves to be a protective factor when dealing with the strains of life.

Research has demonstrated that religiousness and spirituality are associated with decreased levels of depression (Smith et al. 2004), anxiety (Koenig et al. 1993), chronic pain (Kabat-Zinn et al. 1985), and elevated levels of happiness, well-being, and life satisfaction (see Koenig et al. 2001 for review), as well as mental and physical health (Koenig et al. 2001). Furthermore, in a meta-analysis of 49 studies, Ano and Vasconcelles (2005) concluded that positive religious coping was associated with better psychological adjustment to stress. Thus, having a benevolent relationship with the divine appears to provide a protective feature for life's turbulence. There are times, however, when this relationship can also be threatened.

Spiritual Struggles

When faced with tragedy, fundamental assumptions regarding a benevolent divine and notions of a "just world" can be shattered. Specifically, those who search for answers and are unable to find any can be hurled into existential crisis. This form of negative religious coping, also called spiritual struggles, is defined as "a sign of spirituality in tension and in flux" (Pargament et al. 2006, p. 124) and may be fueled by the feelings of alienation from or guilt toward God or a higher power (Exline et al. 2000). Three types of religious and spiritual struggles have been conceptualized and studied: interpersonal, intrapersonal, and divine (Pargament et al. 2005c; Exline 2002).

Interpersonal spiritual struggles refer to spiritual conflicts with friends, family, and/or religious congregations. In contrast, intrapersonal spiritual struggles are marked by personal doubts and questions regarding one's spirituality, faith tradition, or life purpose, or conflicts within oneself about morals, beliefs, and practices. Lastly, divine spiritual struggles are expressions of conflict, questions, and tension in relationship to God, such as feeling abandoned by or angry with the divine. These three types of spiritual struggles can have pervasive effects on individual, social, and physical health and well-being (Bryant and Astin 2008; Pargament et al. 1998a; Exline et al. 2000; Faigin and Pargament 2008). In the same meta-analysis reviewing 49 studies by Ano and Vasconcelles (2005), overall spiritual struggles were related to poor psychological adjustment to stress.

It is important to note that spiritual struggles do not have to be a sign of weak faith or pathology; quite the contrary, they can represent a turning point in life, a fleeting state, or an enduring lifetime experience (Pargament 2007). Furthermore, despite the consistently negative outcomes related to spiritual struggles, some evidence suggests that spiritual struggles can also lead to positive outcomes, such as spiritual- and stress-related growth (Exline 2002; Cole et al. 2008; Pargament et al. 2006).

Resiliency and Religion

Most people use both positive and negative religious coping throughout their lives and, at times, simultaneously. The following review explores some of these resilience factors and their outcomes in adulthood (ages 18–65 years), and in older adulthood (65 years and older).

Resiliency in Adulthood

Adulthood is a tenuous time filled with a multitude of transitions and personal discoveries, and the exploration and deepening of beliefs and behaviors. This phase of life can be filled with monumental growth while also presenting great risk. A large fund of data regarding the impact of religious coping highlights both ends of this spectrum.

Positive Religious Coping in Adulthood

For those dealing with life struggles and traumas, religious coping can have a strong and positive influence. In a meta-analysis of the relationship between religiousness and depression, religiousness was associated with less symptomatology (Smith et al. 2004). In multiple studies, positive methods of spiritual coping have been tied to improvements in health (Pargament et al. 2004), decreased anxiety, greater spiritual health, more positive mood (Wachholtz and Pargament 2005), and lower risk of mortality in a sample of chronically ill military veterans (Reynolds and Nelson 1981).

Spiritual coping may work through a variety of pathways to serve as a source of strength and resilience for adults during times of adversity. Religion can provide a global meaning to otherwise uncontrollable or negative life events (Park et al. 2001).

In particular, religion can provide a frame of reference to help people control, predict, and understand events, as well as enhance self-esteem (Spilka et al. 1997). Specifically, in a review of the literature, Pargament and Park (1995) concluded that people generally use religious resources to promote self-efficacy and active problem-solving rather than helpless dependence and passivity. Further, they asserted that people generally make effective use of their religion in dealing with difficult circumstances, attributing spiritual meaning to these events to diminish their threat. Research suggests that religion and spirituality can promote meaning-making and positive emotions, and enhance spiritual social support for adults coping with stressful life circumstances.

The power of making meaning can provide a great source of strength in the midst of traumatic experiences. Park and Folkman (1997) highlighted that an important component of resilience is the belief that one's life is meaningful and has an ultimate purpose; they acknowledge that religion is a pathway to meaning-making. The power of meaning-making is highlighted by a study of HIV-positive individuals who use benefit finding to reappraise events and ascribe global meaning to a life situation (Carrico et al. 2006). Benefit finding is the process of finding positive outcomes in an otherwise negative experience. In this study, high scores on a measure assessing sense of peace, religious behavior, faith in God, and a compassionate view of others was related to positive appraisal of and finding meaning in having HIV. Participants identified several benefits they received in the process of their HIV diagnosis, such as finding a sense of purpose, learning to accept life's imperfections, and feeling closer to others.

Additionally, positive reappraisal and benefit finding were negatively correlated with depressive symptoms. Furthermore, the negative relationship between spirituality and depressed mood was mediated by positive reappraisal and benefit finding. Thus, spirituality is a method of creating meaning in otherwise grave situations, which can lead to decreased negative affect. Furthermore, research demonstrates that even in arguably the worst of circumstances, such as the tragedy of losing a child, people who have the ability to make meaning have greater resilience, which decreases the negative impact of the grief of the event (Murphy et al. 2003).

Religious coping can promote positive outlook and diminish negative affect, which are both critical components of resiliency (Contrada et al. 2004; Pargament et al. 1994). For example, in a sample of heart surgery patients, those with greater religious beliefs also ascribed to greater optimism and lower levels of hostility (Contrada et al. 2004). Furthermore, in a study of college students' emotional reactions to the Gulf War, spiritually based coping significantly predicted diminished negative emotion, while pleading for divine intervention was related to positive affect (Pargament et al. 1994). Positive spiritual coping is strongly linked with more positive emotions, which are powerful components of building resiliency.

Lastly, religion can bolster resiliency in adults through enhancing spiritual support systems. There are many studies that demonstrate the various ways that religion aids in social support (see Pargament and Cummings 2009 for review). Individuals who utilize secular support networks (e.g., social clubs, intramural sports, etc.) arguably benefit from meeting regularly with others by creating interpersonal bonds. However, research reveals that religious support is unique and can offer notable benefits. For example, in a study by Koenig and colleagues (1992), general religious coping predicted social support in distressed populations across time. Furthermore, in a study of dialysis patients, O'Brien (1982) found that participants who rated their faith as important to them also demonstrated lower levels of alienation and higher levels of social interaction, with greater *quality* of those interactions. In another study of advanced cancer patients, those who scored higher on positive religious coping also exhibited greater perceived support from others (Tarakeshwar et al. 2006). These data support the unique impact of religion on forging, perceiving, and sustaining meaningful relationships with others.

There are differences in the utilization of religious coping based on demographic variables. Historically, religious coping has been found to be more frequent among females, older, black, and married people (Ferraro and Koch 1994). Additionally, prayer is more frequent in African-Americans than Caucasians, as well as in those who are less educated (Bearon and Koenig 1990) and have lower incomes (Gurin et al. 1960). Perhaps it is natural for those who are struggling with life situations or part of a minority group to draw upon religion as a source of strength when other options are limited or appear bleak. Those who are more religious prior to a traumatic event seem to express greater religious resilience (Ai et al. 2004, 2005, 2007), while those who undergo traumatic experiences can also have *stronger*, not weaker, religious beliefs following the event (Falsetti et al. 2003).

These studies support the notion that when people draw on a religion that rests on a benevolent, collaborative view of the divine, their faith can provide them with a powerful resource that can lead to enhanced positive emotions, meaning-making, and social support networks. However, it is important to explore how other religious coping methods can hinder one's growth and grounding during stressful life experiences.

Spiritual Struggles in Adulthood

Multiple studies with college students have underscored the prevalence and potency of struggling with religious issues in early adulthood. Specifically, in a study of 112,232 students from 236 colleges within the USA, Astin and colleagues (2004) found that approximately 50% of college students experience times of doubt or conflict regarding their spirituality or describe themselves as "searching" for better understanding of their spiritual/religious beliefs. This prevalence rate for spiritual struggles has also been corroborated in two other studies of college students (Johnson et al. 2008; Desai 2006).

Spiritual struggles are shown to have wide-reaching potentially harmful effects for young adults, including negative psychological outcomes and addictive behaviors. For example, in a cross-sectional study, religious strife was associated with higher levels of psychological distress, including depression and suicidality, in both clinical (54 adults receiving psychotherapy) and nonclinical (200 college students) samples regardless of the level of religiousness or comfort received from religion

(Exline et al. 2000). Furthermore, spiritual struggles have been connected to more severe levels of psychopathological symptoms. In a recent study of a national cross-sectional sample of people with and without a personal illness, spiritual struggles predicted greater levels of phobic anxiety, depression, paranoid ideation, hostility, obsessive-compulsiveness, and somatization even after controlling for demographic and religious variables (McConnell et al. 2006). These results were corroborated in studies linking religious strife to increased negative mood, lower self-esteem (Pargament et al. 1998b), anxiety (Kooistra and Pargament 1999), and even panic disorder (Trenholm et al. 1998) in adult samples.

Research consistently demonstrates that individuals who reportedly feel unsettled about spiritual matters are more apt to engage in substance use or other addictive behavior. In the aforementioned Astin and colleagues (2004) study that queried 112,232 students across the USA, results indicated that students who scored high on items measuring religious struggles, such as feelings of distance from God, questioning of religious beliefs and feeling unsettled about religious matters, were more likely to drink wine or liquor (65% vs. 48%) and beer (55% vs. 42%) than those reporting low levels of religious struggles. These findings were substantiated in another study investigating whether spiritual struggles were predictive of alcohol problems throughout the first 2 years of college. Johnson and colleagues (2008) queried 1,515 incoming freshmen during the summer before college (Wave 1), and again during the spring of freshman (Wave 2) and sophomore (Wave 3) years regarding their religious/spiritual involvement, view of God, and alcohol consumption. Results from this study indicated that higher religious distress predicted a greater increase in alcohol problems overall. Lastly, in a recent longitudinal study with 90 college freshmen (Faigin and Pargament 2008), results revealed that spiritual struggles predicted an increase in gambling, tobacco use, recreational drug use, prescription drug use, sex, shopping, food starving, work, exercise, and caffeine use. Additionally, specific domains of spiritual struggle (e.g., divine, interpersonal, and intrapersonal) were shown to predict change in addictive behavior over time.

These studies highlight how religious strife can render a person vulnerable to additional negative coping strategies (e.g., drinking, drug use, other addiction) when faced with life's struggles. This understanding underscores the need for increased awareness regarding the *style* of religious coping so that the deleterious outcomes of existential crises can be averted.

Resiliency in Later Years

As our "greatest generation" has entered their eighth and ninth decades of life, there are important insights to be gained about their sources of resiliency. These survivors have struggled through the Great Depression of the 1930s, WWII in the 1940s, threat of nuclear disaster through the 1950s and 1960s, watching their children fight and suffer in the Vietnam war of the 1960s and 1970s, terrorist attacks on the USA in 2001, the resulting wars in Iraq and Afghanistan their grandchildren are fighting in, and now coping with the loss of financial security in 2008–2010. This generation's children also just entered the category of "senior citizen" at age 65.

Positive Religious Coping in the Elderly

The importance of religion increases with age. According to the Pew Forum on Religion and Public Life, 69% of adults 65 years or older cite religion as "very important" in their lives, compared with 45% of adults under 30 years of age (N=34,695; 2008). Research supports that the elderly draw upon their religious beliefs more as they face illness and aging (Reed 1987). Religion may serve as a source of grounding in the face of adversity. In a study of 338 elderly patients admitted to the hospital, when asked an open-ended question regarding their coping resources, over 40% of them spontaneously cited religion (Koenig 1998). To understand the nature of their relationship with the divine, we look to qualitative research to better explain how spirituality and religion serve as a pathway of resilience in old age.

Schwarz and Cottrell (2007) conducted a qualitative study with five elderly adults aged 66–88 involved in occupational therapy to help treat a range of illnesses from clinical depression to spinal stenosis. The researchers conducted multiple in-depth interviews to assess the role of spirituality in rehabilitation and across the lifespan. They found multiple themes pointing to the underlying mechanism of spirituality: it is pivotal in creating meaning and purpose, coping and positive outlook, providing a source of reliance and dependence, consolation and comfort, and hope for recovery in the face of adversity across the lifespan.

The poignant responses of these elderly adults illustrate how spirituality enriches and supports individuals throughout life. For example, an 87-year-old participant indicated the primacy of spirituality as being the "number one thing in life, everything follows after that" (p. 49). Others agreed, indicating that without spirituality, life is devoid of meaning and that spirituality is the reason for living and something to strive toward. Thus, spirituality can be a fundamental aspect of living, one that oftentimes becomes more important as one ages. Another 87-year-old participant underscored the need for spiritual coping in later life: "You just have more problems when you get older and sometimes they do seem quite overwhelming unless you feel like you have some help in shouldering them" (p. 50). Another participant attributed her lifespan resilience to spirituality, which "pulled me out of many, many things that may have disturbed me… [it] is what governs your ability to recover or cope with what you have" (p. 50).

Some participants highlighted the role of spirituality to promote a positive outlook to assist in coping with life's struggles. "Well, it's certainly kept me an optimist all my life in spite of anything that's happened […] I think it's because […] I've had great faith that things were going to turn out alright and I don't let myself get down" (p. 50). This view is shared by others, "You have a more positive attitude if you think you're going to get that spiritual support, it's definitely going to help, it's like 50% of the battle" (p. 50). This positive outlook undoubtedly served as an anchor of support despite the struggles of life.

In terms of spiritual coping, participants described their relationship with the divine as an unyielding resource for coping and that reliance on God increased throughout their lives. One participant stated, "I depend on God a lot by praying, asking for help, for guidance, and He's never forsaken me, He's right there" (p. 51). The divine is viewed as more reliant than people for some; "I've always felt that there was someone to call on for help. As much as you love your family, they cannot always be there for you. They don't have all of the answers" (p. 51).

This reliance on spirituality also provides consolation and comfort throughout life and hopes for recovery during times of illness. "It's a great comfort to me when I have had periods of stress," stated one 88-year-old participant (p. 51). Others stated that "the hope that we have and the reasons why we have the hope is so uplifting, so supporting, you carry that with you afterwards" (p. 52). This important study has provided an in-depth illustration of the ways that spirituality impacts resiliency throughout the lifespan, which is further supported by other empirical data.

Social support is another critical religiously based component of resilience not otherwise noted in the above study. For example, in multiple studies, elderly persons who rely upon religion as a form of resilience in life have lower rates of depression (Koenig et al. 1992; Pressman et al. 1990) and death anxiety (Koenig 1988) than their counterparts who do not access religious coping, even after controlling for social support, history of depression, and demographic variables (Bosworth et al. 2003).

The beneficial outcomes of positive religious coping are further elucidated in a study examining health status of 173 older adults engaged in rehabilitation services (Yohannes et al. 2008). Religious attendance was inversely associated with severity of illness and intrinsic religiousness was associated with less severe depression and older age. Additionally, in a community sample of 836 elderly participants, personal religious practices and intrinsic religiousness were associated with greater perceived coping efficacy (Koenig et al. 1988).

Spiritual Struggles in Elderly Populations

Less effective forms of coping can be a source of distress, particularly among older adults coping with the additional life stressors of illness and aging. For example, in a study by Krause and colleagues (1999), they found that although religious doubt is present in older adults, its impact on general mental health decreases as people age. Building upon this, Galek and colleagues (2007) pinpointed how religious doubt affects mental health across the lifespan. As people age, results indicate religious doubt is associated with psychopathology, such as depression, hostility, general anxiety, obsessive-compulsive, and paranoia symptoms. However, they also found that the magnitude of the relationship between spiritual struggles and mental health decreases as people age.

In a longitudinal study of 268 medically ill, hospitalized, elderly patients, spiritual struggles were shown to be a risk factor for diminished well-being. Pargament and colleagues (2004) investigated whether religious coping was predictive of spiritual outcome, stress-related growth, quality of life, depressed mood, physical, and cognitive functioning. Over the 2 years of the study, negative religious coping was predictive of declines in quality of life, spiritual outcome, Activities of Daily Living (ADLs), and an increase in depressed mood (Pargament et al. 2004).

In another set of analyses using the same dataset, mortality during the follow-up period was assessed as the major outcome variable for the original set of 596 participants. Most importantly, results showed that individuals who endorsed feelings of being unloved by and alienated from God ("Questioned God's love for me," "Wondered whether God had abandoned me"), or felt that the devil was involved in their illness ("Decided the devil made this happen") were 20–30% more likely to die over the 2-year period, even when controlling for physical and mental health, and demographic variables (Pargament et al. 2004). Thus, spiritual struggles clearly have implications not only for the quality of life, physical functioning, and spiritual outcomes, but also for mortality in a sample of medically ill elderly patients.

Practical Applications

As outlined above, researchers have found that religion and spirituality can play distinctive roles in strengthening people as they face traumas, losses, and changes in life (Park and Folkman 1997; Pargament and Cummings 2009). However, as we have noted, some forms of spirituality can impede resiliency. We, therefore, argue that it is critical to understand the *nature* of one's spirituality so that interventions can specifically target mechanisms for growth, while avoiding pitfalls throughout the lifespan. We suggest that the first step for all interventions should involve an explicit spiritual coping assessment (see Pargament 2007) to promote more targeted approaches for each individual.

Adulthood

Building upon knowledge of resiliency in childhood survivors, researchers have developed interventions that adults can apply. Wolin and Wolin (1993) created a model of resiliency that includes spiritual components to transform an individual from a "victim" to a "survivor." They identify traits seen in resilient children, which include: (1) Insight: exploration of the world in order to create meaning about life events; (2) Independence: to transcend self and daily living through participation in spiritual experiences; (3) Relationships: that are compassionate, caring, and affirming as found in religious communities; (4) Initiative: to reach out to the world to save, heal, help, and reconcile to transform the world positively; (5) Creativity: tapping into creative power to generate beauty; (6) Humor: as a transformative force to take oneself lightly (and from a compassionate God's perspective) in the face of adversity; and (7) Morality that promotes spiritual ethics, integrity, and social justice. Models for incorporating these seven components could perhaps bolster a person's ability to reframe their life experiences, create meaning, and cope effectively with traumatic events, even in adulthood.

Additionally, spiritual interventions could be informed by research on the impact of styles of religious coping. Specifically, self-directed religious coping, defined as pursuing personal action without relying upon the divine to solve problems is related to feeling alone and abandoned by God (Pargament et al. 1988). Collaborative religious coping reflects a mutual responsibility involving the person and God to solve the problem; this style of coping is related to an increase in the feelings of control and self-esteem (Pargament et al. 1988). The potency of these methods of coping is highlighted by findings from a study of 142 African-American adolescents. This study found that collaborative religious coping was linked to increased hope and feelings of having reasons to live, while self-directing religious coping was related to an increase in depression, hopelessness, and even suicide attempts (Molock et al. 2006). This study underscores the importance of promoting active and collaborative styles of religious coping in adults to bolster healing in future resilience interventions.

Furthermore, spiritual interventions could be imbued with the tenets of forgiveness and spiritual support to promote resilience. In a sample of 101 adult survivors of childhood sexual abuse, findings reveal that religious forgiveness coping and active surrender coping were related to lower levels of depressed mood, while spiritual support and religious forgiveness coping were components in the resolution of abuse after controlling for demographic variables, cognitive appraisals, support satisfaction, and severity of abuse (Gall 2006).

Some promising efforts to develop interventions in response to these data on the styles of religious coping have already been undertaken. For instance, spiritually sensitive group interventions have been shown to be effective in decreasing depression (Tarakeshwar et al. 2005; Ano 2005), improving spiritual well-being, positive religious coping, and images of God (Murray-Swank and Pargament 2005), decreasing stress and promoting spiritual development and self-control (Ano 2005), increasing private religious practices, daily spiritual experiences, religious coping, decreasing drug use (Avants et al. 2005), decreasing overall psychological distress, negative religious coping, negative affect related to spiritual struggles, stigmatization related to spiritual struggle, and increasing positive affect related to spiritual struggles (Gear et al. 2008). These data suggest that spiritual interventions can have far-reaching and potent implications for adults coping with spiritual struggles.

Older Years

Spiritually integrative interventions on group and individual levels can also be effective for older adults; however, due to the unique life stressors during this stage of life, targeted interventions for geriatrics should also be considered.

Specifically, in 2004 Langer provided a framework for tapping into the spiritual domain to build resilience in older adults. "By acknowledging older adults' resiliency and spiritual resources in light of past and present risk factors, care providers can focus on capabilities, assets, and positive attributes rather than problems and pathologies" (Langer 2004, p. 611). Langer provides a practical framework for conducting strengths counseling to promote the application of spiritual resources in resiliency (e.g., "Can you identify spiritual resources from which you gain strength and energy to overcome some of your stresses/losses?"). The counselor, according to this model, is to draw upon a client's meaning making (or spirituality) to encourage or enhance his or her inherent resiliency and thus provide holistic care (see Langer 2004). This approach is consistent with research on the resilient feature of meaning-making.

Drawing upon the protective feature and prevalence of religious beliefs in older adults, researchers encourage geriatric clinicians to inquire about their patients' religious faith and provide support, particularly when confronted with emotional distress (Bosworth et al. 2003). This approach can help to identify negative divine reappraisals and better identify strengths to build upon in therapy.

Older adults more often draw upon religious coping strategies as they are faced with illness and aging; therefore, special attention to existential crises, concerns about the afterlife, feelings of regret or negative reappraisal of self-worth will be critical to address for this population. Clinicians may want to focus on working through spiritual struggles to promote healing and resilience (see Pargament 2007 for examples).

Additionally, although there is a paucity of outcome data for spiritually sensitive interventions for older adults, there is reason to believe that similar interventions as outlined above for younger adults would also be applicable for those who are older than 65 years old. Future studies could replicate spiritually sensitive interventions designed for younger adults to investigate their efficacy with geriatric adults. This generation would likely benefit from targeted interventions designed to promote positive religious coping, while diminishing the propensity for spiritual struggles to support healing and continued growth throughout the lifespan.

Conclusion

Religion and spirituality are unique and critical resources for coping with the struggles of life; however, they can also contribute to distress if there are struggles inherent in the *method* of spiritual coping. Enhancing knowledge of the utilization of religion and its impact on resilience could prove promising. Furthermore, clinicians could develop targeted interventions to help people work through negative methods of spiritual coping while building upon the positive aspects of religious beliefs. There are many promising studies demonstrating the effectiveness of spiritually sensitive interventions in adults; however, there is a dearth of research on spiritual resiliency interventions with older adults. Future researchers and clinicians could focus on developing targeted spiritual interventions for all ages that draw upon the themes of religious resilience, thus promoting a holistic approach to building resources and enhanced strength in adulthood and aging.

References

Ai, A. L., Park, C. L., Huang, B., Rodgers, W., & Tice, T. N. (2007). Psychosocial mediation of religious coping styles: A study of short-term psychological distress following cardiac surgery. *Personality and Social Psychology Bulletin, 33*(6), 867–882.

Ai, A. L., Peterson, C., Tice, T. N., Bolling, S. F., & Koenig, H. G. (2004). Faith-based and secular pathways to hope and optimism subconstructs in middle-aged and older cardiac patients. *Journal of Health Psychology, 9*(3), 435–450.

Ai, A. L., Tice, T. N., Peterson, C., & Huang, B. (2005). Prayers, spiritual support, and positive attitudes in coping with the September 11 national crisis. *Journal of Personality, 73*(3), 763–791.

Ano, G. G. (2005). *Spiritual struggles between vice and virtue: A brief psychospiritual intervention.* Unpublished doctoral dissertation, Bowling Green State University, Bowling Green, OH.

Ano, G. G., & Vasconcelles, E. B. (2005). Religious coping and psychological adjustment to stress: A meta-analysis. *Journal of Clinical Psychology, 61*, 461–480.

Astin, A. W., Astin, H. S., & Lindholm, J. A. (2004). *The spiritual life of college students: A national study of students' search for meaning and purpose.* University of California, Los Angeles, Spirituality in Higher Education, Entering Freshmen Survey (2004). Retrieved November 15, 2006, from http://www.spirituality.ucla.edu/results/index.html.

Avants, S. K., Beitel, M., & Margolin, A. (2005). Making the shift from 'addict self' to 'spiritual self': Results from a stage I study of spiritual self-schema (3-S) therapy for the treatment of addiction and HIV risk behavior. *Mental Health, Religion & Culture, 8*, 167–177.

Baker, R., & Gorgas, J. (1990, July 19). Crash broke her back, but not her spirit. News Journal (Mansfield OH), p. 5A.

Bearon, L. B., & Koenig, G. (1990). Religious cognitions and use of prayer in health and illness. *The Gerontologist, 30*(2), 249–253.

Bosworth, H. B., Park, K., McQuoid, D. R., Hays, J. C., & Steffens, D. C. (2003). The impact of religious practice and religious coping on geriatric depression. *International Journal of Geriatric Psychiatry, 18*(10), 905–914.

Bryant, A. N., & Astin, H. S. (2008). The correlates of spiritual struggle during the college years. *The Journal of Higher Education, 79*(1), 1–27.

Carrico, A. W., Ironson, G., Antoni, M. H., Lechner, S. C., Duran, R. E., Kumar, M., et al. (2006). A path model of the effects of spirituality on depressive symptoms and 24-h urinary-free cortisol in HIV-positive persons. *Journal of Psychosomatic Research, 61*(1), 51–58.

Cohn, M. A., Fredrickson, B. L., Brown, S. L., Mikels, J. A., & Conway, A. M. (2009). Happiness unpacked: Positive emotions increase life satisfaction by building resilience. *Emotion, 9*(3), 361–368.

Cole, B. S., Hopkins, C. M., Tisak, J., Steel, J. L., & Carr, B. I. (2008). Assessing spiritual growth and spiritual decline following a diagnosis of cancer: Reliability and validity of the spiritual transformation scale. *Psycho-Oncology, 17*(2), 112–121.

Contrada, R. J., Goyal, T. M., Cather, C., Rafalson, L., Idler, E. L., & Krause, T. J. (2004). Psychosocial factors in outcomes of heart surgery: The impact of religious involvement and depressive symptoms. *Health Psychology, 23*(3), 227–238.

D'Aquili, A. B., & Newberg, E. G. (1998). The neuropsychology of spiritual experience. In Koenig, H. G. (Ed.), *Handbook of religion and mental health* (pp. 75–94). San Diego, CA: Academic Press.

Desai, K. M. (2006). *Predictors of growth and spiritual decline following spiritual struggles.* Unpublished master's thesis, Bowling Green State University, Bowling Green, OH.

Dumont, M., & Provost, A. (1999). Resilience in adolescents: Protective role of social support, coping strategies, self-esteem, and social activities on experience of stress and depression. *Journal of Youth and Adolescence, 28*(3), 343–363.

Durkheim, E. (1915). *The elementary forms of religious life: A study in religious sociology.* (trans: Joseph Ward Swain). New York, NY: MacMillan.

Egeland, B., Carlson, E., & Sroufe, L. (1993). Resilience as process. *Development & Psychopathology, 5,* 517–528.

Ellison, C. G., Boardman, J. D., Williams, D. R., & Jackson, J. S. (2001). Religious involvement, stress, and mental health: Findings from the 1995 Detroit area study. *Social Forces, 80*(1), 215–249.

Exline, J. J. (2002). Stumbling blocks on the religious road: Fractured relationships, nagging vices, and the inner struggle to believe. *Psychological Inquiry, 13,* 182–189.

Exline, J. J., Yali, A. M., & Sanderson, W. C. (2000). Guilt, discord, and alienation: The role of religious strain in depression and suicidality. *Journal of Clinical Psychology, 56,* 1481–1496.

Faigin, C. A., & Pargament, K. I. (2008). Filling the spiritual void: Spiritual struggles as a risk factor for addiction. Poster session presented at the 20th annual convention of the Association for Psychological Science, Chicago, IL.

Falsetti, S. A., Resick, P. A., & Davis, J. L. (2003). Changes in religious beliefs following trauma. *Journal of Traumatic Stress, 16*(4), 391–398.

Farley, Y. R. (2007). Making the connection: Spirituality, trauma and resiliency. *Journal of Religion & Spirituality in Social Work, 26*(1), 1–15.

Ferraro, K. F., & Koch, J. R. (1994). Religion and health among Black and White adults: Examining social support and consolation. *Journal for the Scientific Study of Religion, 33,* 362–375.

Florian, V., Mikulincer, M., & Taubman, O. (1995). Does hardiness contribute to mental health during a stressful real-life situation? The roles of appraisal and coping. *Journal of Personality and Social Psychology, 68*(4), 687–695.

Frankl, V. E. (1984). *Man's search for meaning: An introduction to logotherapy.* (Preface: Gordon W. Allport). New York, NY: Washington Square Press.

Freud, S. (1927). *The future of an illusion.* New York, NY: W. W. Norton & Company.

Galek, K., Krause, N., Ellison, C. G., Kudler, T., & Flannelly, K. J. (2007). Religious doubt and mental health across the lifespan. *Journal of Adult Development, 14*(1–2), 1625.

Gall, T. L. (2006). Spirituality and coping with life stress among adult survivors of childhood sexual abuse. *Child Abuse & Neglect, 30*(7), 829–844.

Gear, M. R., Faigin, C. A., Gibbel, M. R., Krumrei, E. J., Oemig, C. K., McCarthy, S. K., & Pargament, K. I. (2008). The winding road: A promising approach to addressing spiritual struggles of college students. *UCLA Spirituality in Higher Education Newsletter, 4*(4), 1–8.

Gurin, G., Veroff, J., & Feld, S. (1960). *Americans view their mental health: A nationwide interview survey.* New York, NY: Basic Books.

Haimes, Y. Y. (2009). On the definition of resilience in systems. *Risk Analysis, 29*(4), 498–501.

James, W. (1961). *The varieties of religious experience.* New York, NY: Simon and Schuster.

Johnson, T. J., Sheets, V., & Kristeller, J. (2008). Identifying mediators of the relationship between religiousness/spirituality and alcohol use. *Journal of Studies on Alcohol and Drugs, 69*(1), 160–170.

Kabat-Zinn, J., Lipworth, L., & Burney, R. (1985). The clinical use of mindfulness meditation for the self-regulation of chronic pain. *Journal of Behavioral Medicine, 8*(2), 163–190.

Kirkpatrick, L. A. (2005). *Attachment, evolution, and the psychology of religion.* New York, NY: The Guilford Press.

King, L. A., King, D. W., Keane, T. M., Fairbank, J. A., Adams, G. A. (1998). Resilience: Recovery factors in post-traumatic stress disorder among female and male Vietnam veterans: Hardiness, postwar social support, and additional stressful life events. *Journal of Personality and Social Psychology, 74*(2), 420-434.

Kobasa, S. C. (1979). Stressful life events, personality, and health: An inquiry into hardiness. *Journal of Personality and Social Psychology, 37*(1), 1–11.

Koenig, H. G. (1998). Religious beliefs and practices of hospitalized medically ill older adults. *International Journal of Geriatric Psychiatry, 13,* 213–224.

Koenig, H. G., Kvale, J. N., & Ferrel, C. (1988). Religion and well-being in later life. *The Gerontologist, 28*(1), 18–28.

Koenig, H. G. (1988). Religious behaviors and death anxiety in later life. *The Hospice Journal, 4*(1), 3–24.

Koenig, H. G., Cohen, H. J., Blazer, D. G., Pieper, C., et al. (1992). Religious coping and depression among elderly, hospitalized medically ill men. *American Journal of Psychiatry, 149*(12), 1693–1700.

Koenig, H. G., Ford, S. M., George, L. K., Blazer, D. G., et al. (1993). Religion and anxiety disorder: An examination and comparison of associations in young, middle-aged, and elderly adults. *Journal of Anxiety Disorders, 7*(4), 321–342.

Koenig, H. G., McCullough, M. E., & Larson, D. B. (2001). *The handbook of religion and health*. New York, NY: Oxford University Press.

Kooistra, W. P., & Pargament, I. (1999). Religious doubting in parochial school adolescents. *Journal of Psychology & Theology, 27*(1), 33–42.

Knight, C. (2007). A resilience framework: Perspectives for educators. *Health Education, 107*(6), 543–555.

Krause, N., Ingersoll-Dayton, B., Ellison, C. G., & Wulff, K. M. (1999). Aging, religious doubt, and psychological well-being. *The Gerontologist, 39*(5), 525–533.

Langer, N. (2004). Resiliency and spirituality: Foundations of strengths perspective counseling with the elderly. *Educational Gerontology, 30*(7), 611–617.

Masten, A. S. (1994). Resilience in individual development: Successful adaptation despite risk and adversity. In Wang, M. C., & Gordon, E. W. (Eds.), *Educational resilience in inner-city America: Challenges and prospects*. Hillsdale, NJ: L. Erlbaum Associates.

Masten, A. S., Hubbard, J. J., Gest, S. D., Tellegen, A., Garmezy, N., & Ramirez, M. (1999). Competence in the context of adversity: Pathways to resilience and maladaptation from childhood to late adolescence. *Development and Psychopathology, 11*(1), 143–169.

McConnell, K. M., Pargament, K. I., Ellison, C. G., Flannelly, K., & Ellison, C. (2006). Examining the links between spiritual struggles and symptoms of psychopathology in a national sample. *Journal of Clinical Psychology, 62*, 1469–1484.

Miller, W. R., & C'de Baca, J. (2001). *Quantum change: When epiphanies and sudden insights transform ordinary lives*. New York, NY: The Guilford Press.

Molock, S. D., Puri, R., Matlin, S., & Barksdale, C. (2006). Relationship between religious coping and suicidal behavior among African American adolescents. *Journal of Black Psychology, 32*, 366–389.

Murphy, S. A., Johnson, L. C., & Lohan, J. (2003). Finding meaning in a child's violent death: A five-year prospective analysis of parents' personal narratives and empirical data. *Death Studies, 27*(5), 381–404.

Murray-Swank, N. A., & Pargament, I. (2005). God, where are you?: Evaluating a spiritually integrated intervention for sexual abuse. *Mental Health, Religion & Culture, 8*(3), 191–203.

O'Brien, M. E. (1982). Religious faith and adjustment to long-term hemodialysis. *Journal of Religion and Health, 21*, 68–80.

Park, C. L., & Folkman, S. (1997). Meaning in the context of stress and coping. *Review of General Psychology, 1*(2), 115–144.

Park, C. L., Folkman, S., & Bostrom, A. (2001). Appraisals of controllability and coping in caregivers and HIV+ men: Testing the goodness-of-fit hypothesis. *Journal of Consulting and Clinical Psychology, 69*(3), 481–488.

Pargament, K. I. (1997). *The psychology of religion and coping: Theory, research, practice*. New York, NY: The Guilford Press.

Pargament, K. I. (2002). Is religion nothing but...? Explaining religion versus explaining religion away. *Psychological Inquiry, 13*(3), 239–244.

Pargament, K. I. (2007). *Spiritually integrated psychotherapy: Understanding and addressing the sacred*. New York, NY: The Guilford Press.

Pargament, K. I., & Cummings, J. (2009). *Anchored by faith: Religion as a resilience factor*.

Pargament, K. I., & Park, L. (1995). Merely a defense? The variety of religious means and ends. *Journal of Social Issues, 51*(2), 13–32.

Pargament, K. I., Ishler, K., Dubow, E., Stanik, P., Rouiller, R., Crowe, P., et al. (1994). Methods of religious coping with the Gulf War: Cross-sectional and longitudinal analyses. *Journal for the Scientific Study, 33*, 347–361.

Pargament, K. I., Kennell, J., Hathaway, W., Grevengoed, N., Newman, J., & Jones, W. (1988). Religion and the problem-solving process: Three styles of coping. *Journal for the Scientific Study of Religion, 27*(1), 90–104.

Pargament, K. I., Smith, B. W., Koenig, H. G., & Perez, L. (1998a). Patterns of positive and negative religious coping with major life stressors. *Journal for the Scientific Study of Religion, 37*, 710–724.

Pargament, K. I., Zinnbauer, B. J., Scott, A. B., Butter, E. M., Zerowin, J., & Stanik, P. (1998b). Red flags and religious coping: Identifying some religious warning signs among people in crisis. *Journal of Clinical Psychology, 54*(1), 77–89.

Pargament, K. I., Koenig, H. G., Tarakeshwar, N., & Hahn, J. (2004). Religious coping methods as predictors of psychological, physical and spiritual outcomes among medically ill elderly patients: A longitudinal study. *Journal of Health Psychology, 9*, 713–730.

Pargament, K. I., Ano, G. G., & Wachholtz, A. B. (2005a). The religious dimension of coping: Advances in theory, research, and practice. In Paloutzian, R. F., & Park, C. L. (Eds.), *Handbook of the psychology of religion and spirituality*. New York, NY: The Guilford Press.

Pargament, K. I., Magyar-Russell, G. M., & Murray-Swank, N. A. (2005b). The sacred and the search for significance: Religion as a unique process, *Journal of Social Issues, 61*(4), 665–687.

Pargament, K. I., Murray-Swank, N. A., Magyar, G. M., & Ano, G. G. (2005c). Spiritual struggle: A phenomenon of interest to psychology and religion. In Miller, W. R., & Delaney, H. D. (Eds.), *Judeo-Christian perspectives on psychology: Human nature, motivation, and change* (pp. 245–268). Washington, DC: American Psychological Association.

Pargament, K. I., Desai, K. M., & McConnell, K. M. (2006). Spirituality: A pathway to posttraumatic growth or decline? In Calhoun, L. G., & Tedeschi, R. G. (Eds.), *Handbook of posttraumatic growth: Research and practice* (pp. 121–137). Mahway, NJ: Lawrence Erlbaum Associates Publishers.

Pressman, P., Lyons, J. S., Larson, D. B., & Strain, J. J. (1990). Religious belief, depression, and ambulation status in elderly women with broken hips. *American Journal of Psychiatry, 147*(6), 758–760

Reed, P. G. (1987). Spirituality and well-being in terminally ill hospitalized adults. *Research in Nursing & Health, 10*(5), 335–344.

Reynolds, D. K., & Nelson, L. (1981). Personality, life situation, and life expectancy. *Suicide and Life-Threatening Behavior, 11*(2), 99–110.

Rizzuto, A. (1979). *The birth of the living God: A psychoanalytic study*. Chicago: University of Chicago Press.

Rutter, M. (1987). Psychosocial resilience and protective mechanisms. *American Journal of Orthopsychiatry, 57*(3), 316–331.

Schooler, C., & Caplan, L. J. (2009). How those who have, thrive: Mechanisms underlying the well-being of the advantaged in later life. In Bosworth, H. B., & Hertzog, C. (Eds.), *Aging and cognition: Research methodologies and empirical advances* (pp. 121–141). Washington, DC: American Psychological Association.

Schwarz, L., & Cottrell, F. (2007). The value of spirituality as perceived by elders in long-term care. *Physical & Occupational Therapy in Geriatrics, 26*(1), 43–62.

Smith, T. B., McCullough, M. E., & Poll, J. (2004). Religiousness and depression: Evidence for a main effect and the moderating influence of stressful life events: Correction to Smith et al. (2003). *Psychological Bulletin, 130*(1), 65.

Spilka, B., Shaver, P. R., & Kirkpatrick, L. A. (1997). A general attribution theory for the psychology of religion. In Spilka, B., & McIntosh, D. (Eds.), *The psychology of religion: Theoretical approaches*. Boulder, CO: Westview Press.

Tarakeshwar, N., Pearce, M. J., & Sikkema, K. J. (2005). Development and implementation of a spiritual coping group intervention for adults living with HIV/AIDS: A pilot study. *Mental Health, Religion & Culture, 8*(3), 179–190.

Tarakeshwar, N., Vanderwerker, L. C., Paulk, E., Pearce, M. J., Kasl, S. V., & Prigerson, H. G. (2006). Religious coping is associated with the quality of life of patients with advanced cancer. *Journal of Palliative Medicine, 9*(3), 646–657.

Trenholm, P., Trent, J., & Compton, W. C. (1998). Negative religious conflict as a predictor of panic disorder. *Journal of Clinical Psychology, 54*(1), 59–65.

Wachholtz, A. B., & Pargament, I. (2005). Is spirituality a critical ingredient of meditation? Comparing the effects of spiritual meditation, secular meditation, and relaxation on spiritual, psychological, cardiac, and pain outcomes. *Journal of Behavioral Medicine, 28*(4), 369–384.

Webster's New Universal Unabridged Dictionary. (2003). China: Barnes & Noble Publishing, Inc. (Original work published The Random House Dictionary of the English Language, the Unabridged Edition (2001)).

Windle, G., Markland, D. A., & Woods, R. T. (2008). Examination of a theoretical model of psychological resilience in older age. *Aging & Mental Health, 12*(3), 285–292.

Wolin, S., & Wolin, S. (1993). *The resilient self.* New York, NY: Villard Books.

Yohannes, A. M., Koenig, H. G., Baldwin, R. C., & Connolly, M. J. (2008). Health behavior, depression and religiosity in older patients admitted to intermediate care. *International Journal of Geriatric Psychiatry, 23*(7), 735–740.

Zinnbauer, B. J., & Pargament, K. I. (2005). Religiousness and spirituality. In Paloutzian, R. F., & Park, C. L. (Eds.), *Handbook of the psychology of religion and spirituality.* New York, NY: The Guilford Press.

Zinnbauer, B. J., Pargament, K. I., Cole, B., Rye, M. S., Butter, E. M., Belavich, T. G., et al. (1997). Religion and spirituality: Unfuzzying the fuzzy. *Journal for the Scientific Study of Religion, 36*(4), 549–564.

Chapter 12
Resilience in Chronic Illness

Ranak B. Trivedi, Hayden B. Bosworth, and George L. Jackson

Our greatest glory is not in never falling, but in rising every time we fall.

Confucius

It is not the size of the dog in the fight; it is the size of the fight in the dog

Mark Twain

I think I can, I think I can...

The Little Engine that Could

Resilience has been written about and valued since time immemorial. Its value is transmitted down generations through adages, mythology, anecdotes, and even children's books. In essence, resilience can be thought of as a process of successfully adapting to maintain or regain emotional well-being in the face of adversity. It does not mean that distress is not experienced; rather, it is a process through which an individual's thoughts and behaviors overcome distress and optimize positive outcomes.

Historically, terms such as "hardiness" or "toughness" have also been used to allude to this construct. The term "resilience" has gained traction as the emphasis has shifted from it being an inherent trait to an ability that can be fostered. Although commonly associated with coping with trauma, catastrophic events, or personal tragedy, increasing attention is being paid to resilience in response to chronic illness. The impetus for this is both the growing number of patients with multiple chronic illnesses (Anderson and Horvath 2004), and the recognition that having a chronic illness can be stressful to manage (Russell et al. 2005). Stress has been shown to impact illness onset and outcomes through deleterious pathophysiological changes (Bairey-Merz et al. 2002; Black and Garbutt 2002; Cacioppo et al. 1998;

R.B. Trivedi (✉)
University of Washington, Seattle, WA, USA
e-mail: Ranak.Trivedi@va.gov

B. Resnick et al. (eds.), *Resilience in Aging: Concepts, Research, and Outcomes*,
DOI 10.1007/978-1-4419-0232-0_12, © Springer Science+Business Media, LLC 2011

Gold et al. 1988) and behavioral changes (DiMatteo et al. 2000, 2002). However, the negative consequences of stress on chronic disease are not inevitable and recent studies have highlighted psychosocial factors that can reduce vulnerability to stress and prevent both psychological and medical comorbidities (Dimsdale 2008). The growing area of resilience aims to capture these factors that may inure chronic illness patients to negative psychological sequelae.

Factors that Enhance Resilience in Chronic Illness

In the context of patients with existing illness, resilience can be thought of as a dynamic process that involves actively coping with experiences of significant adversity (Luthar and Cicchetti 2000). Resilience emerges out of cultural values as well as out of situational contexts (e.g., poverty) to evolve over the life course into highly specific ways of individuals' viewing of the world (Becker and Newsom 2005). The ingredients that shape resilience undoubtedly differ for different groups of people. Nevertheless, certain commonalities appear to transcend the potential variability across individuals and cultures. Data on these factors are summarized below.

Personality Traits

After decades of research on personality traits with negative outcomes, research linking personality characteristics to resilience in physical health has received increasing attention in recent years (Smith and MacKenzie 2006). Personality characteristics that have garnered empirical support include optimism, conscientiousness, and health-related hardiness. *Optimism* can be thought of as a predisposing factor towards positive outcomes expectancies (Scheier and Carver 1987). Optimists tend to have expectations of positive outcomes, unlike their pessimist counterparts. As behavior is often determined by expectancies of outcomes, this model suggests that optimists are more likely to attempt to overcome adversity than pessimists. Patients who score high on optimism report lower incidence of heart disease, faster recovery from cardiac procedures, lower incidence of physical symptoms in HIV/AIDS, and better coping in women with breast cancer (Carver et al. 1993; Kubzansky et al. 2001; Pakenham and Rinaldis 2001; Scheier and Carver 1985; Scheier et al. 1989, 1999). Another personality trait that appears related to resilience is *conscientiousness*, defined as the tendency to act dutifully, aim for achievement, and show self-discipline (McCrae and John 1992). Less studied than optimism, conscientiousness nevertheless is associated with longevity (Friedman et al. 1995) and longer survival in the chronically ill (Christensen et al. 2002). The mechanism for positive relationship between conscientiousness and outcomes may be explained by the fact that individuals high on conscientiousness tend to have higher rates of adherence to treatment regimens. Finally, *health-related hardiness* is the personality characteristic that enables individuals to adapt to health problems through control, commitment, and challenge (Pollock 1989). This trait has been linked with psychosocial adaptation in diabetes, hypertension, and rheumatoid arthritis (Pollock 1986).

Social Support

Perhaps the most widely studied correlate of stress vulnerability is social support. The presence of caring and supportive relationships appears to enhance resilience and facilitate positive outcomes in patients with a wide variety of chronic conditions, including cardiovascular disease (Lett et al., 2005), depression (Fiske et al. 2009), diabetes (White et al. 1992), cancer (Koopman et al. 1998), and renal disease (Dimond 1979). The mechanisms through which social support operates are likely many, but include the presence of emotional support, instrumental support (e.g., practical assistance in actual disease management), higher self-efficacy, lack of isolation, and perceived sense of control (Lett et al. 2005).

Coping Styles

Coping can be thought of as self-conscious effort towards optimal outcomes. In this sense, it is the process through which individuals build or maintain resilience. Resilient patients appear to have coping styles characterized by active engagement, humor, and non-dependency to drugs and alcohol (Schuckit and Smith 2006; Trivedi et al. 2009). In addition, resilient individuals report frequently relying on religion to help cope with adversity (Costanzo et al. 2009). Additional coping factors associated with resilience include the capacity to make realistic plans and take steps to carry them out, a positive view of oneself and confidence in one's ability, skills in communication and problem solving, and the capacity to manage strong feelings and impulses (American Psychological Association 2007). Individuals may also cope using their social support network and through inherent optimism (Trivedi et al. 2008, 2009), highlighting that the various factors determining resilience can be interrelated and overlapping.

Resilience as a Tool for Primary Prevention

Primary prevention is the sine qua non of health care. However, only 2–3% of total health care spending goes for prevention (Woolf 2009). The remaining health care resources are directed toward financing and delivery of medical care with substantially less emphasis on other determinants of health such as behavioral choices, social circumstances, and environmental conditions (Schroeder and Fahey 2007). This is despite the fact that the Center for Disease Control and Prevention recognizes that "increased focus on prevention is not only critical to preserving older individuals' independence and reducing long-term care needs – it is also critical for helping to stem health care costs" (Lang et al. 2006).

Replacing the current emphasis on pathologies and deficits with research examining how people make the most of their lives would enable us to better understand how people persevere despite obstacles. The area of resilience aims to meet precisely these goals. Resilience offers a framework that recognizes the preponderance of positive outcomes in patients with chronic illness and examines their antecedents, such as personality traits, coping styles, and social support. After identifying these antecedents, intervention programs can test whether fostering these can build resilience in a population at-risk for certain illnesses (Luthar and Cicchetti 2000). In this way, resilience offers what research focusing on negative outcomes cannot: the promise of primary prevention.

Attention is turning toward resilience to increase the likelihood of maintaining good health, aging well, and contributing to the vitality of the community. The aging of the population and the increasing prevalence of chronic diseases pose challenges to the US healthcare system. In 2000, 45% of Medicare beneficiaries aged 65 years or older had at least one chronic medical condition, and 21% had multiple chronic conditions (Anderson and Horvath 2002). Healthcare costs for individuals with at least three chronic conditions accounted for 89% of Medicare's annual budget (Anderson and Horvath 2002). There is a growing acknowledgement that burden on healthcare can be reduced only if individuals play an active role in their own healthcare through disease self-management. Self-management consists of activities that promote physical and psychological health; interacting with healthcare providers and adhering to treatment recommendations; monitoring health status and making associated care decisions; and managing the impact of the illness on physical, psychological and social functioning (Bodenheimer et al. 2002; Bosworth et al. 2005). Because resilient patients are more likely to be successful at self-management, monitoring and fostering resilience can have direct implications for disease management.

Current Limitations and Alternate Conceptual Model

A thorough review of the literature suggests that the most common conceptualization of resilience is the ability to have positive psychological outcomes when faced with adversity (Luthar et al. 2000). Resilience is defined as a collection of protective factors that mediate the relationship between a stressful event and positive outcomes (Brooks 2008; Lavretsky and Irwin 2007). In the current conceptualization, resilient individuals may have short-term perturbations of normal functioning, but demonstrate an overall trajectory of healthy functioning and the ability to generate positive experiences (Bonanno 2004). Resilience thus defined is distinct from "recovery," which involves regaining the equilibrium that existed prior to stress (Brooks 2008; Luthar et al. 2000).

We posit that the current conceptualization may be very narrow for patients with chronic illness. First, the current theory of resilience hews very closely with the outdated theory that resilience is a stable trait rather than a modifiable process. Implicit in the theory that resilience is protective is the assumption that these reserves exist and are tested in the face of adversity. If negative outcomes occur, then the individual was non-resilient. By this definition, resilience can only be built before the adverse event occurs and not after. However, because resilience is a two-dimensional construct that requires a stressful event to occur, non-resilient individuals cannot be identified in advance to bolster resilience. Such circular logic may be one of the main reasons why resilience has been difficult to assess or modify in patients with chronic illness.

Second, the current theory of resilience excludes those who display the tenacity to recover after having an initial response of distress. Those who recover are different from those who do not in their ability to return to, and maintain, a state of equilibrium. This is especially relevant to chronically ill patients where disease onset may be defined by an acute event, whether it is a physical event such as a myocardial infarction, or being given a diagnosis of a medical condition, such as diabetes. It is likely that an individual who is "resilient" in the immediate aftermath of a myocardial infarction may experience some distress after going through lengthy cardiac rehabilitation. Similarly, an individual may experience significant loss of emotional well-being immediately following diagnosis with breast cancer but may regain their resiliency while undergoing chemotherapy. In either case, distress may be transient and recovery may occur with time, education, active coping, and habituation. A dichotomy simply based on initial stress response may fail to capture the tenacity of such patients.

Third, the current theory of resilience ignores the potential additive or multiplicative effect of stressors endemic to chronic illness. Facing the challenges of disease management can be harrowing for many patients as they face medical tests, polypharmacy treatments, lifestyle changes, functional impairment, and potential mortality. Furthermore, chronically ill patients are often diagnosed with several chronic conditions and patients who may have a "resilient" response to the initial diagnosis may find their psychological reserves taxed when faced with the sequelae of a second or third diagnosis. In parallel, the increasing disability may lead directly to a reduction in a person's appraised ability to achieve goals, or that their lack of regular engagement in activities leads to decrements in skills and associated lack of self-efficacy (Fiske et al. 2009).

To address these limitations, we propose an alternate conceptualization in which resilience exists on a spectrum and can be fostered at each stage. In our conceptualization, resilience is not only an inherent invulnerability but also the ability to recover from stress. An underlying tenet is that individuals exist in a state of equilibrium and that resilience is the process through which individuals maintain or regain equilibrium over time. Because stress in chronic illness can be additive and can change over time, resiliency can exist on a continuum of stress response and can increase or decrease over time as well. On one end are individuals who, at the given point of assessment, are demonstrating positive psychological well-being and adequate coping. By contrast there are individuals who experience psychological distress but may recover. Within this latter group, we propose two sub-categories: those that may experience subclinical emotional distress but are able to use their own psychosocial resources to recover, and those who experience clinically significant distress that may need professional help.

Therefore, resilience can be conceptualized as a three-level construct which we term primary, secondary, and tertiary resiliences. These are defined as follows:

1. *Primary resilience*: Individuals demonstrating primary resilience do not experience more than *transient* loss of emotional well-being in response to an adverse event, appear to have sufficient resources to ensure optimal outcomes and not likely to experience a specific psychiatric illness.
2. *Secondary resilience*: Individuals demonstrating secondary resilience experience no more than *moderate* loss of emotional well-being and/or subclinical distress after a diagnosis or experiencing a disease, but soon regain equilibrium through own coping resources. These coping resources may be a combination of personality traits, coping styles, and social resources.
3. *Tertiary resilience*: Individuals demonstrating tertiary resilience may experience *significant* loss of emotional well-being when exposed to stress and may develop psychiatric symptoms or illness. These individuals regain equilibrium after a length of time using own resources and/or with professional intervention.

This conceptualization has practical advantages in the clinical management of chronic illness. Recognizing that resilience can change over time can help make providers cognizant of monitoring patients' well-being during treatment. Furthermore, the clinical goals of each level of resilience may be different (Table 12.1). Chronic illness patients who exhibit primary resilience need no more than usual care and monitoring to ensure that they are able to maintain their sense of equilibrium. Those who exhibit secondary resilience may need support and reinforcing of their previous coping, but largely can regain equilibrium on their own. On the other hand, those with tertiary resilience may require professional intervention to prevent further deterioration of well-being, followed by efforts to regain equilibrium. When equilibrium is regained, efforts need to be made to maintain equilibrium. Defining

Table 12.1 Clinical goals corresponding to levels of resilience

Level of resilience	Clinical goals	Methods
Primary resilience	Maintain equilibrium	• Monitor stress response
		• Provide education
		• Augment current resources as needed
Secondary resilience	Regain equilibrium	• Reinforce existing coping resources
		• Provide self-help resources
		• Utilize methods of primary resilience
Tertiary resilience	Stop disequilibrium	• Professional interventions aimed at recovery
		• Utilize methods of secondary and primary resilience

clinical goals in this way offers the added advantage of matching limited resources to patient needs in the most efficient manner.

Once the clinical goals of each level are achieved, patients become more resilient and clinical goals are adjusted accordingly. Imagine a scenario in which a cancer patient experiences significant depressive symptoms when undergoing the arduous treatments of chemotherapy and radiation. The patient begins seeing a mental health professional and is able to inhibit further loss of well-being. Once this is accomplished, the treatment may involve regaining equilibrium that existed prior to cancer diagnosis and treatment. In other words, patients would be exhibiting secondary resilience, where the goals would be to return to the state of equilibrium. Similarly, achieving equilibrium would naturally lead to an intervention aimed at maintaining equilibrium at which point patients would exhibit primary resilience. Therefore, our proposed conceptualization captures the fluid nature of the stress response.

Clinical Management of Resilience

Assessment

An adequate detection and measure of the level of resilience is key to identifying the processes that lead from health to frailty and ultimately to the appearance of disease (Fried et al. 2005; Walston et al. 2006). Although not commonly used in chronic illness, measures that are specific to resilience have been created. Perhaps the most widely used is the Post-traumatic Growth Inventory, also available online at apa.org (Tedeschi and Calhoun 1996). Typically, however, resilience is assessed indirectly, through the assessment of its various correlates, such as quality of life, positive affect, optimism, and coping styles. In addition, depression scales have been used to determine the absence of negative affect as a marker of resilience. In healthcare settings, the interested practitioner may include various self-report measures to measure these constructs. Table 12.2 provides a brief overview of the commonly used measures and the constructs they purport to measure. (For a comprehensive review of commonly used psychosocial scales, we suggest referring to *Measuring Health: A Guide to Rating Scales and Questionnaires* (McDowell 2006) and *Measures of Personality and Social Psychological Attitudes* (Robinson et al. 1991).)

Interventions

Minimizing disruption to the care of persons with chronic disease requires weaving a health care safety net resilient to the stress of illness and to the more personalized disasters such as job loss or loss of one's home (DeSalvo and Kertesz 2007). Various programs and resources can be accessed by both the patient and healthcare providers to improve and maintain resiliency.

Table 12.2 Measures to assess resilience and its correlates

Construct	Scale	Items
Coping	COPE (Carver et al. 1989)	60 items (15 coping styles)
Depressive symptoms	Beck Depression Inventory (Beck et al. 1988)	21 items
Quality of life	Short Form-36 Health Survey (Ware and Sherbourne 1992)	36 items (2 subscales to measure mental and physical components)
	Short Form-12 Health Survey (Ware et al. 1996)	12 items (2 subscales to measure mental and physical components)
Affect	Positive and Negative Affect Scale (PANAS) (Watson et al. 1988)	20 items (10 positive affect items, 10 negative affect items)
Dispositional optimism	Life Orientation Test-Revised (LOT-R) (Scheier and Carver 1987; Scheier et al. 1994)	8 items
Resilience	Post-traumatic Growth Inventory (Tedeschi and Calhoun 1996)	21 items (4 factors: new possibilities, relating to others, personal strength, spiritual change, and appreciation of life)
	Connor-Davidson Resilience Scale (CD-RISC) (Connor and Davidson 2003)	25 items
	Dispositional Resilience Scale 15 (DRS15) (Bartone 2007)	15 Items (3 subscales: communication, challenge, control)

Self-help interventions. Various self-help resources are available to build and maintain resilience. The American Psychological Association online help center at apahelpcenter.org provides a comprehensive overview along with an assessment tool and self-help tips to build and maintain resilience (American Psychological Association 2007). The website highlights key factors that can help sustain resilience, including self-efficacy, setting realistic goals and meeting them, communication and problem-solving skills, and controlling impulsive responses. In addition, the resource focuses on resilience as an ongoing process of growth, providing guidelines for learning from previous life experiences, and actively facing sources of distress (Fig. 12.1).

A key factor in creating, strengthening, and sustaining resilience is the presence of caring and supportive social networks. Fostering such relationships both within and outside of the family is thought to be critical in maintaining well-being through instrumental help, encouragement, and reassurance (Rozanski et al. 2005; White et al. 1992). In patients with chronic illness, this can be particularly challenging if medical conditions limit mobility and lead to isolation. If patients report difficulty in accessing existing social resources or building networks, health care providers can help problem-solve with the patients and their families to ensure patients continue to derive strength from their social networks. Support groups can be helpful venues for building social networks with others experiencing similar stressors. Support groups

1. Make connections.

2. Avoid seeing crises as insurmountable problems.

3. Accept that change is a part of living.

4. Move towards your goals.

5. Take decisive action.

6. Look for opportunities for self discovery.

7. Nurture a positive view of yourself.

8. Keep things in perspective.

9. Maintain a hopeful outlook.

10. Take care of yourself.

    (Source: apahelpcenter.org)

Fig. 12.1 Ten ways to build resilience

allow the sharing of information, ideas, emotions, and can foster a sense of community to replace the isolation often experienced when faced with adversity.

Finally, books and other publications authored by people who have successfully managed adversity can inspire and motivate chronically ill individuals to discover strategies that may optimize outcomes.

Clinical Interventions. Programs that aim to improve emotional well-being in chronically ill patients are still in their infancy. Perhaps the most widely studied are interventions designed using Jon Kabat-Zinn's Mindfulness Based Stress Reduction Program (MBSR). Based on Buddhist practices, mindfulness emphasizes consistent, dispassionate, and non-evaluative moment-to-moment awareness of mental activities (Grossman et al. 2004). The MBSR typically involves 2.5-h weekly sessions for 8–10 weeks and an additional single-day "retreat." A recent meta-analysis evaluated both physical and mental well-being outcomes across a variety of studies and concluded that across a variety of conditions, mindfulness may enhance coping and reduce distress and disability (Grossman et al. 2004). Improvements were seen in mental and physical parameters of health. It should be noted that research in this area still remains sparse; however, these promising results suggest that interventions to promote resiliency can be successful in the chronically ill. Many cities and academic institutions offer MBSR programs through trained professionals. In addition, several online resources are available for those interested in learning more about mindfulness based interventions (e.g., http://www.umassmed.edu/cfm/mbsr/).

Improving physical well-being may be especially important in fostering a sense of emotional well-being in chronic illness. This is typically achieved through a variety of recommended lifestyle changes that may be common across diseases or may be disease specific. For example, patients with most chronic conditions will be advised to increase physical activity, whether it is cardiovascular disease, diabetes, depression, and even pain conditions (American Pain Society 2009; Blumenthal et al. 2000; Boule et al. 2001; Cobb et al. 2006; Green and Pope 2000; Rejeski et al. 1992). Besides improving physical health, exercise has been shown to improve positive effect (Zautra et al. 2008). On the other hand, recommendations may be disease specific, such as following the DASH diet for hypertensive patients (Svetkey et al. 1999) and watching carbohydrate intake in diabetic patients (Diabetes Prevention Program Research Group 2002). Meeting these goals can be challenging and may lead to a loss of well-being as patients attempt to make changes to their existing lifestyles. However, meeting these goals can not only improve physical well-being, it may also potentially foster a sense of mastery, improve self-efficacy, and bolster resilience. An important caveat is that setting reasonable goals and expectations and building on these successes is needed to foster a sense of mastery.

A practical tool that can be utilized by primary care provider and specialists is the 5As construct of behavioral counseling. First adopted from tobacco cessation programs, the 5As represent the steps that a provider team can go through to assess and respond to a given patients' barriers to effective self-management behavior, which might relate to secondary and tertiary resilience issues (Glasgow et al. 2006; Goldstein et al. 2004; Whitlock et al. 2002). The 5As are described below, using exercise as an example:

- *Assess*: Assess disease knowledge (e.g., exercise is important to controlling diabetes), attitudes (e.g., self-efficacy for doing exercise), and preferences (e.g., type of exercise preferred). The provider should address barriers to the desired behavior (e.g., no safe place to walk).
- *Advise*: Provide personalized advice for maintaining or changing behavior; incorporate specific recommendations of behavior change based on personal health risks. For example, it may not be helpful to tell a patient who almost never walks more than a few hundred steps a day to start running a mile a day. It would be more appropriate to advise the patient on how to make gradual increases in exercise.
- *Agree*: There is an extensive literature on the usefulness of collaborative goal setting in improving chronic illness self-management (Goldstein et al. 2004). The provider and patient can discuss realistic goals (e.g., wearing a pedometer and increasing the number of steps walked by 300 over the next 2 weeks). Training in motivational interviewing, which helps the provider elicit talk of change from the patient and respond appropriately, may help the provider in the agreeing process.
- *Assist*: Develop an action plan that responds to the patient's needs and barriers. For example, determining where to obtain a pedometer, where to walk, and where to record steps should be determined. Further, the relationship between the plan and overcoming specific barriers to changes can also be discussed.
- *Arrange*: This step includes specific plans for follow-up to assess the degree of goal achievement and provide needed assistance.

Finally, for complex cases of tertiary resilience, licensed mental health professionals such as clinical psychologists, psychiatrists, and trained nurses can offer counseling, psychotherapeutic interventions, or medications. This level of intervention may be especially important in chronically ill individuals with tertiary resilience who may require strategies for preventing further decline, regaining equilibrium, and maintaining equilibrium. Psychotherapy and psychotropic medications has been found to be an effective intervention for a variety of clinical and subclinical psychiatric issues, including major depressive disorder, depressive symptoms, anxiety, and adjustment disorders. Clinical psychologists effect change through focusing on changing harmful cognitions and behaviors to improve coping and resilience. Within clinical psychology, various specialties exist to tailor interventions to specific populations. For example, clinical psychologists who specialize in treating patients with medical illnesses may be referred to as health psychologists. Health psychologists who specialize in cancer often refer to themselves as psycho-oncologists; likewise those who specialize in heart disease and pain may be known as cardiac psychologists and pain psychologists, respectively.

In addition to individual therapy, patients may be referred to couples or family therapists. Couples' therapists specialize in providing interventions to patients and their significant others. Because significant others are often involved in disease management, this may be a particularly powerful intervention for some chronic illness patients. Family therapists expand the intervention target to include key figures of social network, such as children, to bolster individual response. Using a variety of techniques, these specialists can help improve patients' functioning within their own social context and optimize positive outcomes.

Organizing Chronic Illness Care to Address Resilience

Healthcare providers cannot be expected to suddenly be able to address issues of resilience and support on top of the many other issues that need to be addressed in often brief visits. Such changes in care require properly organized healthcare organizations. The Wagner Chronic Care Model (CCM) provides a roadmap for such a system (Coleman et al. 2009; Wagner 1998; Wagner et al. 2001a, b). The CCM postulates that patient outcomes would be enhanced in healthcare systems organized for chronic illness management. Specifically, delivery systems that provide self-management support (e.g., 5As), are organized around integrated teams whose members have specifically described roles (e.g., nurse that does initial assessment and negotiation of self-management goals that are reinforced by a physician), utilize tools to support evidence-based guidelines (e.g., reminders to providers, discussion of guidelines with patients, etc.), and include clinical information systems (e.g., computerized reminders, patient registries, etc.) are more likely to have "productive interactions between informed, activated patients and prepared proactive practice teams." Further, these organizations should be connected to community resources that may help patients reach their goals. For example, improving social support may include a working knowledge of how to refer patients to local community centers. Healthcare systems utilizing more elements of the CCM or making changes aimed at improving multiple CCM elements have generally experienced better chronic illness care processes and outcomes (Coleman et al. 2009). Healthcare organizations seeking to assess the degree to which patients perceive use of techniques suggested by the Chronic Care Model utilized the Patient Assessment of Chronic Illness Care (PACIC) (Glasgow et al. 2006, 2004). An expanded version of the PACIC also allows organizations to assess the degree to which providers practice the 5As of brief patient behavior described above.

Of special importance to addressing issues of resilience, there has been an increasing effort to include clinical psychologists, psychiatrists, and other mental health professionals in primary care teams. Often co-located in the same office as physicians, these professionals can address both issues related to traditional mental illness (e.g., providing psychotherapy) or behavioral issues of chronic illness care (e.g., providing, brief, targeted counseling) (Frank et al. 2004). Advantages of this approach are primary prevention to improve and maintain resilience at the time of chronic illness diagnosis and on an ongoing basis; secondary prevention through early detection of lower resilience; and tertiary prevention through active interventions and outside referrals where necessary. The integration of mental health into traditionally medical settings can assist in developing an ongoing relationship between a patient and provider team that addresses the broad range of patient biopsychosocial needs and coordinates related services. This notion of integrated primary care is congruent with the Chronic Care Model and renewed attempts at the development of primary care medical homes which have the goal of developing an ongoing relationship between a patient and provider team that addresses the broad range of patient biopsychosocial needs and coordinates related services (Reid et al. 2009).

Summary and Discussion

Resilience in chronic illness is an area in much need of empirical evidence and much of the current literature derives implicitly from related areas, such as coping in chronic illness. The majority of the literature emphasizes resiliency as an inherent invulnerability to stress. We argue that the current definition may be too restrictive and ignores the experiences of patients with chronic illness. We propose a conceptual model that extends the concept of resilience to individuals who can recover from emotional setbacks that are common to chronically ill patients. In this model, patients can be characterized as exhibiting primary, secondary, and tertiary resilience. Each level of resilience denotes a place on the spectrum of resilience. According to this model, appropriate interventions at each stage have the potential to move the individual towards primary resilience and positive outcomes. Pragmatically, this model allows clinicians to tailor interventions so that limited resources are allocated most efficiently.

Resilience can be both built and maintained through the proactive efforts of patients using self-help resources. These are available in the forms of books, online resources, and support groups, and healthcare providers are encouraged to acquaint their patients with these resources to optimize positive outcomes. In addition, we provide an overview of tools that healthcare professionals can use in their practice to assess and address primary and secondary resilience in their practices. To address tertiary resilience, it is recommended that patients seek professional help from a mental health expert, such as clinical psychologists, psychiatrists, and other professionals. Many specialists are available that can provide interventions based on the type of chronic illness that patients may suffer and who can involve patients' own social networks in the interventions. Provision of such services requires appropriately organized healthcare systems to address comprehensive biopsychosocial needs of the patients.

Future Directions

The importance of examining resilience in chronic disease is likely to grow with the growing prevalence of chronic disease. Studies in the twentieth century have significantly expanded our understanding of psychopathology and its impact on adverse disease outcomes. The twenty-first century should bring a greater understanding of factors that not only buffer against negative outcomes, but also enhance recovery from distressed states.

We advance a new conceptualization of resilience as a step towards meeting these goals. However, our model needs to be validated and refined through rigorous empirical studies before it can gain wider acceptance. The growing impetus to integrate mental health services in traditional medical setting should be sustained and capitalized upon. Conducting quality research that demonstrates the superiority of these models against more traditional medical healthcare delivery systems will be a necessary catalyst to important policy changes in healthcare delivery. Enhancing resilience through fundamental changes in healthcare research and delivery has the potential of preventing disease onset and exacerbation, and improving the vitality of the growing population of chronic illness patients.

References

American Pain Society. (2009). Retrieved October 29, 2009, from http://www.ampainsoc.org/

American Psychological Association. (2007). *The road to resilience.* Retrieved October 16, 2009, from http://apahelpcenter.org/featuredtopics/feature.php?id=6

Anderson, G., & Horvath, J. (2002). *Chronic conditions: making the case for ongoing care.* Princeton, NJ.

Anderson, G., & Horvath, J. (2004). The growing burden of chronic disease in America. *Public Health Reports, 119*, 263–270.

Bairey-Merz, C. N., Dwyer, J., Nordstrom, C. K., Walton, K. G., Salerno, J. W., & Schneider, R. H. (2002). Psychosocial stress and cardiovascular disease: pathophysiological links. *Behavioral Medicine, 27*, 141–147.

Bartone, P. T. (2007). Test-retest reliability of the dispositional resilience scale-15, a brief hardiness scale. *Psychological Reports, 101*(3 Pt 1), 943–944.

Beck, A. T., Steer, R. A., & Carbin, M. G. (1988). Psychometric properties of the Beck Depression Inventory: twenty-five years of evaluation. *Clinical Psychology Review, 8*(1), 77–100.

Becker, G., & Newsom, E. (2005). Resilience in the face of serious illness among chronically ill African Americans in later life. *The Journals of Gerontology. Series B, Psychological Sciences and Social Sciences, 60*(4), S214–S223.

Black, P. H., & Garbutt, L. D. (2002). Stress, inflammation and cardiovascular disease. *Journal of Psychosomatic Research, 52*, 1–23.

Blumenthal, J. A., Sherwood, A., Gullette, E. C. D., Babyak, M., Waugh, R., Georgiades, A., et al. (2000). Exercise and weight loss reduce blood pressure in men and women with mild hypertension. *Archives of Internal Medicine, 160*, 1947–1958.

Bodenheimer, T., Lorig, K., Holman, H., & Grumbach, K. (2002). Patient self-management of chronic disease in primary care. *JAMA: The Journal of the American Medical Association, 288*(19), 2469–2475.

Bonanno, G. A. (2004). Loss, trauma, and human resilience: have we underestimated the human capacity to thrive after extremely aversive events? *American Psychologist, 59*(1), 20–28.

Bosworth, H. B., Olsen, M. K., & Oddone, E. Z. (2005). Improving blood pressure control by tailored feedback to patients and clinicians. *American Heart Journal, 149*(5), 795–803.

Boule, N. G., Haddad, E., Kenny, G. P., Wells, G. A., & Sigal, R. J. (2001). Effects of exercise on glycemic control and body mass in type 2 diabetes mellitus: a meta-analysis of controlled clinical trials. *JAMA: The Journal of the American Medical Association, 286*, 1218–1227.

Brooks, M. V. (2008). Health-related hardiness in individuals with chronic illnesses. *Clinical Nursing Research, 17*(2), 98–117.

Cacioppo, J. T., Berntson, G. G., Malarkey, W. B., Kiecolt-Glaser, J. K., Sheridan, J. F., Poehlmann, K. M., et al. (1998). Autonomic, neuroendocrine, and immune responses to psychological stress: the reactivity hypothesis. *Annals of New York Academy of Sciences, 840*, 664–673.

Carver, C. S., Scheier, M. F., & Weintraub, J. K. (1989). Assessing coping strategies: a theoretically based approach. *Journal of Personality and Social Psychology, 56*(2), 267–283.

Carver, C. S., Pozo, C., Harris, S. D., Noriega, V., Scheier, M. F., Robinson, D. S., et al. (1993). How coping mediates the effect of optimism on distress: a study of women with early stage breast cancer. *Journal of Personality and Social Psychology, 65*(2), 375–390.

Christensen, A. J., Ehlers, S. L., Wiebe, J. S., Moran, P. J., Raichle, K., Ferneyhough, K., et al. (2002). Patient personality and mortality: a 4-year prospective examination of chronic renal insufficiency. *Health Psychology, 21*(4), 315–320.

Cobb, S. L., Brown, D. J., & Davis, L. L. (2006). Effective interventions for lifestyle change after myocardial infarction or coronary artery revascularization. *Journal of the American Academy of Nurse Practitioners, 18*(1), 31–39.

Coleman, K., Austin, B. T., Brach, C., & Wagner, E. H. (2009). Evidence on the Chronic Care Model in the new millennium. *Health affairs (Project Hope), 28*(1), 75–85.

Connor, K. M., & Davidson, J. R. (2003). Development of a new resilience scale: the Connor–Davidson Resilience Scale (CD-RISC). *Depression & Anxiety, 18*(2), 76–82.

Costanzo, E. S., Ryff, C. D., & Singer, B. H. (2009). Psychosocial adjustment among cancer survivors: findings from a national survey of health and well-being. *Health Psychology, 28*(2), 147–156.

DeSalvo, K. B., & Kertesz, S. (2007). Creating a more resilient safety net for persons with chronic disease: beyond the "medical home". *Journal of General Internal Medicine, 22*(9), 1377–1379.

Diabetes Prevention Program Research Group. (2002). Reduction in the incidence of Type 2 diabetes with lifestyle intervention or metformin. *New England Journal of Medicine, 346*, 393–403.

DiMatteo, M. R., Giordani, P. J., Lepper, H. S., & Croghan, T. W. (2002). Patient adherence and medical treatment outcomes: a meta-analysis. *Medical Care, 40*(9), 794–811.

DiMatteo, M. R., Lepper, H. S., & Croghan, T. W. (2000). Depression is a risk factor for noncompliance with medical treatment: meta-analysis of the effects of anxiety and depression on patient adherence. *Archives of Internal Medicine, 160*(14), 2101–2107.

Dimond, M. (1979). Social support and adaptation to chronic illness: the case of maintenance hemodialysis. *Research in Nursing & Health, 2*(3), 101–108.

Dimsdale, J. E. (2008). Psychological stress and cardiovascular disease. *Journal of the American College of Cardiology*, *51*(13), 1237–1246.

Fiske, A., Wetherell, J. L., & Gatz, M. (2009). Depression in older adults. *Annual Reviews in Clinical Psychology*, *5*, 363–389.

Frank, R. G., McDaniel, S. H., Bray, J. H., & Heldring, M. (2004). *Primary care psychology*. Washington, DC: American Psychological Association.

Fried, L. P., Hadley, E. C., Walston, J. D., Newman, A. B., Guralnik, J. M., Studenski, S., et al. (2005). From bedside to bench: research agenda for frailty. *Science of Aging Knowledge Environment*, *2005*(31), pe24.

Friedman, H. S., Tucker, J. S., Schwartz, J. E., Martin, L. R., Tomlinson-Keasey, C., Wingard, D. L., et al. (1995). Childhood conscientiousness and longevity: health behaviors and cause of death. *Journal of Personality and Social Psychology*, *68*(4), 696–703.

Glasgow, R. E., Emont, S., & Miller, D. C. (2006). Assessing delivery of the five 'As' for patient-centered counseling. *Health Promotion International*, *21*(3), 245–255.

Glasgow, R. E., Goldstein, M. G., Ockene, J. K., & Pronk, N. P. (2004). Translating what we have learned into practice. Principles and hypotheses for interventions addressing multiple behaviors in primary care. *American Journal of Preventive Medicine*, *27*(2 Suppl), 88–101.

Gold, P. W., Goodwin, F. K., & Chrousos, G. P. (1988). Clinical and biochemical manifestations of depression: relation to the neurobiology of stress. (First of two parts). *New England Journal of Medicine*, *319*(7), 348–353.

Goldstein, M. G., Whitlock, E. P., & DePue, J. (2004). Multiple behavioral risk factor interventions in primary care. Summary of research evidence. *American Journal of Preventive Medicine*, *27*(2 Suppl), 61–79.

Green, C. A., & Pope, C. R. (2000). Depressive symptoms, health promotion, and health risk behaviors. *American Journal of Health Promotion*, *15*(1), 29–34.

Grossman, P., Niemann, L., Schmidt, S., & Walach, H. (2004). Mindfulness-based stress reduction and health benefits: a meta-analysis. *Journal of Psychosomatic Research*, *57*(1), 35–43.

Koopman, C., Hermanson, K., Diamond, S., Angell, K., & Spiegel, D. (1998). Social support, life stress, pain and emotional adjustment to advanced breast cancer. *Psychooncology*, *7*(2), 101–111.

Kubzansky, L. D., Sparrow, D., Vokonas, P., & Kawachi, I. (2001). Is the glass half empty or half full? A prospective study of optimism and coronary heart disease in the normative aging study. *Psychosomatic Medicine*, *63*(6), 910–916.

Lang, J. E., Anderson, L., LoGerfo, J., Sharkey, J., Belansky, E., Bryant, L., et al. (2006). The Prevention Research Centers Healthy Aging Research Network. *Preventing Chronic Disease*, *3*(1), A17.

Lavretsky, H., & Irwin, M. R. (2007). Resilience and aging. *Aging and Health*, *2*(3), 309–323.

Lett, H. S., Blumenthal, J. A., Babyak, M. A., Strauman, T. J., Robins, C., & Sherwood, A. (2005). Social support and coronary heart disease: epidemiologic evidence and implications for treatment. *Psychosomatic Medicine*, *67*(6), 869–878.

Luthar, S. S., & Cicchetti, D. (2000). The construct of resilience: implications for interventions and social policies. *Development and Psychopathology*, *12*, 857–885.

Luthar, S. S., Cicchetti, D., & Becker, B. (2000). The construct of resilience: a critical evaluation and guidelines for future work. *Child Development*, *71*(3), 543–562.

McCrae, R. R., & John, O. P. (1992). An introduction to the five-factor model and its applications. *Journal of Personality*, *60*(2), 175–215.

McDowell, I. (2006). *Measuring health: a guide to rating scales and questionnaires* (3rd ed.). New York, NY: Oxford University Press, Inc.

Miller, W. R., & Rose, G. S. (2009). Toward a theory of motivational interviewing. *American Psychologist*, *64*(6), 527–537.

Pakenham, K. I., & Rinaldis, M. (2001). The role of illness, resources, appraisal, and coping strategies in adjustment to HIV/AIDS: the direct and buffering effects. *Journal of Behavioral Medicine*, *24*(3), 259–279.

Pollock, S. E. (1986). Human responses to chronic illness: physiologic and psychosocial adaptation. *Nursing Research*, *35*(2), 90–95.

Pollock, S. E. (1989). The hardiness characteristic: a motivating factor in adaptation. *Advances in Nursing Science, 11*(2), 53–62.

Reid, R. J., Fishman, P. A., Yu, O., Ross, T. R., Tufano, J. T., Soman, M. P., et al. (2009). Patient-centered medical home demonstration: a prospective, quasi-experimental, before and after evaluation. *American Journal of Managed Care, 15*(9), e71–e87.

Rejeski, W. J., Thompson, A., Brubaker, P. H., & Miller, H. S. (1992). Acute exercise: buffering psychosocial stress responses in women. *Health Psychology, 11*, 355–362.

Robinson, J. P., Shaver, P. R., & Wrightsman, L. S. (Eds.). (1991). *Measures of personality and social psychological attitudes* (Vol. 1). San Deigo, CA: Elsevier.

Rozanski, A., Blumenthal, J. A., Davidson, K. W., Saab, P. G., & Kubzansky, L. (2005). The epidemiology, pathophysiology, and management of psychosocial risk factors in cardiac practice: the emerging field of behavioral cardiology. *Journal of the American College of Cardiology, 45*(5), 637–651.

Russell, L. B., Suh, D. C., & Safford, M. A. (2005). Time requirements for diabetes self-management: too much for many? *Journal of Family Practice, 54*(1), 52–56.

Scheier, M., & Carver, C. S. (1985). Optimism, coping, and health: assessment and implications of generalized outcome expectancies. *Health Psychology, 4*, 219–247.

Scheier, M., & Carver, C. S. (1987). Dispositional optimism and physical well-being: the influence of generalized outcome expectancies on health. *Journal of Personality, 55*, 169–210.

Scheier, M. F., Matthews, K. A., Owens, J. F., Magovern, G. J., Sr., Lefebvre, R. C., Abbott, R. A., et al. (1989). Dispositional optimism and recovery from coronary artery bypass surgery: the beneficial effects on physical and psychological well-being. *Journal of Personality and Social Psychology, 57*(6), 1024–1040.

Scheier, M. F., Carver, C. S., & Bridges, M. W. (1994). Distinguishing optimism from neuroticism (and trait anxiety, self-mastery, and self-esteem): a reevaluation of the Life Orientation Test. *Journal of Personality and Social Psychology, 67*(6), 1063–1078.

Scheier, M. F., Matthews, K. A., Owens, J. F., Schulz, R., Bridges, M. W., Magovern, G. J., et al. (1999). Optimism and rehospitalization after coronary artery bypass graft surgery. *Archives of Internal Medicine, 159*, 829–835.

Schroeder, K., & Fahey, T. (2007). Improving adherence to drugs for hypertension. [Editorial]. *British Medical Journal, 335*(7628), 1002–1003.

Schuckit, M. A., & Smith, T. L. (2006). The relationship of behavioural undercontrol to alcoholism in higher-functioning adults. *Drug and Alcohol Review, 25*(5), 393–402.

Smith, T. W., & MacKenzie, J. (2006). Personality and risk of physical illness. *Annual Reviews in Clinical Psychology, 2*, 435–467.

Svetkey, L. P., Sacks, F. M., Obarzanek, E., Vollmer, W. M., Appel, L. J., Lin, P. H., et al. (1999). The DASH Diet, Sodium Intake and Blood Pressure Trial (DASH-sodium): rationale and design. DASH-Sodium Collaborative Research Group. *Journal of the American Dietetic Association, 99*(8 Suppl), S96–S104.

Tedeschi, R. G., & Calhoun, L. G. (1996). The posttraumatic growth inventory: measuring the positive legacy of trauma. *Journal of Traumatic Stress, 9*(3), 455–471.

Trivedi, R. B., Ayotte, B., Edelman, D., & Bosworth, H. B. (2008). The association of emotional well-being and marital status with treatment adherence among patients with hypertension. *Journal of Behavioral Medicine, 31*(6), 489–497.

Trivedi, R. B., Blumenthal, J. A., O'Connor, C., Adams, K., Hinderliter, A., Dupree, C., et al. (2009). Coping styles in heart failure patients with depressive symptoms. *Journal of Psychosomatic Research, 67*(4), 339–346.

Wagner, E. H. (1998). Chronic disease management: what will it take to improve care for chronic illness? *Effective clinical practice: ECP, 1*(1), 2–4.

Wagner, E. H., Austin, B. T., Davis, C., Hindmarsh, M., Schaefer, J., & Bonomi, A. (2001a). Improving chronic illness care: translating evidence into action. *Health affairs (Project Hope), 20*(6), 64–78.

Wagner, E. H., Glasgow, R. E., Davis, C., Bonomi, A. E., Provost, L., McCulloch, D., et al. (2001b). Quality improvement in chronic illness care: a collaborative approach. *The Joint Commission Journal on Quality Improvement, 27*(2), 63–80.

Walston, J., Hadley, E. C., Ferrucci, L., Guralnik, J. M., Newman, A. B., Studenski, S. A., et al. (2006). Research agenda for frailty in older adults: toward a better understanding of physiology and etiology: summary from the American Geriatrics Society/National Institute on Aging Research Conference on Frailty in Older Adults. *Journal of the American Geriatric Society, 54*(6), 991–1001.

Ware, J. E., Jr., & Sherbourne, C. D. (1992). The MOS 36-item short-form health survey (SF-36). I. Conceptual framework and item selection. *Medical Care, 30*(6), 473–483.

Ware, J., Jr., Kosinski, M., & Keller, S. D. (1996). A 12-Item Short-Form Health Survey: construction of scales and preliminary tests of reliability and validity. *Medical Care, 34*(3), 220–233.

Watson, D., Clark, L. A., & Tellegen, A. (1988). Development and validation of brief measures of positive and negative affect: the PANAS scales. *Journal of Personality and Social Psychology, 54*, 1063–1070.

White, N. E., Richter, J. M., & Fry, C. (1992). Coping, social support, and adaptation to chronic illness. *Western Journal of Nursing Research, 14*(2), 211–224.

Whitlock, E. P., Orleans, C. T., Pender, N., & Allan, J. (2002). Evaluating primary care behavioral counseling interventions: an evidence-based approach. *American journal of preventive medicine, 22*(4), 267–284.

Woolf, S. H. (2009). A closer look at the economic argument for disease prevention. *JAMA: The Journal of the American Medical Association, 301*(5), 536–538.

Zautra, A. J., Hall, J. S., & Murray, K. E. (2008). Resilience: a new integrative approach to health and mental health research. *Health Psychology Review, 2*(1), 41–64.

Chapter 13
The Relationship Between Resilience and Motivation

Barbara Resnick

The word "resilience" comes from the Latin word "salire," which means to spring up and the word "resilire" which means to spring back. Resilience, therefore, refers to the capacity to spring back from a physical, emotional, financial, or social challenge. Being resilient indicates that the individual has the human ability to adapt in the face of tragedy, trauma, adversity, hardship, and ongoing significant life stressors (Newman 2005). Resilient individuals tend to manifest adaptive behavior, especially with regard to social functioning, morale, and somatic health (Wagnild and Young 1993), and are less likely to succumb to illness (Caplan 1990; O'Connell and Mayo 1998). Resilience, as a component of the individual's personality, develops and changes over time through ongoing experiences with the physical and social environment (Glantz and Johnson 1999; Hegney et al. 2007). Resilience can, therefore, be perceived as a dynamic process that is influenced by life events and challenges (Grotberg 2003; Hardy et al. 2002, 2004). Increasingly, there is evidence that resilience is related to motivation, specifically the motivation to age successfully (Harris 2008) and recover from physical or psychological traumatic events (Charmey 2004; Chow et al. 2007; Sanders et al. 2008).

Older women who have successfully recovered from orthopedic or other stressful events describe themselves as resilient and determined (Resnick et al. 2005; Travis and McAuley 1998) and tend to have better function, mood, and quality of life than those who are less resilient (Hardy et al. 2004). Resilience has also been associated with adjustments following the diagnosis of dementia (Harris 2008), widowhood (Rossi et al. 2007), management of chronic pain (Karoly and Ruehlman 2006), and overall adjustment to the stressors associated with aging (Ong et al. 2006).

Types of Resilience

Resilience has been differentiated into health resilience (Sanders et al. 2008), psychological resilience (Boardman et al. 2008), emotional resilience (Chow et al. 2007), and dispositional resilience (Rossi et al. 2007). Health resilience is the capacity to

B. Resnick (✉)
University of Maryland, Baltimore, MD, USA
e-mail: barbresnick@gmail.com

B. Resnick et al. (eds.), *Resilience in Aging: Concepts, Research, and Outcomes*,
DOI 10.1007/978-1-4419-0232-0_13, © Springer Science+Business Media, LLC 2011

maintain good health in the face of significant adversity. Psychological resilience is focused on being able to maintain a positive affect regardless of the situation. Emotional resilience is described as the ability to maintain the separation between positive and negative emotion in times of stress. Dispositional resilience incorporates three personality characteristics including commitment to others, a sense of control over outcomes, and a willingness to learn from the current situation. All of these different types of resilience reflect being able to maintain a positive attitude and endure through any variety of health related, emotional, or social challenges. Moreover, it is anticipated that resilience translates across areas of physical and mental health.

Factors that Influence Resilience

Many factors or qualities within individuals have been associated with resilience (Table 13.1). These include such things as positive interpersonal relationships, incorporating social connectedness with a willingness to extend oneself to others, strong internal resources, having an optimistic or positive affect, keeping things in perspective, setting goals and taking steps to achieve those goals, high self-esteem, high self-efficacy, determination, and spirituality which includes purpose of life, religiousness or a belief in a higher power, creativity, humor, and a sense of curiosity (Boardman et al. 2008; Bonanno et al. 2007; Hegney et al. 2007; Kinsel 2005; Tedeschi and Kilmer 2005).

Positive Interpersonal Relationships

Interpersonal relationships include interactions with a network of family, friends, colleagues, and other acquaintances for enjoyment, or to provide psychological or physical assistance for in return. Involvement in interpersonal relationships and activities, whether receiving or giving the help, serves as a psychological buffer

Table 13.1 Resilient qualities or traits commonly noted in older adults

Positive interpersonal relationships
Strong self-efficacy
Positive self-esteem
A sense of purpose
Spirituality
Ability to use humor
Creativity
Acceptance of changes (physical and mental)
Maintaining a positive attitude
Ability to identify and utilize resources
Self-determination
Optimism

against stress, anxiety, or depression which commonly occurs with aging. Interpersonal activities also help individuals cope with losses, maintain a sense of belonging, and strengthen self-esteem and self-efficacy.

Strong Internal Resources: Self-Efficacy, Self-Esteem, Determination, Problem Solving

Self-efficacy, which is described in detail below, is the belief in one's ability to organize and execute a course of action to achieve a specific outcome, and is thereby relevant to resilience. Different than self-efficacy, self-esteem is reflective of one's appraisal of his or her self-worth. Individuals who have a positive self-worth, accept and like themselves, and refrain from being "too hard on themselves" tend to be resilient and psychologically successful (Byles and Pachana 2006). The ability to accept oneself is particularly important in aging due to the many physical and mental changes that can occur, as well as the role losses. With age, for example, the older individual may note impairments in his or her ability to go up the stairs, carry grocery bags, complete a crossword puzzle, or remember how to get to a daughter's home. These changes can be devastating unless one has the resilience to accept the change and appreciate what he or she is still able to do. Self-esteem need not, however, decline with age despite the commonly experienced physical and mental changes that occur such as declines in strength and memory. Rather, self-esteem can be strengthened by helping older adults to recall prior successes and by exposing them to situations in which they can exceed and excel.

Determination, or hardiness, which may in part be a personality trait, can be strengthened by helping the older individual to focus on his or her abilities, current opportunities, and use of resources. Determined individuals tend to be more confident in their ability to cope and to take advantage of the resources, internal and external, that help them to adjust, accept, and cope with the challenges encountered in life. Strengthening determination and hardiness can be done by helping the individual to problem solve and stay focused on the positive rather than the negative – the "I can" versus "I can't" perspective. It is also helpful to remind the older adult how he or she handled stressful situations in the past and re-invigorate those prior strengths and abilities.

Optimism, Positivism, and Keeping Things in Perspective

Repeatedly it has been noted that focusing on positive outcomes and avoiding a focus on negative facts is critical to resilience (Greene and Graham 2009; Harris 2008). Positive emotions and the use of humor are recommended as a way to help eliminate, or cancel out, the impact of negative emotions. Older adults can be helped to manage negative emotions and negativism in the face of challenges, and to stay focused on positive events and feelings that may be occurring at the same time.

Spirituality

Spirituality, considered broadly, includes a sense of self and purpose, creativity, humor, and a curiosity and willingness to learn and experience new things. With regard to resilience spirituality is conceptualized more broadly. Spirituality includes establishing a sense of connection to others and a purpose. Spiritual activities that are reflective of resilience include such things as marching for world peace, exploring creative endeavors and taking art classes, and trying new activities (e.g, learning to play an instrument or speak a foreign language).

Motivation

Motivation, as previously described, is based on an inner urge rather than stimulated in response to adversity or challenge. Motivation refers to the need, drive, or desire to act in a certain way to achieve a certain end. Motivation is different from compliance in that compliance refers to doing what others want or ask rather than being truly motivated and driven by an inner desire. Ideally, health care providers want older adults to be motivated to comply with behaviors that are known to be effective in preventing disease and disability and improving overall health and quality of life.

Motivation is generally behavior or activity specific. An older adult may be motivated to spend the day lying in bed or to engage in physical activity, to learn a new language or creative skill, to take a prescribed medication or to skip the medication. Motivation has been conceptualized as a uni-dimensional concept focused on intrinsic personality components as well as a multidimensional concept that is influenced by many variables both intrinsic and extrinsic to the individual. The extrinsic factors include such things as social interactions with friends, family, and health care providers and the environment.

Factors that Influence Motivation

To comprehensively consider the many factors that influence motivation in older adults it is helpful to use a model of motivation (Fig. 13.1). As with resilience, these factors include traits of the individual as well as external resources that can be used to strengthen motivation in any given area. This model is based on social cognitive theory as well as empirical findings (Albright et al. 2005; Damush et al. 2005; Netz and Raviv 2004; Wilcox et al. 2005). According to social cognitive theory (Bandura 1997), human motivation and action are regulated by forethought. This cognitive control of behavior is based on two types of expectations: (1) self-efficacy expectations, which are the individuals' beliefs in their capabilities to perform a course of action to attain a desired outcome and (2) outcome expectancies, which are the beliefs that a certain consequence will be produced by personal action.

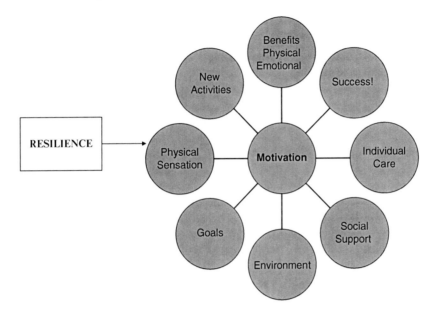

Fig. 13.1 A model of motivation and the relationship between resilience and motivation

Beliefs, both in relationship to outcomes (outcome expectations) and with regard to what older adults believe they are capable of doing (self-efficacy expectations), have been noted to influence motivation to engage in health promoting behaviors (Dohnke et al. 2005; McAuley et al. 2006; Resnick et al. 2008c). The benefits experienced by the individual such as improvement in blood pressure, ability to walk a longer distance without getting short of breath, or the improvement in mood associated with physical activity or adherence to a medication are critical to motivation in older adults. Pleasant or unpleasant physical sensations experienced by older adults are particularly relevant to motivation as with age there is a tendency to focus on immediate benefits (e.g., feeling good after exercising) associated with a behavior rather than remaining motivated to engage in the behavior for a long-term benefit (e.g., weight loss, decreased cardiovascular disease). Conversely, pain associated with an activity such as walking or climbing the stairs, or the belief that performing these activities will result in pain, will decrease the older adults motivation to engage in the activity. Alternating these beliefs and/or eliminating the negative sensations associated with the activity are critical to strengthening motivation and engaging the individual in the given activity.

Successful completion of an activity, particularly if this is done without experiencing unpleasant sensations, is one of the most effective ways to strengthen older adults' beliefs in their ability to perform the behavior and thereby increase motivation to continue to engage in the behavior. Being able, for example, to walk for 30 min or complete a dance class will increase the likelihood that the individual will return to the class another time and continue to engage in the activity.

Enhancing Motivation

Individualized care and demonstrating caring has an important influence on the older adults' motivation to perform a given activity. Individualized care includes recognizing individual differences and needs, using kindness and humor, empowering older adults to take an active part in their care, providing gentle verbal persuasion to perform an activity, positive reinforcement after performing (Resnick et al. 2006b, 2008a; Wilcox et al. 2005), and knowing when to confront the individual about his or her harmful health behaviors (e.g., not taking prophylactic medication or engaging in regular activity). An essential component of individualized care is letting the individual know *exactly* what it is recommended. This may be simple written instructions about what exercise program to engage in or what medication to take, why it is important, and exactly how the activity should be done or the medication should be taken. At each care interaction, it is critical to re-evaluate how the individual is doing with the behavior of interest. Checking with the individual and re-evaluating progress demonstrates that the provider cares about whether or not the activity is performed. Individualized care may initially be effective because the older adult simply wants to reciprocate for the care given to him or her by doing what the health care provider or family member requests (e.g., doing a certain exercise). Once the behavior is initiated, however, it is likely that the older individual will experience the benefit(s) associated with the behavior and thus continue to adhere for reasons beyond initial reciprocity for care received.

Social support networks including family, friends, peers, and health care providers are important determinants of behavior (Jackson 2006; Kim and Sobal 2004; Thrasher et al. 2004). Repeatedly, motivation to exercise, for example, has been found to be influenced by the social milieu of the individual and/or the care setting. Social interactions can alter recovery trajectories by disrupting the progression of functional limitations to disability. The influence of any member of the individual's social network, however, can have a positive or negative influence depending on his/her philosophy and beliefs related to activity of interest. Social supports can directly serve as powerful external motivators by (1) providing encouragement; (2) helping the older adult feel cared for and cared about; and (3) helping to establish goals such as regaining self-care abilities, and being able to return home alone. Social supports can also indirectly impact motivation by strengthening the individual's beliefs in his or her ability to participate in rehabilitation activities, for example, or engaging in a regular exercise program.

The environment can also influence motivation. Environments that offer opportunities for physical activity (e.g., parks or wide open clutter free hallways), access to staircases, or heart healthy food options can increase motivation to adhere to the recommended activity (Booth et al. 2000). The ability to develop personal goals and evaluate one's performance toward that goal can influence motivation to engage in a given behavior (Bandura 1997). Articulated goals give older adults something to work toward, and help motivate them to adhere to a specific health promoting activity. Short-term goals provide the older individual with exactly what he or she should do on a daily basis (e.g., walk for 20 min; do ten sit to stands). Long-term goals focus on what the individual wants to achieve such as being able to ambulate without an assistive device, being able to care for oneself, being able to walk to the grocery store, or to go on a trip. Goals are most effective when they are (1) related to a specific behavior; (2) challenging, but realistically attainable; and (3) achievable in the near future (Bandura 1997).

Exposure to new and different activities, such as Tai Chi classes or creative art classes, tends to motivate older adults to adhere to these classes and be willing to expand and try additional new activities (Resnick et al. 2005). Lastly, the individual's personality and self-determination have an important influence on motivation. Older adults report that it is their own personality, that is, determination, and their own firm resolutions and adherence to those resolutions, that motivates them to perform specific tasks (King et al. 1992).

Relationship Between Motivation and Resilience

Similarities Between Motivation and Resilience

There are some similar factors that are associated with both resilience and motivation such as determination, self-efficacy, being open and willing to experience new things, and social supports. The capacity to be resilient and/or motivated is present in everyone and choices are made in the face of routine and challenging situations to be motivated and/or resilient. Motivation related to engaging in physical activities is high in some people while others are highly motivated to sit in a chair or lie in a bed. Conversely, some older adults are motivated to take classes in a senior center while others refuse to even consider this and are motivated to sit daily and watch television alone. Some individuals are resilient with regard to physical challenges but cannot cope with challenges associated with finances or cognitive changes. Both resilience and motivation can be strengthened through appropriate interventions and exposure to life experiences. Strengthening factors that influence motivation and resilience such as self-efficacy, self-esteem, positive relationships with others, sense of purpose, and learning to keep things in perspective are all ways in which older adults can strengthen motivation and resilience (Bandura 1997; Newman 2005; Tedeschi and Kilmer 2005). Thus, there are traits and characteristics of individuals associated with resilience and motivation as well as external factors that can impact resilience and motivation as individuals respond to challenges or activities within their lives.

Differences Between Motivation and Resilience

Resilience, unlike motivation, relies on the individual experiencing a life challenge or some type of adversity. These challenges may be developmental challenges such as those associated with normal aging (e.g., vision changes), or they maybe social and/or economic challenges such as those experienced by the loss of employment, the loss of a spouse, or a move into an assisted living facility. Conversely, motivation is not dependent on an adverse event or challenge; rather motivation is a necessary component for all activity. Routine personal care activities such as bathing and dressing require motivation, as do making plans to have dinner with a friend or play cards. Resilience would be required, however, when the individual is faced with bathing and dressing challenges following a wrist fracture. It is only when an activity does not occur that questions are raised as to the level of motivation of the individual. Resilience is a process of coping with stressors, adversity, change, or opportunity. The individual is forced to pass through stages of biopsychospiritual homeostasis (i.e., adaptation physically, mentally, and spiritually to a set of circumstances), disruption, and finally reintegration. Resilience, or successful reintegration, involves coping with the adversity such that there is personal growth, an increase in knowledge and self-understanding, and an increased strength of his or her resilient qualities. Unfortunately, resilient reintegration does not always occur. Some individuals may recover from a challenge with a permanent loss, such as the loss of function due to a stroke. These individuals may give up hope of recovery and may not return to a state of optimal homeostasis. There is also the possibility that dysfunctional reintegration will occur and the individual might resort to use of alcohol or other destructive behaviors, become depressed, and isolate him or herself as a way to cope with the challenge.

Interaction of Motivation and Resilience

The current work in resilience theory and understanding of this concept is focused on the individuals' response to challenges and the use of resilience. It is believed that all individuals have the innate ability to return to homeostasis successfully and to transform, change, and grow, regardless of age (Werner and Smith 1992). The individual must summon the motivation, in the face of adversity, to be resilient. Thus, motivation may be present independent of resilience, but resilience depends on the individual being motivated to successfully reintegrate. Resilient reintegration requires increased energy, or motivation, for resilience to successfully occur.

Empirical Evidence of the Relationship Between Motivation and Resilience

Prior research has repeatedly demonstrated that resilience, or the factors that are reflective of resilience such as vitality and extraversion, were predictive of the factors that are generally conceptualized as indicative of motivation such as self-efficacy, physical activity, and active coping (Engel et al. 2004; Fredrickson 2001; Ingledew et al. 2004). Moreover, there is evidence that motivation serves as a mediator for resilience in older adults. As part of the KNEE study (Wright et al.

2008), a longitudinal intervention study aimed at reducing levels of pain and disability in a sample of community dwelling older adults with knee osteoarthritis, participants completed a comprehensive baseline survey including multiple psychosocial measures such as negative and positive affect, self-efficacy, and health status, as well as reports of physical activity. The sample included 275 older adults with degenerative joint disease. Resilience was conceptualized in this study as positive affect, vitality, and extraversion. Motivation was conceptualized as self-efficacy and measured using the arthritis self-efficacy scale which addresses self-efficacy for function, pain management, and the ability to control other arthritis symptoms. The relationship between resilience, motivation, and physical activity was tested using structural equation modeling. As hypothesized, resilience was mediated by self-efficacy and thus resilience was indirectly related to function through self-efficacy.

In a study that included 163 older adults living in a continuing care retirement community, the mediating effects of motivation on resilience and the impact of motivation and resilience on physical activity were also tested (Resnick and D'Adamo manuscript submitted). Data were collected for this study as part of an annual health promotion survey and residents completed interviews that included measures of physical activity (Dipietro et al. 1993), self-efficacy related to physical activity (Resnick and Jenkins 2000), and the 14-item Resilience Scale (Wagnild 2009). As demonstrated in the KNEE study, the relationship between resilience and physical activity was mediated by self-efficacy (Resnick and D'Adamo manuscript submitted).

These studies provide some empirical support for the premise that resiliency is present in everyone but when faced with a challenge, at least a physical or functional challenge, motivation is needed so that physical recovery or predetermined goals (e.g., being able to walk a certain distance) can be achieved. Both resiliency and motivation are necessary for optimal recovery to occur. Understanding the similarities and differences between these two concepts and their relationships provides important background for the development of appropriate interventions to innervate resilience and strengthen motivation and thereby improve recovery across a variety of clinical situations.

Practical Applications of Resilience

Assessment of Resilience

Increasingly resilience is believed to be a human ability that can be developed over time. Older adults, by virtue of surviving through decades of life experiences, tend to be resilient (Nygren et al. 2005). These individuals have lived through losses including physical changes such as declines in vision, hearing, or physical abilities, social losses such as loss of parents, siblings, spouses, and in some cases children, and role-related losses. Although they may not have been successfully resilient in all of these experiences, they have accrued some positive experiences in which they were resilient and motivated and thus recovered from the challenge experienced. Thus, when working with older adults it is particularly helpful to explore prior challenges and establish strengths with regard to recovery that suggest resilience and motivation.

Talking with individuals about past experiences may be the most comprehensive way to establish prior evidence of resilience. However, the stories provided may be difficult to interpret. As an alternative to a qualitative assessment of resilience, scales reflecting individual correlates of resilience such as self-efficacy, coping, optimism, vitality, or self-esteem can be utilized. Table 13.2 provides examples of

Table 13.2 Measures of resilience used among older adults

Measure	Description
The 25- and 14-item Resilience Scale (Wagnild and Young 1993)	The 25- and 14-item Resilience Scale was developed as a general measure of resilience for adults across the lifespan. Initially, the measure included 25 items reflecting five interrelated components that constitute resilience: Equanimity reflecting the ability to "go with the flow"; perseverance or determination; self-reliance reflecting a belief in one's ability to manage; meaningfulness or a belief that life has meaning; and existential aloneness or a sense of uniqueness. Participants respond by either agreeing or disagreeing with the statements on a scale of 1 (disagree) to 7 (agree). The responses are summed and a higher score reflects stronger resilience. Prior research has demonstrated evidence of internal consistency (alpha coefficient of 0.91), test–retest reliability, and construct validity of the measure based on a significant correlation between resilience and life satisfaction, morale, and depression when used with older adults (Wagnild and Young 1993)
The Resilience Scale (Hardy et al. 2004)	To complete the resilience scale participants identify the most stressful life event they experienced in the past 5 years and respond to a series of nine questions about their response to that event. There was evidence of internal consistency with an alpha coefficient of 0.70, and test–retest r eliability with an intraclass correlation of coefficient of 0.57. Validity was based on a significant correlation between resilience and having few depressive symptoms, and good to excellent self-rate(d?) health (Hardy et al. 2004).
Dispositional Resilience Scale (DRS) (Rossi et al. 2007; Friborg et al. 1997)	The DRS is a 45-item questionnaire that includes 15 commitment, 15 control, and 15 challenge items. There is a 4-point scale response used to rate participant agreement with items ranging from 1 (completely true) to 4 (not at all true). A total dispositional resilience score is created based on responses. The original DRS was modified to be appropriate for older adults (Rossi et al. 2007). There was evidence of internal consistency with an alpha of 0.83, and validity based on a statistically significant relationship between sense of coherence and Hopkins symptom checklist, and a statistically significant difference in Dispositional Resilience among patients and healthy volunteers (Friborg et al. 1997)

some of the more commonly used measures reflective of resilience. In addition, there are several measures that address different aspects of resilience including dispositional resilience, physical resilience, psychological resilience, or a measure of general resilience. These measures can be completed during a clinical assessment of a patient to gain insight as to the strength of his or her resilience.

Interventions to Strengthen Resilience

Interventions to stimulate and build resilience are focused in three areas: (1) developing disposition attributes of the individual such as vigor, optimism, and physical robustness; (2) improving socialization practices; and (3) strengthening self-efficacy, self-esteem, and motivation through interpersonal interactions as well as experiences.

These three areas are not necessarily mutually exclusive and the interventions that can strengthen physical robustness may improve socialization practices and strengthen self-efficacy. For example, encouraging an older adult to participate in a dance class because he or she enjoys dance and has previously excelled in this activity may also increase socialization and strengthen self-efficacy and self-esteem.

It is important not to oversimplify interventions to strengthen resilience or ignore the larger context in which the individual lives. For example, recommending participation in a dance class for an individual who lives in a community in which such activity is considered frivolous or an insufficient source of physical activity may result in decreasing self-esteem and can have a negative impact on resilience. Thus, multifaceted approaches to optimizing resilience are needed. Risk-oriented strategies should be considered with all interventions to help assure that older adults are not exposed to experiences that might decrease resilience. Environmental interventions such as chairs, beds, and toilets that facilitate successful transfers are needed to assure that resilience is not undermined. Social networking systems that help disseminate opportunities for successful activities and increase reach to older adults are likewise important and useful interventions to consider when trying to strengthen resilience. The Strength-Focused and Meaning-Oriented Approach to Resilience and Transformation (SMART) Intervention (Chan et al. 2006) is another example of a multifaceted approach to strengthen resilience in response to trauma that incorporated Eastern spiritual teaching, physical techniques such as yoga, and psycho-education that promoted meaning reconstruction.

Interventions to Strengthen Motivation

Motivation is necessary for resilience to be activated following a challenge. Although it may be difficult to motivate older adults to engage in certain activities (e.g., exercise, medication adherence), there is evidence to support that interventions, particularly those based on the theory of self-efficacy, are effective (King et al. 2007; Resnick et al. 2007, 2008b). Likewise, effective interventions include those that are guided by a social ecological model (Fleury and Lee 2006; Gregson et al. 2003) which considers intrapersonal, interpersonal, environmental factors and policy.

Table 13.3 describes specific interventions that can be used to motivate older adults to engage in specific activities. First and foremost, it is critical to establish whose motives are being addressed in the motivational interaction. If goals are established without the input of the older individual it is not likely he or she will be willing to participate in the activities needed to achieve the goal. For individuals who are cognitively impaired and cannot articulate goals, it is useful to review old records and speak with families, friends, and caregivers who have known the individual previously. Goals can then be developed based on their prior life and accomplishments (Galik et al. 2008). Further it is important that the goals established be realistic and achievable so as to assure feelings of success.

Demonstrations of caring on the part of the interventionist are central to motivating older adults. Care can be demonstrated by behaviors and activities perceived by the individual as expressions of love, attention, concern, respect, and support (Boynton and Boynton 2005; Resnick et al. 2005). Another important aspect of caring is setting some guidelines or limits with regard to behaviors. This does not relate to punishment or threats. Rather, it is focused on being firm and informing the individual of the activity they need to do and why they need to do it. For example, an older individual may need to get up and walk to the bathroom to prevent skin breakdown, optimize continence, and regain strength and function.

Examining the setting in which behaviors are expected to occur is also important to motivation. Simple interventions such as eliminating background noise and speaking slow, low, and loud can help with the communication that is needed between an older adult and the interventionist. Altering the physical environment so that the older individual can perform successfully is an important first step in motivation. Continued alteration in the environment maybe needed, however, to assure that physically the individual is challenged in such a way as to optimize function and provide the ongoing goals for motivation. For example, initially motivating an older adult to be independent with toileting might mean putting a commode chair right by the bedside. Once successful, the distance between the bed and commode could be extended with an ultimate goal being to walk all the way to the bathroom.

Addressing outcome expectations associated with an activity, particularly the immediate unpleasant sensation that may be occurring is critical to motivation in older adults. Sensations such as fear of falling or fear of exacerbating underlying medical problems, pain, and shortness of breath or fatigue associated with an activity are likely to decrease motivation to engage in the activity. Interventions to overcome these sensations such as graded activity or graded exposure treatments (Jong et al. 2005; George et al. 2008) have been shown to increase individuals' willingness to persist with an exercise program. Graded activity starts by finding out how much activity the individual can do before the unpleasant sensation occurs (e.g., pain or fear). The training starts at that level of exercise or activity. The individual is

Table 13.3 Interventions to strengthen motivation

Focus of intervention	Examples of intervention techniques
Beliefs	Interventions to strengthen efficacy beliefs are as follows:
	1. Verbal encouragement of capability to perform
	2. Expose older adult to role models (similar to others who successfully perform the activity)
	3. Decrease unpleasant sensations associated with the activity
	4. Encourage actual performance/practice of the activity
	5. Educate about the benefits of the behavior and reinforce and underline those benefits
	6. Teach realistic beliefs
	7. Relate behavior to outcomes (e.g., exercise reduces blood pressure and causes weight loss)
Elimination of unpleasant sensations (e.g., pain, fear)	1. Facilitate appropriate use of pain medications to relieve discomfort
	2. Use alternative measures such as heat/ice to relieve pain associated with the activity
	3. Cognitive behavioral therapy:
	(a) Explore thoughts and feelings related to sensations
	(b) Help patient develop a more realistic attitude to the pain, that is, pain will not cause further bone damage
	(c) Relaxation and distraction techniques
	(d) Graded exposure to overcome fear of falling
Individualized care	1. Demonstrating kindness and caring to the patient
	2. Use of humor
	3. Positive reinforcement following a desired behavior
	4. Recognition of individual needs and differences such as setting a rest period or providing a favorite snack
	5. Clearly and simply write out/inform patient of what activity is recommended
Social supports	1. Evaluate the presence and adequacy of social network
	2. Teach significant other(s) to verbally encourage/reinforce the desired behavior
	3. Use social supports as a source of goal identification
Goal identification	1. Develop appropriate realistic goals with the older adult
	2. Set goals that can be met in a short time frame (daily or weekly) as well as a long range goal to work toward
	3. Set goals that are challenging but attainable
	4. Set goals that are clear and specific
	5. Identify and use rewards that have meaning to the individual
Successful performance	1. Review prior times challenges overcome and skills and techniques utilized
	2. Expose the individual to activities in which he or she can be successful
	3. Continue to build challenges into the activity so that new successes can be incorporated

guided in a way that will help build tolerance to the unpleasant sensation by slowly increasing duration, intensity, and frequency of the exercise or activity that was noted to cause the pain or the fear. In contrast, graded exposure treatment involves presenting the individual with anxiety-producing material (e.g., having him or her engage in an activity that causes pain) for a long enough time to decrease the intensity of their emotional reaction. Ultimately, the feared situation no longer results in the individual becoming anxious or avoiding the activity.

Managing Apathy

Apathy or a lack of interest, concern, or emotion has been conceptualized as the opposite of motivation (Marin 1991). Although not pervasive among all older adults, apathy is common particularly among those with dementia and depression (Marin 1991). Interventions include the use of pharmacological agents including amantadine, amphetamine, bromocriptine, bupropion, methylphenidate, and selegiline (Marin et al. 1995), cholinesterase inhibitors (Whyte et al. 2008), and selective serontonic reuptake inhibitors (Padala et al. 2007), and focus on structure and stimulation such that the individual is encouraged to engage in activities that he or she can easily do successfully. It may be necessary to persistently encourage and actually accompany the apathetic individual to an activity and provide one-on-one encouragement to keep them engaged.

Conclusion

Resilience and motivation are related but separate concepts and together serve as keys to successful aging. Resilience emphasizes the older individual's capacity to respond to a challenge or adversity and motivation provides the impetus to engage in the behaviors needed to recover. A focus on resilience and motivation is an innovative way to optimize aging and buffer many physical and psychosocial losses. Helping older adults sustain their resilient characteristics and implementing motivational intervention in times of physical, emotional, social, or economic crises can result in helping the individual through the challenging situation and facilitating personal growth beyond the immediate event through the posttraumatic or postchallenge period.

References

Albright CL, Pruitt L, Castro C, Gonzalez A, Woo S, & King AC (2005). Modifying physical activity in a multiethnic sample of low-income women: One-year results from the IMPACT (Increasing Motivation for Physical ACTivity) project. *Annals of Behavioral Medicine, 30*(3), 191–200.

Bandura A (1997). *Self-efficacy: The exercise of control*. New York: W.H. Freeman and Company.

Boardman JD, Blalock CL, & Button TM (2008). Sex differences in the heritability of resilience. *Twin Research and Human Genetics, 11*(1), 12–27.

Bonanno GA, Galea S, Bucciarelli A, & Vlahov D (2007). What predicts psychological resilience after disaster? The role of demographics, resources, and life stress. *Death Studies, 31*(10), 863–883.

Booth ML, Owen N, Bauman A, Clavisi O, & Leslie E (2000). Social-cognitive and perceived environment influences associated with physical activity in older Australians. *Preventive Medicine, 31*(1), 15–22.

Boynton M & Boynton CA (2005). *The educator's guide to preventing and solving discipline problems*. Alexandria, VA: The Association for Supervision and Curriculum Development.

Byles JE & Pachana N (2006). Social circumstances, social support, ageing and health: Findings from the Australian Longitudinal Study on Women's Health (2006). Available at http://en.scientificcommons.org/n_pachana. Last accessed June 2009.

Caplan G (1990). Loss, stress, and mental health. *Community mental health journal, 26*, 27–48.

Chan CL, Chan TH, & Ng SM (2006). The Strength-focused and Meaning-Oriented Approach to Resilience and Transformation (SMART): A body-mind-spirit approach to trauma management. *Social Work Health Care, 43*(2), 9–36.

Charmey DS (2004). Psychobiological mechanisms of resilience and vulnerability: Implications for successful adaptation to extreme stress. *American Journal of Psychiatry, 16*(1), 195–216.

Chow SM, Hamagani F, & Nesselroade JR (2007). Age differences in dynamical emotion-cognition linkages. *Psychol Aging. 22*(4), 765–780.

Damush T, Perkins SM, Mikesky AE, Roberts M, & O'Dea J (2005). Motivational factors influencing older adults diagnosed with knee osteoarthritis to join and maintain an exercise program. *Journal of Aging and Physical Activity, 13*(1), 45–60.

de Jong JR, Vlaeyen J, Onghena P, Goossens ME, Geilen M, & Mulder H (2005). Fear of movement/(re)injury in chronic low back pain: Education or exposure in vivo as mediator to fear reduction? *Clinical Journal of Pain, 21*(1), 9–17.

Dipietro L, Caspersen CJ, Ostfeld AM, & Nadel ER (1993). A survey for assessing physical activity among older adults. *Medicine Science Sports and Exercise, 25*(5), 628–642.

Dohnke B, Knäuper B, & Müller-Fahrnow W (2005). Perceived self-efficacy gained from, and health effects of, a rehabilitation program after hip joint replacement. *Arthritis and Rheumatism, 53*(4), 585–592.

Engel C, Hamilton NA, Potter P, & Zautra AJ (2004). Impact of two types of expectancy on recovery from total knee replacement surgery in adults with osteoarthritis. *Behavioral Medicine, 30*, 113–123.

Fleury J & Lee SM (2006). The social ecological model and physical activity in African American women. *American Journal of Community Psychology, 1*, 1–8.

Fredrickson BL (2001). The role of positive emotions in positive psychology. The broaden-and-build theory of positive emotions. *American Psychologist, 563*, 218–226.

Friborg O, Hjemdal O, Rosenvinge JH, & Matinussen M (1997). A new rating scale for adult resilience: What are the central protective resources behind healthy adjustment? *International Journal of Methods in Psychiatric Research, 12*(2), 65–76.

Galik EM, Resnick B, Gruber-Baldini A, Nahm ES, Pearson K, & Pretzer-Aboff I (2008). Pilot testing of the restorative care intervention for the cognitively impaired. *Journal of the American Medical Directors Association, 9*(7), 516–522.

George SZ, Zeppieri G Jr, Cere AL, Cere MR, Borut MS, Hodges MJ, et al. (2008). A randomized trial of behavioral physical therapy interventions for acute and sub-acute low back pain. *Pain, 140*(1), 145–157.

Glantz M & Johnson J (1999). *Resliience and Development Positive Life Adaptations*. New York: Kluwer Academic Press.

Greene RR & Graham SA (2009). Role of resilience among Nazi Holocaust survivors: A strength-based paradigm for understanding survivorship. *Family and Community Health, 32*(1 suppl), S75–S82.

Gregson J, Foerster S, Orr R, Jones L, Benedict J, Clark B, et al. (2003). System, environment and policy changes: Using the social ecological model as a framework for evaluating nutrition education and social marketing programs with low income audiences. *Journal of Nutrition Education, 33*, S4–S15.

Grotberg EH (2003). *Resilience for today: Gaining strength from adversity.* Wesport, CT: Praeger.

Hardy S, Concato J, & Gill TM (2004). Resilience of community-dwelling older persons. *Journal of the American Geriatrics Society, 52*(2), 257–262.

Harris PB (2008). Another wrinkle in the debate about successful aging: The undervalued concept of resilience and the lived experience of dementia. *International Journal of Aging and Human Development, 67*(1), 43–61.

Hegney DG, Buikstra E, Baker P, Rogers-Clark C, Pearce S, Ross H, et al. (2007). Individual resilience in rural people: A Queensland study, Australia. *Rural and Remote health, 7*(4), 620–625.

Ingledew DK, Markland D, & Sheppard KE (2004). Personality and self-determination of exercise behavior. *Personality and Individual Differences, 368*, 1921–1932.

Jackson T (2006). Relationships between perceived close social support and health practices within community samples of American women and men. *Journal of Psychology, 40*(3), 229–246.

Karoly P, & Ruehlman LS (2006). Psychological "resilience" and its correlates in chronic pain: findings from a national community sample. *Pain. 123*(1–2), 90–97.

Kim KH & Sobal J (2004). Religion, social support, fat intake and physical activity. *Public Health and Nutrition, 7*(6), 773–781.

King AC, Friedman R, Marcus B, Castro C, Napolitano M, Ahn D, et al. (2007). Ongoing physical activity advice by humans versus computers: The Community Health Advice by Telephone (CHAT) trial. *Health Psychology, 26*(6), 718–727.

King A, Blair SN, Bild D, Dishman R, Dubbert P, Marcus B, Oldridge N, Paffenbarger R, Powell K, & Yeager K (1992). Determinants of physical activity and interventions in adults. *Medicine and Science in Sports and Exercise, 24*, 3221–3223.

Kinsel B (2005). Resilience as adaptation in older women. *Journal of Women and Aging, 17*(3), 23–39.

Marin RS (1991). Apathy: A neuropsychiatric syndrome. *J Neuropsychiatry and Clinical Neurosciences, 3*(3), 243–254.

Marin RS, Fogel BS, Hawkins J, Duffy J, & Krupp B (1995). Apathy: A treatable syndrome. *Journal of Neuropsychiatry and Clinical Neurosciences, 7*, 23–30.

McAuley E, Konopack JF, Motl RW, Morris KS, Doerksen SE, & Rosengren KR (2006). Physical activity and quality of life in older adults: Influence of health status and self-efficacy. *Annals of Behavioral Medicine, 31*, 99–103.

Netz Y & Raviv S (2004). Age differences in motivational orientation toward physical activity: An application of social-cognitive theory. *Journal of Psychology, 138*(1), 35–48.

Newman R (2005). APA's resilience initiative. *Professional Psychology: Research and Practice, 36*(2), 227–229.

Nygren B, Jonsen E, Gustafson Y, Norberg A, & Lundman B (2005). Resilience, sense of coherence, purpose in life and self-transcendence in relation to perceived physical and mental health among the oldest old. *Aging & Mental Health, 9*(4), 354–362.

O'Connell R, & Mayo J (1998). The role of social factors in affective disorders: a review. *Hospital and community Psychiatry, 39*, 842–851.

Ong AD, Bergeman CS, Bisconti TL, & Wallace KA (2006). Psychological resilience, positive emotions, and successful adaptation to stress in later life. *J Pers Soc Psychol, 91*(4), 730–749.

Padala PR, Burke W, & Bhatia SC (2007). Modafinil therapy for apathy in an elderly patient. *Annals of Pharmacotherapy, 41*(2), 346–349.

Resnick B & D'Adamo C. (In press). Wellness Center Use and Factors Associated with Physical Activity Among Older Adults in A CCRC Setting. Rehabilitation Nursing.

Resnick B & Jenkins L (2000). Testing the reliability and validity of the self-efficacy for exercise scale. *Nursing Research, 49*(3), 154–159.

Resnick B, Vogel A, & Luisi D (2006b). Motivating minority older adults to exercise. *Cultural Diversity and Ethnic Minority Psychology, 3,* 17–21.

Resnick B, Orwig D, Yu-Yahiro J, Hawkes W, Shardell M, Hebel J, et al. (2007). Testing the effectiveness of the exercise plus program in older women post-hip fracture. *Annals of Behavioral Medicine, 34*(1), 67–76.

Resnick B, Orwig D, Zimmerman S, Simpson M, & Magaziner J (2005). The Exercise Plus Program for Older Women Post Hip Fracture: Participant Perspectives. *The Gerontologist, 45*(4), 539–544.

Resnick B, Petzer-Aboff I, Galik E, Russ K, Cayo J, Simpson M, et al. (2008a). Barriers and benefits to implementing a restorative care intervention in nursing homes. *Journal of the American Medical Directors Association, 9*(2), 102–108.

Resnick B, Luisi D, & Vogel A (2008b). Testing the Senior Exercise Self-efficacy Pilot Project (SESEP) for use with urban dwelling minority older adults. *Public Health Nursing, 25*(3), 221–234.

Resnick B, Michael K, Shaughnessy M, Nahm ES, Kobunek S, & Sorkin J, et al. (2008c). Inflated perceptions of physical activity after stroke: Pairing self-report with physiologic measures. *Journal of Physical Activity and Health, 5*(2), 308–318.

Rossi NE, Bisconti TL, & Bergeman CS (2007). The role of dispositional resilience in regaining life satisfaction after the loss of a spouse. *Death Studies, 31*(10), 863–883.

Sanders AE, Lim S, & Sohn W (2008). Resilience to urban poverty: Theoretical and empirical considerations for population health. *Am J Public Health. 98*(6), 1101–1106.

Tedeschi RG & Kilmer RP (2005). Assessing strengths, resilience, and growth to guide clinical interventions. *Professional Psychology: Research and Practice, 36*(3), 230–237.

Thrasher JF, Campbell MK, & Oates V (2004). Behavior-specific social support for healthy behaviors among African American church members: Applying optimal matching theory. *Health Education and Behavior, 31*(2), 193–205.

Travis SS, & McAuley WJ (1998). Mentally restorative experiences supporting rehabilitation of high functioning elders recovering from hip surgery. *J Adv Nurs, 27*(5), 977–985.

Wagnild GM (2009). The Resilience Scale User's Guide. Available for purchase at www.resiliencecenter.com. Last accessed June 2009.

Wagnild G & Young H (1993). Development and psychometric evaluation of the resilience scale. *Journal of Nursing Measurement, 1*(2), 165–177.

Werner E & Smith R (1992). *Overcoming the odds: High risk children from birth to adulthood.* Ithaca, NY: Cornell University Press.

Whyte EM, Lenze EJ, Butters M, Skidmore E, Koenig K, Dew MA, et al. (2008). An open-label pilot study of acetylcholinesterase inhibitors to promote functional recovery in elderly cognitively impaired stroke patients. *Cerebrovascular Diseases, 26*(3), 317–321.

Wilcox S, Oberrecht L, Bopp M, Kammermann S, & McElmurray, C (2005). A qualitative study of exercise in older African American and white women in rural South Carolina: Perceptions, barriers, and motivations. *Journal of Women and Aging, 17*(1–2), 37–53.

Wright LJ, Zautra AJ, & Going S (2008). Adaptation to early knee osteoarthritis: The role of risk, resilience, and disease severity on pain and physical functioning. *Annals of Behavioral Medicine, 36*(1), 70–80.

Chapter 14
The Association Between Resilience and Survival Among Chinese Elderly*

Ke Shen and Yi Zeng

Introduction

Resilience, a psychological construct, has been defined differently in extant theoretical writings. Luthar et al. (2000) characterized resilience as a dynamic process encompassing positive adaptation within the context of significant adversity. Lamond et al. (2009) stated that resilience connoted the ability to adapt positively to adversity, or in other words, the ability to bounce back from negative events by using positive emotions to cope (Tugade et al. 2004). The former definition viewed resilience as a dynamic process, whereas the latter regarded it as a personality trait. In this paper, we adopt the second definition.

As researchers and clinicians have become more interested in resilience in recent decades, there is an increasing need for high quality measures of this construct. Wagnild and Young (1993) proposed the 25-item Resilience Scale (RS), representing two factors of resilience: personal competence and acceptance of self and life. More recently, Friborg et al. (2003) developed the 45-item Resilience Scale for Adults (RSA). It aimed to measure the presence of protective resources that promote adult resilience such as personal competence, social competence, family coherence, social support, and personal structure. Connor and Davidson (2003) have developed the 25-item Connor–Davidson Resilience Scale (CD-RISC). In contrast to the RSA, the CD-RISC focused on qualifying resilience itself, and covered five dimensions of resilience including personal competence, tolerance of negative affect and stress-related growth, acceptance of changes, personal control and spiritual orientation. Although particular measurement of resilience for the elderly has not received sufficient attention yet, the RS and the CD-RISC have both been verified to be appropriate for use among older people (Wagnild 2003; Lamond et al. 2009).

*A shorter version of the contents of this chapter was published in Demographic Research 23(5) 105–116. doi: 10.4054/DemRes.2010.23.5

K. Shen (✉)
Peking University, Beijing, China
e-mail: shenke.ccerpku@yahoo.com.cn

A growing focus on healthy aging and the availability of validated resilience scale tools have prompted researchers to investigate the role of resilience in health and survival in a multidisciplinary framework. Resilience scores were demonstrated to be positively correlated with mental health and physical functioning of the elderly (Wagnild 2003; Hardy et al. 2002), as well as with self-rated successful aging (Lamond et al. 2009). Other studies explored how resilience ameliorated the negative effect of adverse events such as loss of a loved one on health and well-being. Windle et al. (2008) discovered that psychological resilience moderated the negative effect of chronic illness on subjective well-being among the elderly aged 60+. Reker (2008) tentatively applied the latent construct approach and structural equation modeling, and found that resilience, either partially or fully, mediated the impact of stress on subjective well-being and physical health of the elderly.

Furthermore, several researchers have been engaged in exploring the mechanism through which resilience exerted a positive impact on survival and health. One possible channel was that resilient elderly were more likely to experience positive emotions (Masten 2001; Ong et al. 2006), and positive emotions were found to promote health and longevity (Levy et al. 2002; Giltay et al. 2004).

However, several limitations confined the development of research on resilience in aging. Above all, most of the prior studies were based on small samples, with especially limited numbers of oldest-old subjects, which restricted the estimation efficiency. Wagnild (2003) evaluated the Resilience Scale in a sample of 43 older adults and Nygren et al. (2005) reexamined the same scale in a sample of 125 Swedish oldest-old aged 85 years and older. Reker's work (2008) was based on a sample of 146 older adults. Lamond et al. (2009) made use of a larger sample of 1,395 community-dwelling elderly aged between 60 and 91 years old; but, all of the subjects were women, which hindered the generalization of the results among the whole population. Windle et al. (2008) utilized a random sample of 1,847 people aged between 50 and 90 from rural and urban areas in England, Wales, and Scotland. In both these studies, the people older than 90 years were not included, even though the fast aging of the elderly population called for more attention to the oldest-old.

Second, many studies were cross-sectional (Hardy et al. 2002; Windle et al. 2008; Lamond et al. 2009), and the few longitudinal designs were conducted to test the psychometric properties of resilience scales such as test–retest correlations (Friborg et al. 2003). Thus, they can only justify the correlation between resilience and current physical/psychological health. Whether resilience is associated with long-term health benefits, especially mortality risk, is not yet explored. A notable exception is the study by Surtees et al. (2006). They applied partial correlation analysis to show that a slower capacity to adapt to the consequences of adverse experience was associated with increased mortality after adjustment for age and sex. However, the authors did not control for initial health status and socio-economic characteristics of the elderly, which may confound the impacts of resilience on survival.

This chapter made use of the 2002–2005 Chinese Longitudinal Healthy Longevity Survey (CLHLS) dataset, covering 16,064 Chinese elderly aged 65 and older. The CLHLS was initiated to meet the needs of scientific research on the oldest-old (older than 80 years) in the 1998 baseline survey, and further expanded to also cover the young-old aged 65–79 years in the 2002 and 2005 survey.

The purpose of our study is to explore the impact of total resilience scores as well as each resilience indicator on the mortality risks of Chinese elderly.

Our research is unique in two aspects. First, the longitudinal survey has investigated the elderly with a sufficiently large proportion of oldest-old individuals, and also collected more information on demographic and socio-economic characteristics and health status of this population. This provided us with a good opportunity to separate the effect of resilience on survival from other confounding effects, and to produce more efficient estimates. Second, we addressed resilience and survival in a developing country, China, whereas almost all previous studies on this topic dealt with developed countries. It was realized that resilience factors vary among different developmental and environmental contexts (Fraser et al. 2004), and it is worth examining the resilience scale and its impact on longevity in China.

Data

The data used in this paper were from the Chinese Longitudinal Healthy Longevity Survey (CLHLS). This survey was carried out in 1998, 2000, 2002, 2005, and 2008–2009 in randomly selected half of the countries/cities in 22 Chinese provinces, covering 85% of the total population in China (Zeng et al. 2008). The 1998 baseline and the 2000 follow-up wave interviewed the oldest-old aged 80 and older only; since the 2002 wave, younger elderly aged 65–79 were also included in the sample. Gu and Zeng (2004) have conducted a careful evaluation (such as reliability coefficients and factor analysis) and shown that the data quality of this survey was reasonably good.

This study was based on the 2002–2005 longitudinal sample to explore the impact of resilience on survival among the elderly aged 65+ over a 3-year interval. Those who survived to be interviewed in the 2005 survey were considered as censored. We excluded elderly individuals who were lost to follow-up in the 2005 survey and individuals who had missing information on the year of death or the month of death. We further dropped the cases that had incomplete information on ethnicity, marital status, education, and activities of daily living (ADL). The final sample size of the valid cases used in this study was 13,800 elderly, consisting of 5,686 men (41.20%) and 8,114 women (58.80%).

Measurements

Resilience

Indicators of resilience in this paper were derived based on the framework of the Connor–Davidson Resilience Scale (CD-RISC, Connor and Davidson 2003). CD-RISC was a 25-item scale involving personal competence, tolerance of negative affect and stress-related growth, acceptance of changes, personal control and spiritual orientation. Of the total 25 items, we used 7 available items to measure resilience (Table 14.1). There are three reasons why we only have 7 items. First reason was cultural relevance, namely, only a few Chinese elderly are Christians, thus items such as "sometime fate or God can help" in CD-RISC were not suitable. Second, our research objects were people aged above 65, so items like "you work to attain your goals" and "prefer to take the lead in problem solving" were not suitable. Third, the CLHLS is study focusing on various factors which may affect healthy longevity rather than a special study focusing on psychology, and thus we cannot include too many items in the questionnaire. We asked respondents whether the statements fit with them (denoted as 1) or not (denoted as 0). Thus, total resilience scores ranged from 0 to 7, with higher scores reflecting greater resilience.

The rate of missing values on item 1, item 2, item 3, item 4, and item 7 was 10.84, 10.17, 10.21, 10.31, and 10.91%, respectively. Items 5 and 6 had complete information. We found that those interviewees with a missing value for the variables mostly had poor mental health and physical capacity. Thus, we did not conduct imputation for each of these variables, and instead treated the group with a missing value as a separate category of "missing" (Zeng et al. 2007).

Socio-Demographic Variables

As shown in Table 14.2, age, race (Han or minority), current residence (urban or rural), primary occupation before age 60 (non-manual job or manual job), education (literate or illiterate), and marital status (currently married or not) were included as socio-demographic controls.

Health Status

As the follow-up mortality risk was highly correlated with the initial health status, we controlled for two dimensions of health status in 2002: physical capacity and mental well-being. Physical capacity was measured by ADL, consisting of six items such as eating, dressing, indoor transferring, using toilet, bathing, and continence. Following the studies by Guralnik et al. (1994) and Zeng et al. (2007), if the elderly can complete all six activities without others' assistance, he/she was classified as "ADL independent"; if the elderly needed help in at least one activity, he/she was classified as "ADL dependent."

Mental well-being was measured by the Mini-Mental State Examination (MMSE) questionnaire, which was adapted to Chinese cultural context. The questionnaire included 24 items regarding orientation, registration, attention, calculation, recall, and language, with a total score ranging from 0 to 30. The same cutoffs as the MMSE international standard were used to define a total score of 24 and above as "normal mental health" and a score below 24 as "impaired mental health."

Table 14.1 Measures of resilience: statements concerning self-reported resilience

Item	Relevant part of the CLHLS questionnaire			Summarized and dichotomized item statements		
	Questions asked	Codes	Item statements	Yes	No	Missing
1	Do you feel the older you get, the more useless you are?	0.always; 1.often; 2.sometimes; 3.seldom; 4. never	I don't feel the older you get, the more useless I am.	4,542 (32.91)	7,761 (56.24)	1,497 (10.85)
2	Do you always look on the bright side of things?	4.always; 3.often; 2.sometimes; 1.seldom; 0. never	I always look on the bright side of things.	11,785 (85.40)	611 (4.43)	1,404 (10.17)
3	Do you often feel fearful or anxious?	0.always; 1.often; 2.sometimes; 3.seldom; 4. never	I don't often feel fearful or anxious.	9,015 (65.33)	3,375 (24.46)	1,410 (10.22)
4	Do you often feel lonely and isolated?	0.always; 1.often; 2.sometimes; 3.seldom; 4. never	I don't often feel lonely or isolated	8,310 (60.22)	4,067 (29.47)	1,423 (10.31)
5	To whom do you usually talk most frequently in daily life?	1. Family members/friends/ neighbors/ social workers/ caregivers; 0. Nobody.	I talk frequently to family members or friends in daily life	12,463 (90.31)	1,337 (9.69)	0
6	Who do you ask first for help when you have problems/difficulties?	1. Family members/friends/ neighbors/ social workers/ caregivers; 0. Nobody.	when I have problems, I can turn to my family or friends for help	12,873 (93.28)	927 (6.72)	0
7	Can you make your own decisions concerning your personal affairs?	4.always; 3.often; 2.sometimes; 1.seldom; 0. never	I can make my own decisions concerning my personal affairs	10,287 (74.54)	2,006 (14.54)	1,507 (10.92)

Notes: (1) We dichotomized the answers of each of the seven questions in two categories "Yes" and "No" of the item statements. For Items 1, 3, and 4, the scores 0,1, and 2 are grouped as "No", and the scores 3 and 4 are grouped as "Yes". For Items 2 and 7, the scores 0 and 1 are grouped as "No", and the scores 2, 3, and 4 are grouped as "Yes". For Items 5 and 6, the code 0 is "No" and the codes 1 is "Yes".
(2) In the columns of "Yes" and "No", the numbers which are not within the parentheses are the number of respondents, and their percentages are presented in parentheses.
(3) Missing cases include those who are unable to answer.

Table 14.2 Descriptive statistics of the potentially confounding variables

Confounding variables	Number	Percent
Socio-demographic characteristics		
Mean age	86.40	–
Gender		
Male	5,896	42.72
Female	7,904	57.28
Race		
Han	12,956	93.88
Minority	844	6.12
Current residence		
Urban	5,941	43.05
Rural	7,859	56.95
Education		
Literate	8,637	62.59
Illiterate	5,163	37.41
Primary occupation before age 60		
Non-manual job	1,110	8.04
Manual job	12,690	91.96
Marital status		
Currently married	4,081	29.57
Divorced, widowed, never married	9,719	70.43
Initial health status		
Activities of daily living		
Independent	9,697	70.27
Dependent	4,103	29.73
MMSE		
Good	8,160	59.13
Impaired	5,640	40.87

Note: Variables are measured at the 2002 interview

Methods

We calculated the Pearson correlation coefficients between individual items and the total score of the resilience scale, and evaluated the internal consistency of the resilience scale using Cronbach's alpha statistic. Principal component analysis (PCA) with varimax rotation was conducted to assess the factor composition of the resilience scale among Chinese elderly. Principle component analysis, a common form of factor analysis, aimed to transform these seven possibly correlated items into a smaller number of uncorrelated factors. Varimax rotation was to make the PCA results as easy as possible to identify each item with a single factor and thus to facilitate the interpretation of factors.

We estimated a Cox proportional hazards regression model controlling for the potential confounding factors to explore the association between resilience and survival of the elderly. Survival time from the 2002 survey to the time of death (for those who died) or to the 2005 survey (for those censored) was measured in years (with decimal points).[1] In the survival analyses, we included seven resilience indicators and the total score of resilience separately, to examine the impact of each individual item as well as the overall impact of resilience. To better understand how the impact of resilience on mortality is moderated by other confounding variables, we adopted a stepwise method. Model 1 only included seven resilience indicators or the total resilience score; Model 2 controlled for socio-demographic variables. Model 3 further adjusted for initial physical and mental health.

Results

Sample Characteristics

As shown in Table 14.1, of the 13,800 elderly individuals who had complete information on key variables, 33% did not consider that the older they get, the more useless they are, and 85% always tended to look on the bright side of things. About two thirds did not often feel fearful, anxious, lonely, or isolated. More than 90% talked frequently to their family and friends, or turned to them for help when needed. 75% of the elderly were in control of their personal affairs.

Table 14.2 presented that the mean age of the participants was 86.4 years (sd = 11.69). Most of the elderly were Han (93.9%). 43% resided in urban areas. 37.4% had at least 1 year of schooling. Only 8% held a non-manual job before age 60. Nearly 30% were currently married, and the remaining elderly were widowed. 70.3% were ADL independent, and about half of the elderly had good mental health.

Properties of the Resilience Scale

The mean total score of seven resilience indicators in our sample was 5.43 (sd = 1.28).[2] Item-total correlations (correlations between individual item scores and total scores) ranged from $r = 0.29$ ("when I have problems, I can turn to my family or friends for help") to $r = 0.69$ ("I do not often feel lonely or isolated"), which was considered appropriate (Munro 2005). Because of the small number of items, the Chronbach's α for the scale was 0.478, indicating moderate and acceptable internal consistency.

---

[1] For those died: survival time = (year of death-2002) + (month of death − month of the 2002 survey)/12; For those censored: survival time = (2005–2002) + (month of the 2005 survey − month of the 2002 survey).

[2] We only considered 11,938 cases with complete information on seven resilience indicators to examine the psychometric properties.

Table 14.3 Factors and factor loading of the seven-item resilience scale

Item	Factors and item statements	Eigenvalue	Variance explained (%)	Factor loading
	Factor 1: self-approval, calmness, and sociability	1.78	24.7%	
1	I don't feel the older I get, the more useless I am	–	–	0.65
3	I don't often feel fearful or anxious	–	–	0.78
4	I don't often feel lonely or isolated	–	–	0.79
	Factor 2: close relationship with family and friends	1.30	18.9%	
5	I talk frequently to family members or friends in daily life	–	–	0.78
6	when I have problems, I can turn to my family or friends for help	–	–	0.81
	Factor 3: optimism and control of own life.	1.01	14.8%	
2	I always look on the bright side of things	–	–	0.38
7	I can make my own decisions concerning my personal affairs	–	–	0.93

A principal component analysis with varimax rotation was conducted to transform the seven resilience measures into a smaller number of uncorrelated factors. This procedure generated three uncorrelated factors with eigenvalues ≥1, explaining 58.4% of the total variance. The factor loadings (the correlation coefficients between the items and factors) ranged from 0.38 to 0.93. These factors could be interpreted as follows: Factor 1 containing three items reflecting self-approval, calmness, and sociability; Factor 2 containing three items corresponding to close relationship with family and friends; and Factor 3 including two items related to optimism and control of own life (Table 14.3).

Results of Survival Analyses

Impact of Seven Resilience Indicators on Mortality Risk of the Elderly

Tables 14.4 and 14.5 contained hazard ratios of the effects of seven resilience indicators and total resilience scores on mortality at old ages, which were the focus of this chapter. Without controlling for any confounding factors, those who didn't feel the older they got, the more useless they became had 22.4% lower mortality risk at old ages (Model 1). The effect of this resilience indicator was ameliorated after adjusting for socio-demographic characteristics and initial health status (Models 2 and 3), but remained significant at the $p < 0.01$ level. Those who had missing values on this indicator were faced with significantly higher mortality risks in Model 1. However, after controlling for other covariates, there was no significant difference in mortality between those with and without missing values.

Having an eye on the bright side of things raised the mortality risk by 14% in Model 1 but was only marginally significant at the 0.1 level. When the other potentially

Table 14.4 Hazard ratios of the effects of seven resilience indicators on mortality risk

	Model 1	Model 2	Model 3
Resilience measurements			
I don't feel the older I get, the more useless I am (no)	0.776***	0.849***	0.894***
Missing (no)	1.280***	1.029	0.982
I always look on the bright side of things (no)	1.140*	1.021	1.049
Missing (no)	1.411***	1.177	1.145
I do not often feel fearful or anxious (no)	0.920**	0.887***	0.931**
Missing (no)	0.970	0.911	0.937
I do not often feel lonely or isolated (no)	0.807***	0.910***	0.932**
Missing (no)	1.195	1.105	1.039
I talk frequently to family members or friends in daily life (no)	0.722***	0.880***	0.939
When I have problems, I can turn to my family or friends for help (no)	0.947	0.914*	0.919
I can make my own decisions concerning my personal affairs (no)	0.723***	0.881***	0.920**
Missing (no)	1.519***	1.185*	1.126
Socio-demographic characteristics			
Age	–	1.067***	1.054***
Male (female)	–	1.298***	1.378***
Han (minority)	–	1.200***	1.076
Urban (rural)	–	1.004	0.984
Literate (illiterate)	–	1.026	1.0517
Non-manual job (manual job)	–	0.894*	0.908
Currently married (divorced, widowed, never married)	–	0.759***	0.759***
Initial health status			
Independent ADL (dependent)	–	–	0.619***
Good MMSE (impaired)	–	–	0.705***
Observation	13,800		

Note: $*p < 0.1$; $**p < 0.05$; $***p < 0.01$

confounding factors were added to the model (Models 2 and 3), the coefficient lost its marginal significance. The significant difference in mortality between those with and without missing values on this indicator diminished after we controlled for other covariates.

Not feeling fearful or anxious significantly reduced the mortality risk by 6.9–11.3%. Those elderly who did not feel lonely or isolated were also faced with 6.8–19.3% lower mortality risk. The mortality risks of the elderly with missing information on these two indicators were not significantly different from the elderly with complete information.

Talking frequently to family members or friends in daily life reduced the 3-year mortality risk by 27.8%. When socio-demographic characteristics were added in Model 2, the effect shrank to 12% lower mortality risk. After further controlling for initial physical and psychological health in Model 3, the effect was no longer

Table 14.5 Hazard ratios of the effects of total resilience scores on mortality risk

	Model 1 (all elders)	Model 2 (all elders)	Model 3 (all elders)	Model 4 (young-old)	Model 5 (oldest-old)
Total resilience score					
≥6 (<6)	0.647***	0.772***	0.845***	0.800***	0.870***
Missing (<6)	2.082***	1.278***	1.085**	1.353**	1.107***
Socio-demographic characteristics					
Age	–	1.068***	1.054***	1.077***	1.039***
Male (female)	–	1.288***	1.376***	1.303***	1.327***
Han (minority)	–	1.196***	1.073	0.898	1.117
Urban (rural)	–	0.998	0.980	0.897	0.986
Literate (illiterate)	–	1.024	1.051	1.125	1.032
Non-manual job (manual job)	–	0.889*	0.906	0.921	0.908
Currently married (divorced, widowed, or never married)	–	0.757***	0.757***	0.823***	0.803***
Initial health status					
Independent ADL (dependent)	–	–	0.614***	0.473***	0.637***
Good MMSE (impaired)	–	–	0.694***	0.582***	0.736***
Observations	13,800	13,800	13,800	5,990	7,810

Note: *p < 0.1; **p < 0.05; ***p < 0.01

significant. Turning to family members or friends for help had insignificant effect on mortality in Models 1 and 3. Self decision-making reduced the mortality risk by 27.7%. When controlling for socio-demographic characteristics and health status, those in control of personal affairs were faced with 9.1% lower mortality risk.

Regarding socio-demographic controls, female elderly had significantly lower mortality risks, consistent with many prior studies. Race, current residence, and education had no significant impact on mortality when the socio-demographic characteristics and initial health statuses were controlled for. Marriage was an important indicator for longevity. Those who were currently married were faced with 24.1% lower mortality risk than those who were divorced, widowed, or never married. Good health status, both physical and mental, significantly reduced mortality risk at old ages.

Impact of Total Resilience Scores on Mortality Risk of the Elderly

For those with complete information on seven resilience indicators, we computed their total resilience scores. Scores higher or equal to 6 were denoted as 1, reflecting higher resilience; scores lower than 6 were denoted as 0, reflecting lower resilience. For those respondents who had missing values on at least one resilience indicator, we treated them as a separate category of "missing" and did not do any imputation.

In the Cox proportional hazard model without controlling for any covariates, the elderly with higher resilience were faced with 35.3% lower mortality risk. Models 2 and 3 show that part of the effect of resilience was moderated by socio-demographic characteristics and initial health status. After adjusting for various covariates including the initial health, higher resilience reduced mortality risk at old ages by 15.5% (Model 3). In Model 1, the respondents with missing values on total resilience scores had about twice higher mortality risks than those with low resilience scores. After controlling for other confounding factors, the effect shrank to 8.5–27.8%.

In order to explore the relationship between resilience and survival among the oldest-old which was seldom examined in previous research, we further conducted survival analyses among the young-old (aged between 65 and 84) and oldest-old (aged 85 and older) separately (Models 4 and 5). The effect of high resilience on mortality was a bit smaller for the oldest-old, but remained significant at the 0.01 level.

The effects of socio-demographic characteristics and initial health status were similar to the estimates presented in Table 14.4.

Discussion and Conclusions

The present study was unique as it explored the association between resilience and longevity at old ages based on a large panel data with a sufficiently large subsample of the oldest-old in China, a developing country. Exploratory principal components analysis indicated that the resilience scale applied to Chinese elderly contained three dimensions: self-approval, calmness, and sociability; close relationship with family and friends; and optimism and control of own life. Survival analyses showed that most of the resilience indicators had significantly positive impacts on longevity of the elderly. Furthermore, we summed these seven resilience indicators to construct a total resilience measure. It was demonstrated that after controlling for socio-demographic characteristics and initial health status, higher resilience significantly reduced the risk of mortality, and the effect of total resilience among the young-old was a bit larger than the effect among the oldest-old.

Why was resilience positively associated with survival at old ages in China? One possible explanation was that resilience was positively correlated with better physical and psychological health, and better health status lowered the mortality risk. As shown in our survival analyses, the effect of each resilience indicator as well as the effect of total resilience score on the mortality risk substantially shrank after variables of initial health status were included in the model. Prior investigations also lent support to this explanation; for instance, Wagnild (2003) and Lamond et al. (2009) indicated that resilience had a positive association with physical and cognitive function. Ong et al. (2006) have demonstrated that resilient individuals were more likely to hold positive emotions, which promoted both resistance to and recovery from stress, and thus probably contributed to better health and longevity. However, due to data limitation, we were unable to explore the detailed mechanisms on how resilience worked.

The findings presented in this paper should be interpreted with caution given the limitations of our study. First, as the CLHLS was a demographic survey focusing on determinants of healthy longevity such as demographic characteristics, socio-economic status, life style and health status of the elderly, we did not have as many resilience indicators as other psychological surveys. Although the original Connor–Davidson resilience scale had 25 items, we only analyzed 7 of the items because of data limitations. Future research that collects the whole C-D resilience scale could improve our understanding of the association between resilience and mortality. Second, we only have examined the association between resilience and mortality, rather than the causal relationship between them. More detailed data and advanced methods such as instrumental analysis are called for to explore the causal relationship.

In conclusion, the present study provided evidence to support the conclusion that better resilience tended to reduce mortality risk among the young-old and oldest-old in a developing country. Thus, policy makers may need to take measures to promote resilience. The developed countries have formulated some resilience training programs, including organizing group activities, encouraging individual expressions and so on (Waite and Richardson 2004). The governments and societies in developing countries including China could learn from these matured training programs and adapt them to their own social and cultural contexts. These efforts would have long-term effects on the well-being and longevity of the elderly.

References

Connor, K.M., and Davidson, J.R. (2003). Development of a new resilience scale: the Connor–Davidson Resilience Scale (CD-RISC). *Depression and Anxiety*, 18, 76–82.

Fraser, M.W., Kirby, L.D., and Smokowski, P.R. (2004). Risk and resilience in childhood. In M.W. Fraser (Ed.), *Risk and resilience in childhood: An ecological perspective* (2nd ed., pp.13–66). Washington, DC: NASW.

Friborg, O., Hjemdal, O., Rosenvinge, J.H., and Martinussen, M. (2003). A new rating scale for adult resilience: what are the central protective resources behind healthy adjustment? *International Journal of Methods in Psychiatric Research*, 12(2), 65–76.

Giltay, E.J., Geleijnse, J.M., Zitman, F.G., Hoekstra, T., and Schouten, E.G. (2004). Dispositional optimism and all-cause and cardiovascular mortality in a prospective cohort of elderly Dutch men and women. *Archives of General Psychiatry*, 61, 1126–1135.

Gu, D., and Zeng, Y. (2004). Data quality assessment of the CLHLS 1998, 2000, and 2002 waves. In Zeng, Y., Liu, Y., Zhang, C. and Xiao, Z. (eds.), *Analyses of the Determinants of Healthy Longevity* (pp. 4–22). Beijing: Peking University Press.

Guralnik, J.M., Simonsick, E.M., Ferrucci, L., Glynn, R.J., Berkman, L.F., Blazer, D.G., Scherr, P.A., and Wallace, R.B. (1994). A short physical performance battery assessing lower extremity function: association with self-reported disability and prediction of mortality and nursing home addition. *Journal of Gerontology: Medical Sciences*, 49(2), M85–M94.

Hardy, S.E., Concato, J., and Gill, T.M. (2002). Stressful life events among community-living older persons. *Journal of General Internal Medicine*, 17, 832–838.

Lamond, A.J., Depp, C.A., Allison, M., Langer, R., Reichstadt, J., Moore, D.J., Golshan, S., Ganiats, T.G., and Jeste, D.V. (2009). Measurement and predictors of resilience among community-dwelling older women. *Journal of Psychiatric Research*, 43, 148–154.

Levy, B.R., Slade, M.D., and Kasl, S.V. (2002). Longitudinal benefit of positive self perceptions of aging on functional health. *Journals of Gerontology Series B-Psychological Sciences and Social Sciences*, 57, 409–417.

Luthar, S.S., Cicchetti, D., and Becker, B. (2000). The construct of resilience: a critical evaluation and guidelines for future work. *Child Development*, 71, 543.

Masten, A.S. (2001). Ordinary magic: resilience processes in development. *American Psychologist*, 56, 227–238.

Munro, B.H. (2005). *Statistical Methods for Health Care Research* (5th edn). Philadelphia: Lippincott Williams & Wilkins.

Nygren, B., Alex, L., Jonsen, E., Gustafson, Y., Norberg, A., and Lundman, B. (2005). Resilience, sense of coherence, purpose in life and self-transcendence in relation to perceived physical and mental health among the oldest old. *Aging and Mental Health*, 9, 354–362.

Ong, A.D., Bergeman, C.S., Bisconti, T.L., and Wallace, K.A. (2006). Psychological resilience, positive emotions and stressful adaptation to stress in later life. *Journal of Personality and Social Psychology*, 91(4), 730–749.

Reker, G. (2008). Resilience as a mediator of stressful life events and subjective wellbeing, existential regret, and physical health in older adults. *The Gerontologist*, 48, 114.

Surtees, P.G., Wainwright, N.W.J., and Khaw, K. (2006). Resilience, misfortune, and mortality: evidence that sense of coherence is a marker of social stress adaptive capacity. *Journal of Psychosomatic Research*, 61, 221–227

Tugade, M.M., Fredrickson, B.L., and Barrett, L.F. (2004). Psychological resilience and positive emotional granularity: examining the benefits of positive emotions on coping and health. *Journal of Personality*, 72(6), 1161–1190.

Wagnild, G. (2003). Resilience and successful aging: comparison among low and high income older adults. *Journal of Gerontology Nursing*, 29, 42–49.

Wagnild, G.M., and Young, H.M. (1993). Development and psychometric evaluation of the Resilience Scale. *Journal of Nursing Measurement*, 1(2), 165–178.

Waite, P.J., and Richardson, G.E. (2004). Determining the efficacy of resiliency training in the work site. *Journal of Allied Health*, 33(3), 178–183.

Windle, G., Woods, R., and Markland, D. (2008). The effect of psychological resilience on the relationship between chronic illness and subjective well-being. *The Gerontologist*, 48, 179.

Zeng, Yi., Gu, D., and Land, K.C. (2007). The association of childhood socioeconomic conditions with healthy longevity at the oldest-old age in China. *Demography*, 44 (3), 497–518.

Zeng, Y., Poston, D., Vlosky, D.A., and Gu, D. (eds.). (2008). *Healthy Longevity in China: Demographic, Socioeconomic, and Psychological Dimensions*. Dordrecht: Springer.

Chapter 15
Fostering Resilience in Dementia Through Narratives: Contributions of Multimedia Technologies

Barbara Purves, Marie Y. Savundranayagam, Elizabeth Kelson, Arlene Astell, and Alison Phinney

This chapter brings together recent innovative uses of multimedia tools to explore narratives of people with a diagnosis of dementia. The foundations for this work are located in an understanding of the concepts of resilience and well-being and the role of narrative-based reminiscence in fostering resilience, especially as applied to people with dementia. The work collected here focuses on supporting people with a diagnosis, their families, and their communities. We begin with a discussion of the conceptual foundations underpinning this research.

Resilience and Well-Being

The concept of resilience has a long history in the study of human development, emerging initially from research on child development and arriving more recently in the gerontological literature. Although resilience has been described as a personal attribute, it has been more recently interpreted as a dynamic process (Ryff and Singer 2008). While there are various definitions of this process in the literature on aging, central features include the presence of life challenges or adversity, and the maintenance or regaining of physical health and psychological well-being. It has been argued that the concept of resilience may be preferable to the notion of successful aging as a way of emphasizing positive aspects of health (Harris 2008), specifically because it can accommodate adversity as central to the process. This argument rings true in the case of people with dementia, especially given that conceptualizations of dementia and successful aging within current public discourses are not entirely compatible; resilience, on the other hand, encourages a focus on well-being that reminds us of the possibility of positive outcomes despite dementia (Harris 2008). This assertion also encourages a closer examination of the concept of well-being, including well-being in the context of dementia across all levels of severity.

B. Purves (✉)
University of British Columbia, Vancouver, BC, Canada
e-mail: purves@audiospeech.ubc.ca

B. Resnick et al. (eds.), *Resilience in Aging: Concepts, Research, and Outcomes*,
DOI 10.1007/978-1-4419-0232-0_15, © Springer Science+Business Media, LLC 2011

231

We take as our starting-point for this examination the work of Ryff and Singer (2008), who base their definitions on theoretical concepts of well-being articulated in Aristotle's descriptions of eudaimonic (versus hedonic) happiness, in the work of philosophers such as John Stuart Mill and Bertrand Russell, and also in the work of twentieth century humanistic psychologists such as Frankl, Rogers, and Maslow. Drawing on these foundations, Ryff and Singer propose six dimensions of well-being including: (1) self-acceptance, involving awareness and acceptance of one's personal strengths and weaknesses, (2) positive relations with others, acknowledged as a central feature of a positive, well-lived life, (3) personal growth, involving the continued development of personal potential, (4) a sense of purpose in life, including the search for meaning in adversity, (5) environmental mastery, involving the ability to find or create an environment that fits one's personal needs, including the ability to control and manipulate that environment, and (6) and autonomy, arguably the most western of all dimensions, which emphasizes qualities such as self-determination and independence (Ryff and Singer 2008, pp. 20–23).

In recent years, there has been increasing evidence to support claims that many people with dementia continue to live meaningful lives with a sense of purpose, maintaining a sense of autonomy and environmental mastery, as well as positive relations with others, and demonstrating ongoing personal growth. Autobiographical accounts of living with dementia (e.g. Henderson and Andrews 1998), as well as the findings of predominantly qualitative research studies and the emergence of self-advocacy groups (see Harris 2008) all indicate such resilience. Much of this evidence, however, focuses on individuals in earlier stages of dementia. Interpretation of what constitutes well-being becomes more complex with increasing severity of dementia.

Kitwood (1997) wrote extensively about well-being in people with dementia claiming that the inevitable losses associated with dementia cause these individuals become increasingly dependent on others to support their well-being, primarily through recognition and support of their unique personhood, which incorporates their life history, values, and personal preferences. His now-famous definition of personhood as "a standing or status that is bestowed upon one human being, by others, in the context of relationship and social being" (Kitwood 1997, p. 8) is primarily a relational one, and as such it is very consistent with Ryff and Singer's dimension of positive relations with others as a source of well-being. Indeed, Ryff and Singer (1998) suggest that while the relative importance of each dimension may be different across cultures, this relational dimension of well-being may be the most universal. However, Kitwood's insistence on the importance of others in supporting the well-being of persons with dementia goes beyond envisioning positive relations with others as a single dimension of well-being; instead, he suggests that it is through the informed intervention of others, creating a supportive social environment, that the person with dementia can realize and demonstrate other dimensions of well-being, even into more severe stages of dementia. Although Kitwood's work has been criticized for lacking sufficient evidence for such claims (Baldwin and Capstick 2007), supportive evidence can be found in the work of others, which illustrates, for example, the capacity of people with more severe dementia to seek meaning in their circumstances or to exploit opportunities for creative work (Sabat 2001).

Although Kitwood's work explores a relationally based concept of well-being in persons with dementia, it fails to adequately address the issue of well-being in others within their social networks; indeed, the concept of relational care arose in part out of such criticisms (Baldwin and Capstick 2007; Hellström et al. 2005). Yet, if resilience and well-being for persons with dementia are increasingly located in their social networks of family, formal carers, and community, the resilience and well-being of others within those networks are also of central concern, a point that is addressed in a growing body of literature on this topic (Gaugler et al. 2007; Ortiz et al. 1999).

Fostering Resilience Through Narrative

We are narrative beings, with our very selves constituted through the stories told by and about us. It is not surprising, then, that narrative has been identified as a therapeutic tool to support resilience in those coming to terms with adversity (Caldwell 2005; Neimeyer and Levitt 2001). But how can this tool be adapted for those with dementia, especially when increasing cognitive losses can fragment the performance of meaningful narratives? The value of drawing on the unique life histories of people with dementia to enhance care practice has been generally acknowledged; most often this has involved seeking biographical information from those familiar with the person with dementia. More recently, however, there is growing attention to ways in which carers can support the person with dementia as teller of his or her own narrative, finding ways to understand that narrative, however, fragmented (e.g. Hydén and Örluv 2009; Sabat 2001). Reminiscence activities are another form of narrative therapy for individuals with dementia, with some evidence to support their use. Woods (1994), for instance, demonstrated that reminiscence activities offer people who have dementia the opportunities for more successful social interaction, providing not only positive experiences for persons with dementia, but also helping carers for persons with dementia in institutional settings appreciate the unique experiences and life histories of those persons (see also Hagens et al. 2003). Reminiscence activities do not always lead, however, to successful interactions (Woods and McKiernan 1995), creating the risk of frustration for both persons with dementia and their conversation partners.

In this chapter, we describe three innovative approaches to engaging narrative as a therapeutic device; these draw on the foregoing literature, but also broaden the scope of exploration to include the role of family, friend, and community relationships in fostering resilience. Each of these three approaches draws on multimedia technologies, capitalizing not only on their potential to create new ways of engaging in narrative constructions, but also, as Caldwell (2005) suggests, their ability to generate legacies for families and communities.

In addition, all three approaches acknowledge the importance of social relationships as a source of well-being by seeking ways to foster that well-being both in persons with dementia and those caring for them. Finally, each of the three approaches draws in some way on narratives that are grounded by a sense of place and community, emphasizing narratives as joint constructions that maintain and strengthen relationships.

Narrative Approaches

Fostering Resilience Within Families by Enhancing Personhood

Resilience requires an inner strength that can come from relationships that are affirming. This is especially true for families who struggle to maintain relationships in the face of chronic illnesses, such as dementia, that affect cognitive and communicative abilities. As discussed earlier, a key approach to fostering resilience for persons with dementia involves supporting and enhancing their personhood. However, because personhood is a relational concept that necessitates consideration not only of persons with dementia but also those who care for them, it is important to examine *shared* activities that involve both family caregivers and individuals with dementia. Current research findings on shared activities suggest that although both parties may work together on activities, family caregivers tend to deal with their emotions alone, which consequently may hinder their own coping or adaptation (Hellström et al. 2005). Therefore, it is critical to examine the ways in which collaborative activities promote the sharing of experiences and emotions for both parties.

One example of a collaborative activity that enhanced personhood is StoryCorps' *Memory Loss Initiative*, which was a national interviewing project in the United States that gathered oral histories of individuals with early stage memory loss by encouraging participants to focus on emotion-based memories. The goal of the Memory Loss Initiative was to support and encourage people with illnesses such as Alzheimer's disease, vascular dementia, and mild cognitive impairment (MCI) to share their stories with family and friends. Conversations were recorded in a booth that was outfitted with equipment for producing a broadcast-quality CD, which was given to participants and also archived at the Library of Congress with participants' permission. Each booth was operated by a StoryCorps facilitator who received training on how to communicate with individuals with cognitive-communicative impairments. The training focused on memory and communication impairments, as well as language-based strategies that elicit communication, such as asking questions that were emotion- or experience-focused instead of questions that focused on specific dates (Kensinger et al. 2004; Small and Perry 2005). In cases where storytellers with memory loss did not have a family member who could conduct the interview, facilitators completed the interview.

A recent study investigated the impact of StoryCorps' Memory Loss Initiative on storytellers with memory loss and their family members (Savundranayagam et al. in press). StoryCorps interviews related to the Memory Loss Initiative took place at several sites in three cities (Milwaukee, Chicago, and New York). Follow-up telephone interviews were conducted with 42 persons with memory loss, along with 27 family members who participated in the StoryCorps interviews. The interviews were analyzed using the process of constant comparative analysis to identify themes that emerged from the conversations.

Findings revealed that the StoryCorps experience was a meaningful activity that offered opportunities for feeling comfort and acceptance, for enjoying precious moments with one another, for reflection and engagement in meaningful conversations, for re-affirming both the selfhood of individuals with memory loss and their relationships with family members, for leaving a legacy for future generations within families, and for being part of national history. Given that the purpose of the StoryCorps interview was to share stories and life histories, family members tended to choose personhood-affirming topics that addressed personal preferences, family and intimate relationships, and educational and occupational history. These topics were more likely to elicit conversations than questions that tested the individual with memory loss because the focus was on emotions surrounding the topics listed above (Kensinger et al. 2004). Moreover, the StoryCorps facilitators and family members created a positive social environment by perceiving the experience as an opportunity to showcase the stories of individuals with memory loss. This was especially apparent in the comments about legacies; if individuals with memory loss did not experience a positive social environment, they would not have commented on the importance of the present moment or on the value of their legacies. Both the choice to interview and the act of interviewing acknowledged the worth of the person.

The study findings also illustrated that enhancing personhood, which has most often been viewed in terms of the *individual* with memory loss, is in fact about strengthening reciprocity in relationships. Relationships can easily be taken for granted, but even more so when disease process and disease management threaten to take precedence. By re-affirming and validating the person with memory loss, family members were able to value their existing relationship. Unlike collaborative activities where the focus is solely on the person with memory loss, an emotion-based oral storytelling experience, such as StoryCorps, offers a meaningful way to collectively reflect on past memories and begin a personhood-affirming dialogue. This dialogue allows family members to share their emotions about caregiving directly with the individual suffering from memory loss, instead of processing them alone, which is a prevalent caregiver practice (Hellström et al. 2005). This dialogue also allows persons with memory loss a chance to share emotions based on family stories.

The StoryCorps approach, which focuses on emotion-based conversations, creates new possibilities for family caregivers to foster resilience using personhood-enhancing conversations. It teaches family members that communication is not about answering questions correctly. It is about experiencing shared activities that celebrate relationships. In doing so, the relationship identity of both the storyteller with memory loss and his or her family member is maintained. StoryCorps' Memory Loss Initiative was a powerful experience that acknowledged the personhood of both storytellers with memory loss and their family members (Savundranayagam et al. in press); as both parties began to appreciate the present moment in addition to past histories, they were actively involved in creating legacies that will impact their existing and future relationships.

Fostering Resilience Within Care Settings: Visual Life Stories

Visual Life Stories (*VLS*) is a photo-based biographical tool designed for a study exploring how familiarizing long-term care (LTC) staff with residents' life stories can support personhood and contribute to person-centered dementia care. Kelson's concept of *VLS* is based on a definition of life story as a "personal narrative that thematically links events" occurring in a person's lifetime (de Medeiros 2005, p. 6). In her qualitative pilot study conducted in Canada, Kelson (2006) created *VLS* of two LTC residents with dementia. Each was in the form of a 13-minute DVD presentation about the person's life that had been produced, based on the resident's personal photographs, through guided conversations with the resident and his or her family. This photo-based biographical tool was designed to support person-centered care by providing formal caregivers and nursing home volunteers with information about the residents' life histories.

Kelson conducted her study in two phases. The first phase involved conversational interviews with each resident with dementia and his or her family members. These discussions were based on the viewing of their family photographs. As other studies have found, the use of visual prompts in this study supported residents' ability to recall and share their life stories. In reflecting on their photographs, resident participants frequently added to the familial accounts of the experiences depicted in the photos, which included childhood photos, wedding and holiday shots, family celebrations, and photos of friends. In the second phase, draft *VLS* presentations were developed and brought back to participants for clarification and approval. Resident responses to viewing of their *VLS* revealed how the presentation allowed them the opportunity to re-connect with the emotions embedded in the photographs and to re-visit aspects of their past selves. For example, Claire commented: *"You've taken me, taken me in my thoughts, deeply," "Happy memories, happy memories," and "I was lost when he went, but for the time we were married, we were very happy."* The other resident participant, Jack, also reflected on his life, *"You forget what a good life you've had,"* and recollected identity: *"I like to tinker with machinery."*

Participating family members expressed enjoying the opportunity to view photos with their relative, to reminisce, and to re-live family history and shared memories. Family members' participation was integral to *VLS* production and might be seen as a positive vehicle to support family involvement in care by drawing on the expertise that can come from their intimate knowledge of their relative. Interestingly, family members also noted how the *VLS* might have helped smooth their relative's transition into care, which had been difficult for both participants.

Following completion of the *VLS*, four focus groups involving 26 staff members in the two long-term care facilities were conducted. Participants viewed and discussed the feasibility and therapeutic value of the *VLS*. Content analysis of the textual data generated in these sessions led to the identification of the following five themes.

Knowing the Resident. The majority of staff expressed the importance of knowing the resident in order to provide person-centered care. Staff noted how they learned new information about the resident through the *VLS*, information that represented key aspects of the resident's identity, such as a favorite pastime, family structures, personal preferences, and other information that impacted the resident in the present.

Comments shared during the focus groups revealed staff insights regarding the potential of the *VLS* to affirm the personhood of residents with dementia. For example, one manager commented on the continuity of the resident's personhood: *"It [VLS] shows who they were and is a reminder of truly who they still are."*

A nurse noted how *VLS* led to a shift in focus from the resident in the present to the resident over time:

> *If you walked upstairs right now and you see Claire walking by you'll think of her more as the person she used to be instead of the person she is right in front of you and less of the dementia and more of her history.*

Staff comments revealed their enthusiasm for the potential of the *VLS* to support them in their specific roles within the care team. They discussed the possibility of it helping to create a more positive social environment by supporting more effective, meaningful communication in care, citing examples of both informal and formal resident/staff interactions (e.g. meeting a resident in the hall or bathing a resident). Moreover, responses indicated an appreciation for the qualitative difference between visual presentations of residents' life stories versus facilities' current use of text-based documents (i.e. two-page summaries) left in resident charts. As one staff member said, *"Pictures tell a lot that's true."*

They want everybody to know everything on the first day. Staff shared how family members often expected them to know a great deal about their relative's life history, beginning at the time of admission. This expectation created a level of stress for both staff and family carers, and it led the majority of staff to conclude that families would support the addition of the *VLS* to care delivery.

Effects of Macro-Level Policies. Across all four focus groups, management staff referred to changes in healthcare policy that have negatively impacted their ability to gather comprehensive, accurate biographical information on residents prior to admission. Other changes regarding eligibility for care have resulted in residents being admitted at a lower functional level with more significant cognitive challenges. These policy outcomes serve to highlight the potential role of the *VLS* to assist residents who are increasingly unable to present biographical information to formal caregivers without assistance. According to one manager, *"...we used to be able to get quite reliable information from the resident themselves, now virtually, you can't really..."*

Effects of Micro-Level Demands. Staff offered important insights into organizational level challenges that created barriers to their ability to deliver person-centered care. Staff shared their perceptions of increasing workloads, high resident to staff ratios, rising care levels, and significant time constraints, captured in one aide's comment that *"We're always racing against the clock."* In the long-term care facilities studied, care aides did not attend care plan meetings where residents' social lives were discussed, nor did they generally have access to the resident charts. This meant that front line staff had little alternative but to receive their information about residents' lives from the residents themselves. Given that the resident population is increasingly challenged in their ability to communicate, this approach seems problematic. Care staff felt that a brief accessible tool like the *VLS* would effectively reduce some of these organizational barriers.

In conclusion, this pilot study suggests that the development and sharing of *VLS* support resilience in LTC settings, in large part by allowing staff to see beyond the labels of "resident" and "dementia," interacting instead with the *person* in light of his or her unique life story. Clearly, staff members want to better understand the people they provide care for and *VLS* represents a possible means to this end. Given the receptiveness of staff to the presentation of residents' histories in a *VLS* format, the potential of this tool to support personhood and well-being amongst LTC residents appears to be promising.

Fostering Resilience Through Shared Histories

Social reminiscence (Cohen and Taylor 1998) refers to the activity of recollecting and sharing personal memories in a one-to-one or group setting. In dementia care, reminiscence is popular as a relatively simple group activity that takes advantage of the typically well-preserved long-term memories of older people with dementia as their memory for recent events is progressively undermined. Old photographs, artifacts, and music are commonly used to prompt recollections among group members and provide an enjoyable way for them to pass the time.

Reminiscence also has the potential to facilitate and support communication and the development of relationships between people with dementia and those who care for them. This may be particularly true when conversational topics are drawn from shared histories, relevant in some way to all participants. The extent to which group reminiscence activities as compared with individual sessions fulfill this potential for building relationships remains, however, an empirical question; it is unusual for reminiscence to take place as a one-to-one activity in most dementia care facilities. This may be due in part to staffing levels and limited time available for staff to find stimuli to support conversation on an individual basis, but it could also be due to challenges in maintaining ongoing one-to-one conversation with persons with dementia.

The Computer Interactive Reminiscence and Conversation Aid (CIRCA) project in Dundee, Scotland, set out to provide an easy-to-use computer system that can draw on the shared history of participants to support one-to-one interactions between caregivers and people with a diagnosis of dementia (Alm et al. 2004). CIRCA contains a database of approximately 600 media files, including digitized photos, music, and film clips. It incorporates touch-screen technology, making it easy to use both for persons with dementia and their caregivers; either one of the conversation partners, who sit together in front of the computer screen, can select an item that may prompt a recollection or comment. These responses then form the basis of conversation between people with dementia and caregivers as they share their stories and experiences.

CIRCA requires no previous computing experience; there is no mouse or keyboard, and no training is required to start using the program. Upon starting CIRCA, the users are offered three themes to choose from, such as, for example, Entertainment, Recreation, and People and Events. Users make a selection by touching one of the three themes appearing on the screen. Within this theme, users are then offered a further choice between photographs, videos, or music. A key feature of the program is that each time it is opened, media are randomly accessed from the database files so that only a subset of files are available (for example, only three of seven possible themes will be available in any one session). This feature ensures greater equality between the interactants; neither participant can predetermine what media will be accessed.

A second feature of the CIRCA program is that the files draw on generic rather than personal media from a time period associated with long-term memories, thus highlighting the shared history of a community. The CIRCA program developed in Dundee was designed primarily for Dundee seniors, either locally (as in, for example, photographs of a typical Dundee street scene from the 1950s) or more globally (as in short film clips from mainstream movies such as *Casablanca*, or popular songs from the 1940s such as *Siegfried Line*). In fact, the program captured the shared history of Dundee so well that the local Science Centre has included it as a kiosk exhibit intended to promote intergenerational activities for a target audience of primary school students who frequently attend with their grandparents.

In a series of studies, the CIRCA system has proved easy to use and provides an enjoyable shared activity that can promote well-being both for people with dementia and their caregivers. Analysis of the interactions during CIRCA sessions (as compared with interactions during traditional reminiscence sessions) showed that for people with dementia, even relatively severe dementia, CIRCA provides the opportunity to make choices and engage as an equal partner in a one-to-one conversation with a caregiver. Such opportunities are consistent with dimensions of well-being including autonomy, environmental mastery, and positive relations.

Evaluation of CIRCA identified three major outcomes for care staff: (1) staff saw the people with dementia in a new light; (2) staff re-evaluated their perceptions and expectations of their interactions with people with dementia; and (3) using the computer to run one-to-one sessions improved staff feelings of competence as caregivers (Astell et al. 2009). CIRCA also provided opportunities for enhanced well-being, for both staff members and people with dementia, through improved positive relations.

These findings support the use of social reminiscence as an engaging one-to-one activity for people with dementia and caregivers. Both caregivers and people with dementia enjoy participating in CIRCA sessions and the evidence suggests that this engagement facilitates communication and strengthens relationships. Additionally, the findings from the CIRCA project highlight the utility of generic (as opposed to personal) materials as prompts for reminiscence in dementia care, as the CIRCA contents successfully elicited recollection and sharing of personal memories by people with dementia and caregivers.

Discussion

In this chapter, we considered the question of how narrative can be leveraged as a tool to support resilience for people affected by dementia, their families, and communities. Through StoryCorps, persons with dementia and their family members were supported to engage together in meaningful conversations through which they co-constructed stories from the past, but in so doing they were also sustaining and strengthening their relationships in the present and contributing to the collective stories of the nation. *Visual Life Stories* also provided an opportunity for persons with dementia and their families to work together toward the construction of a personal history narrative, but with the intent of sharing it within a residential community. By providing a basis for understanding the person with dementia, this tool potentially enables better person-centered care, thus supporting well-being and quality of life for everyone involved – residents, family members, and care staff alike. CIRCA is also designed for use primarily within a care environment, but draws more on the narratives of a community than on individual life stories to support meaningful conversation between persons with dementia and their caregivers.

While each of these tools brings something unique to an overall project, there are important similarities to consider as well. The most obvious of these is the fact that each one is made possible in part because of the opportunities afforded by digital media. The technology itself should not be overlooked for its role in supporting resilience through narrative. There is a very real sense in which history is brought to life through the recorded voice, through photographs, film, and music. So much of our life's narrative is beyond language (Baldwin 2009), and with these technologies we are better equipped to harness the power of personal stories. With these technologies at our disposal, we not only have better ways to elicit and convey narratives, allowing us to overcome some of the barriers posed by illness such as dementia, but we also have better ways to share these narratives with others, over time and across place.

Of course, just because we can, does it mean that we should? Dawn Brooker was very astute in her observation that "filing cabinets in care facilities around the world are full of information about people's lives, but still care staff will not know even the rudimentary facts" (Brooker 2004, p. 220). If these sorts of tools are to be just one more depository of information that is stored away, never to be used in any meaningful way, then why make the effort? By way of answering this question, we want to argue that these kinds of tools are different in more than merely technical ways. They are not just different ways of getting at and sharing the information, but rather they rely on technology that is supporting a different way of engaging around these narratives, and it is this question of how we might engage around the narrative that makes a difference.

First, these technologies are not offering narrative as a simple strategy to be taken up by family members and care providers to help support the person with dementia, but rather are offering a way of creating an *interactional environment* (O'Connor et al. 2007) that itself supports the well-being of everyone involved. The findings of Kelson's study regarding how care staff responded to *VLS* suggest that the focus groups were in and of themselves an important part of the tool. The benefit was not just in the information conveyed through the *VLS*, but was also in the opportunity to talk about it together as a community of practice who share the goal of providing better person-centered care. Similarly, CIRCA is a tool whose primary purpose is to create an environment for supporting meaningful interactions between people with dementia and their care partners.

Second, the matter of history is obviously an important thread in all of this work. In some way, each of these projects takes on the task of drawing out stories from the past. But in each case, it is not just the individual narratives that are important, but also the shared histories that have shaped who we are and how we are in the world. Engaging around shared histories is made possible in part because of the opportunities afforded by the different media. The significance of the technology itself should not be overlooked. These digital tools seem to have some way of extending the reach of these stories – they are no longer "merely" personal, some kind of possession of the individual, but rather are something to which we all belong in some way. StoryCorps is perhaps the best example of this, with its goal of not only creating stories for families to share, but also bringing together these stories of a nation into a collective whole. In different ways, all three projects described in this chapter demonstrate how history can be brought into a communal space where people can engage with each other, sharing common histories and bridging the cultural and generational divides that separate us.

Next Steps

When it comes to technology, questions about next steps are often of the technical sort, e.g. "How do we make it better?" But as health and social scientists, our priority should be to ask: "What counts as better?" Certainly if we are to consider this question from an individual perspective, Ryff and Singer's framework of resilience may provide some important direction. Although these kinds of multimedia-based tools have not been subjected to extensive research, there is evidence in these preliminary studies to suggest that they may support particular aspects of resilience both for people with dementia and those who care for them, sustaining positive relations with others, sense of life purpose, and environmental mastery. Further research to explore this application of multimedia tools in greater depth would contribute to a more nuanced understanding of the relationship between narrative and resilience in the context of dementia.

While it is important to consider the benefits of such tools for the individuals involved, this early work suggests that we also need to ask questions to help us understand the context in which these kinds of technologies emerge and used in everyday practice, and about the impact they might have on the broader community. For example, how does the socio-political milieu of residential care (or indeed the broader healthcare system) affect the potential of these kinds of technologies? Kelson's findings suggest that the need for something like *VLS* emerges with the shifting socio-political climate of residential care that has made it more difficult to get to know residents. Is it possible that as healthcare environments become increasingly depersonalized and fast-paced there will be increased pressure to produce technologies that support social engagement? This broader contextual view highlights the importance of moving beyond the individual level ask how narrative, especially given the opportunities afforded by new technologies, can be leveraged to support something we might rightfully call *community* resilience. These three projects have each, in different ways, directed us to consider the idea that communities can be strengthened to better accommodate the challenges of aging and dementia. Further research will be needed to explore how emerging technologies can build on ideas of narrative to help create these possibilities.

References

Alm, N., Astell, A., Ellis, M., Dye, R., Gowans, G., & Campbell, J. (2004) A cognitive prosthesis and communication support for people with dementia. *Neuropsychological Rehabilitation, 14*(1–2), 117–134.

Astell, A. J., Alm, N., Gowans, G., Ellis, M., Dye, R., & Vaughan, P. (2009) Involving older people with dementia and their carers in designing computer-based support systems: Some methodological considerations. *Universal Access in the Information Society, 8*(1), 49–59.

Baldwin, C. (2009) Narrative and decision-making. In D. O'Connor & B. Purves (Eds.), *Decision-making, personhood, and dementia: exploring the interface* (pp. 25–36). London: Jessica Kingsley.

Baldwin, C. & Capstick, A. (Eds.). (2007) *Tom Kitwood on dementia: a reader and critical commentary*. Maidenhead, UK, New York: Open University Press.

Brooker, D. (2004) What is person-centred care in dementia? *Reviews in Clinical Gerontology, 13*, 215–222.

Caldwell, R.L. (2005) At the confluence of memory and meaning - life review with older adults and families: Using narrative therapy and the expressive arts to re-member and re-author stories of resilience. *The Family Journal, 13*(2), 172–175.

Cohen, G., & Taylor, S. (1998) Reminiscence and aging. *Ageing and Society, 18*, 601–610.

de Medeiros, K. (2005) The complementary self: Multiple perspectives on the aging person. *Journal of Aging Studies, 19*, 1–13.

Gaugler, J.E., Kane, R.L., & Newcomer, R. (2007) Resilience and transitions from dementia caregiving. *Journal of Gerontology: Psychological Sciences, 62B*(1), 38–44.

Hagens, C., Beaman, A., & Ryan, E.B. (2003) Reminiscing, poetry writing, and remembering boxes: Personhood-centered communication with cognitively impaired older adults. *Activities, Adaptation, & Aging, 27*(3/4), 97–112.

Harris, P.B. (2008) Another wrinkle in the debate about successful aging: The undervalued concept of resilience and the lived experience of dementia. *International Journal of Aging and Human Development, 67*(1), 43–61.

Hellström, I., Nolan, M., & Lundh, U. (2005) 'We do things together:' A case study of 'couplehood' in dementia. *Dementia, 4*(1), 7–22.

Henderson, C.S., & Andrews, N. (1998) *Partial view*. Dallas, TX: South Methodist University Press.

Hydén, L.-C., & Örluv, L. (2009) Narrative and identity in Alzheimer's disease: A case study. *Journal of Aging Studies, 23*, 205–214.

Kelson, E. (2006) *Supporting personhood within dementia care: The therapeutic potential of personal photographs*. Unpublished master's thesis, Simon Fraser University, Vancouver, British Columbia, Canada.

Kensinger, E.A., Anderson, A., Growdon, J.H., & Corkin, S. (2004) Effects of Alzheimer disease on memory for verbal information. *Neuropsychologia, 42*, 792–800.

Kitwood, T. (1997) *Dementia reconsidered*. Buckingham, UK: Open University Press.

Neimeyer, R. A., & Levitt, H. (2001) Coping and coherence: A narrative perspective on resilience. In C. R. Snyder (Ed.), *Coping with stress: Effective people and processes* (pp. 47–67) Oxford: Oxford University Press.

O'Connor, D., Phinney, A., Smith, A., Small, J., Purves, B., Perry, J., Drance, E., Donnelly, M., Chaudhury, H., & Beattie, B. L. (2007) Personhood in dementia care: Developing a research agenda for broadening the vision. *Dementia, 6,* 121–142.

Ortiz, A., Simmons, J., & Hinton, W.L. (1999) Locations of remorse and homelands of resilience: Notes on grief and sense of loss of place of Latino and Irish-American caregivers of demented elders. *Culture, Medicine, and Psychiatry, 23,* 477–500.

Ryff, C.D., & Singer, B. (1998) The contours of positive human health. *Psychological Inquiry, 9*(1), 1–28.

Ryff, C.D., & Singer, B. (2008) Know thyself and become what you are: A eudaimonic approach to psychological well-being. *Journal of Happiness Studies, 9,* 13–39.

Sabat, S. (2001) *The experience of Alzheimer's disease: Life through a tangled veil.* Oxford, UK, Malden, MA: Blackwell.

Savundranayagam, M.Y., Dilley, L.J., & Basting, A. (in press) StoryCorps Memory Loss Initiative: Enhancing personhood for storytellers with memory loss. *Dementia: The International Journal of Social Research and Practice.*

Small, J.A., & Perry, J. (2005) Do you remember? How caregivers question their spouses who have Alzheimer's disease and the impact on communication. *Journal of Speech, Language, and Hearing Research, 48*(1), 125–136.

Woods, B. (1994) Management of memory impairment in older people with dementia. *International Review of Psychiatry, 6*(2/3), 153–161.

Woods, R. T., & McKiernan, F. (1995) Evaluating the impact of reminiscence on older people with dementia. In B.K. Haight & J. Webster (Eds.), *Art and science of reminiscing: Theory, research, methods, and applications* (pp. 233–242). Washington DC: Taylor and Francis.

Chapter 16
Building Resilience in Mild Cognitive Impairment and Early-Stage Dementia: Innovative Approaches to Intervention and Outcome Evaluation

Linda Clare, Glynda J. Kinsella, Rebecca Logsdon, Carol Whitlatch, and Steven H. Zarit

The onset of dementia presents many challenges, but people with dementia (PWD) and their family members bring an array of coping resources to bear on their situations. We now understand that dementia reflects an interplay between biology, individual psychology and social context (Kitwood 1997). Personal psychology, supportive relationships, and contexts can play a crucial role in helping individuals and families manage the impact of dementia-related changes on everyday life, confirming the value of promoting well-being and quality of life for people with dementia and their family members or care partners. This also holds true for people who develop mild cognitive impairment (MCI), which in many cases will progress to dementia.

Resilience in the face of late life cognitive impairment can operate on a number of levels. A range of psychosocial and lifestyle factors, including lifelong level of cognitive, social and physical activity, and size and complexity of social networks, may delay the onset of cognitive disability for some individuals (Fratiglioni et al. 2004; Wilson et al. 2002). The cognitive reserve hypothesis suggests that complex mental activity over the lifespan builds a capacity that may help individuals compensate for neural dysfunction, delaying the onset of difficulties or slowing progression (Stern et al. 2003). Once cognitive difficulties have developed, a degree of plasticity is still retained, and people with dementia or MCI still have some capacity for new learning and behavior change (Fernández-Ballesteros et al. 2003). Experience gained throughout life also contributes to the development of psychological resilience in terms of resources for coping with challenges and difficulties. People who develop MCI or dementia have a personal history and a wealth of life experience which has shaped their capacity for coping effectively with the resulting challenges (Kitwood 1997). The nature of relationships with family members and the degree of integration within a supportive social network will also influence resilience, as will social circumstances and social context.

Research on the subjective experience of dementia or MCI suggests those affected are not passive sufferers, but active agents engaged in finding ways to live with, and manage the effects of these conditions (Clare 2003; Lingler et al. 2006). Scholars increasingly acknowledge that PWD, despite cognitive losses, have both the capability

L. Clare (✉)
Bangor University, Bangor, UK
e-mail: l.clare@bangor.ac.uk

B. Resnick et al. (eds.), *Resilience in Aging: Concepts, Research, and Outcomes,*
DOI 10.1007/978-1-4419-0232-0_16, © Springer Science+Business Media, LLC 2011

and desire to participate in interventions. PWD with mild to moderate cognitive loss retain a sense of self, are able to participate actively in the intervention process, often have a keen awareness of their diagnosis and its implications, and have the ability to voice their preferences and choices about care (Downs 1997; Dresser and Whitehouse 1994; Whitlatch et al. 2005). Improvements in medical technology have led to more accurate and early diagnosis of dementia and MCI, providing the opportunity for intervention at a time when cognitive loss and the resulting stress are in their earliest stages (Whitlatch et al. 2006). In these early stages, psychological and psychosocial interventions aim to build resources for coping that will not only provide immediate benefits but also continue to support well-being as the condition progresses.

Family members of persons with dementia also face a host of threats and challenges, and many types of intervention strategies are available to help family members cope with the changing nature of their relatives' dementia. However, interventions that target both the family caregiver and his/her relative with dementia as a dyad are still relatively rare. This lack of a dyadic focus is not because dyadic strategies have been shown to be ineffective, but because dyadic research and intervention design has lagged far behind research focusing separately on PWD or family caregivers. Yet the early period of dementia provides a unique and timely opportunity for PWD and family caregivers to work together to understand the diagnosis and the challenges that may develop as a result (Robinson et al. 2005; Whitlatch and Feinberg 2003; Whitlatch et al. 2006; Zarit et al. 2004), and to develop effective ways of coping.

Identifying the factors that support or limit resilience and coping provides a basis for developing interventions, whether for individuals or for dyads, that can help promote coping and adjustment and facilitate management of the condition. This chapter presents four examples of innovative approaches to intervention that aim to support resilience, coping and adjustment, and ultimately enhance the quality of life for people with MCI or early-stage dementia (PWD). Cognitive intervention for people with MCI aims to improve memory functioning in everyday situations and reduce memory-related disability through a 5-week group program. Support groups for people with early-stage dementia aim to help PWD and their families cope with the psychological and social changes that the diagnosis brings. Cognitive rehabilitation for people with early-stage Alzheimer's disease focuses on improving everyday functioning and reducing functional disability by targeting personally relevant and meaningful rehabilitation goals in the real-life setting. While primarily focused on the PWD, caregivers also participate where available. Early diagnosis dyadic intervention focuses on PWD–caregiver dyads, helping them work together to explore care values and preferences and the impact of dementia on their relationship, with the goal of reducing stress in both partners over the longer-term.

Cognitive Intervention for People with MCI

The onset of dementia often emerges over several years before clinical diagnosis, and MCI refers to that condition in which self-report of cognitive difficulty can be confirmed in neuropsychological assessment but fails to reach criteria for a diagnosis of Alzheimer's disease (AD) (Petersen 2004). Given the increased risk of MCI sufferers developing AD, development of cognitive interventions to assist this population is important. Several recent randomized trials have investigated the benefits of memory training in healthy older adults (e.g. Willis et al. 2006), and positive effects have been reported even at a 5-year follow-up (Willis et al. 2006). However, study of the response of persons with MCI to memory intervention has been very limited, and debate persists regarding whether or not participants with MCI can benefit from cognitive training (Belleville 2008; Troyer et al. 2008). Furthermore, although improvements can be achieved on memory tasks in a clinic setting, it remains to be demonstrated whether daily functioning is concurrently improved. This is important as the memory deficits associated with MCI are troublesome in everyday life.

Memory of course has several dimensions, and training may address one or more of these processes. One promising component for intervention is prospective memory which refers to that component of memory that allows us to remember to carry out delayed intentions at the appropriate time; for example, remembering to prune the roses in early winter or returning a book to a friend when you next see her. Many everyday activities rely on prospective memory and complaints amongst older adults are most frequently about prospective memory errors (Einstein and McDaniel 2005). To comprehensively evaluate cognitive interventions for older adults with progressive memory loss, outcome measures that index memory performance in everyday activities are a necessary addition to standard clinical tests for memory impairment. Prospective memory assessment can provide a useful approach to measurement of everyday memory competence.

In a recent study (Kinsella et al. 2009) these arguments were pursued through evaluation of an early cognitive intervention for older adults diagnosed with MCI. Rather than attempting to change the underlying memory impairment (performance on clinical memory tests), the primary aim was to minimize memory disability in everyday life (prospective memory errors) by increasing knowledge and use of specific strategies to prevent failures of prospective memory. A sample of participants with MCI were randomly allocated to an intervention group ($n = 22$) and a waiting list control group ($n = 22$). The intervention consisted of a 5-week memory group providing information about memory and memory strategies. Assessments were conducted pre- and post-intervention and at 4-month follow-up. Overall, the study results were encouraging for the value of early intervention. Participants who received intervention demonstrated significant gains in actual performance of everyday memory as measured by prospective memory tasks (their memory disability was reduced). Prospective memory in everyday life depends on a complex interaction of planning and attention skills as well as retrieval of the to-be-remembered information (Einstein et al. 2005); for example, remembering to ring the plumber sometime in the afternoon requires forming a plan of how to remember (linking the intention with a plan to ring after lunch) and recalling who it is that you have to ring (placing the plumber's business card by the telephone to remind you that it is the plumber and not the hairdresser that needs contacting). Thus, there are multiple opportunities for people with MCI to apply cognitive strategies in order to compensate for impairments in memory.

However, although study participants demonstrated improvement in objective performance on prospective memory tasks, this improvement was not replicated in the frequency of self-reported memory failures in everyday life, which remained relatively unchanged across assessments. This suggests the possibility that although participants can improve their performance on prospective memory tasks, this may not generalize to actual everyday tasks; and yet, patient testimony did not support this interpretation. For example, one participant described having learnt through application of strategies how to remember to self-administer her diabetic regime reliably so that she no longer required home nursing involvement; another participant reported his success in developing a mnemonic for remembering the rotation schedule for summer watering of his garden sections. An alternative explanation is provided by a substantial body of research which reports little relationship between self-appraisal and objective memory performance (Johansson et al. 1997; Troyer and Rich 2002). It is frequently reported that memory questionnaires are liable to be confounded by subjective memory beliefs or negative stereotypes about age-related memory (Troyer et al. 2008; Troyer and Rich 2002). In other words, there can be a time-lag between changing behavior (actual performance in everyday situations) and capacity for accurate self-appraisal of that change.

As compared with waitlist controls, the intervention group displayed more knowledge and actual use of memory strategies immediately following intervention, and the advantage of improved knowledge of memory strategies remained at follow-up. Nevertheless, self-report of actual strategy use in everyday activities had dissipated by 4-month follow-up, suggesting a need to investigate the use of ongoing booster sessions as part of successful cognitive interventions for healthy older adults (Willis et al. 2006).

Although prospective memory may provide a useful means for determining outcome following cognitive intervention, this approach also presents a methodological challenge. A central problem relates to establishing appropriate tasks that continue to be ecologically valid and yet reliably assessable. Nevertheless, prospective memory as an outcome measurement offers a potentially useful approach to evaluating everyday memory and response to cognitive intervention.

A Support Group Program for People with Early-Stage Dementia

With the advent of sensitive diagnostic procedures, Alzheimer's disease and other dementias are being diagnosed in their earliest stages. Although early diagnosis provides opportunities for treatment, decision making, and planning (Gauthier 2002), it also conveys potentially negative consequences, including both affective and interpersonal changes (Phinney 2002). Early-stage support groups for individuals with dementia have been developed to help these individuals and their families cope with the psychological and social changes that the diagnosis brings

(Snyder et al. 1994; Yale 1995; Zarit et al. 2004). These groups vary in format, level of cognitive impairment of participants, inclusion of family members, and number and content of sessions. All groups, however, share a common goal of improving quality of life for individuals with dementia and their families.

Prior studies indicate that early-stage support groups are a promising approach to early-stage care, but outcomes have been mixed. As is common in any new area of clinical research, early studies are limited by small samples, lack of control groups, and lack of standardized outcome measures. Each prior study has concluded that randomized controlled trials with objective outcomes assessments are needed to evaluate the efficacy of these groups. To address this need for empirical investigations of early-stage support groups, the Northwest Research Group on Aging at the University of Washington School of Nursing and the Alzheimer's Association Western and Central Washington State Chapter (AAW) collaborated on a controlled randomized trial, to evaluate the efficacy of the AAW Chapter's Early Stage Memory Loss Seminar Program (ESML) as compared to a wait list control condition (WL).

ESML is a structured support group program developed and used by the AAW since 1995, following a written manual developed in collaboration with Lisa Snyder, MSW, ACSW. ESML sessions average 90 min in duration, and meet weekly for 8–9 weeks. Each session includes both individuals with early-stage dementia and a family member or partner, who meet together for part of the session, and separately for part of the session. Session topics include: coping with memory problems; information on dementia diagnosis, treatment, and research; the impact of diagnosis on social and family relationships; legal and financial considerations; safety concerns; health issues; and planning for the future. At each session, some didactic information is presented, and a trained facilitator leads a discussion of the session topic and/or other concerns that participants raise. More details about these sessions are provided elsewhere (Logsdon et al. 2006).

WL participants received written educational materials that are routinely provided by the AAW, and AAW staff provided their typical telephone support and information about local referral sources as needed. After their follow-up assessment, people randomized to WL were invited to participate in the next available ESML seminar within their community.

We randomly assigned 142 dyads (PWD and their family care partners) to ESML ($n = 96$) or WL ($n = 46$), and assessed outcomes of both the person with dementia and the care partner at baseline, post-treatment (2 months), and follow-up (6 months). Participants were required to: (a) have a diagnosis of dementia; (b) have an MMSE score of 18 or higher; (c) be aware of their memory loss and able to communicate verbally; (d) be able to participate independently in a group setting; (e) have no significant history of severe mental illness that would impede their ability to take part; and (f) have a family care partner (husband, wife, or other adult family member) who agreed to participate in the study. At baseline, mean age of participants was 75 years, and mean MMSE score was 23. Eighty percent of care partners (mean age 68 years) were spouses, 14% were adult children, and the rest were other relatives or friends. Primary outcome measures included: overall quality of life, depression, perceived stress, self-efficacy, communication between participant and care partner, and frequency of and care partner distress concerning memory and behavior problems.

Of 142 dyads that began the study, 136 (96%) completed post-treatment assessments and 88% completed 6-month assessments. At baseline, ESML and WL participants did not differ significantly on any of the outcome measures, and there was no difference in completion rates between the two groups. At both post treatment and 6 months, PWD in the ESML groups had significantly better quality of life, social functioning, depression and family communication than PWD in the WL control group. There were no significant differences in care partner outcomes between ESML and WL groups, although there was a trend for decreased distress over PWD memory-related problems in the ESML care partners compared to those in the WL condition.

Early-stage dementia support groups are becoming more widespread as individuals are being diagnosed earlier and are recognizing the need for education, support, and sharing of experiences. This randomized controlled clinical trial found statistically significant improvement in quality of life, social functioning, depression, and family communication for participants in the ESML seminars, compared to those on the WL. Care partners reported decreased distress about memory-related behavioral changes.

Although these results are promising, we must acknowledge that they may not generalize to everyone. For example, individuals with early onset dementia (age 35–65 years) face a different set of problems than those with later onset, and may not feel they fit into the typical early-stage group. Most of the dyads in these groups were married couples, and consequently most care partners who participated in this study were spouses. Adult child care partners or dyads with other relationships may respond differently to these support groups. Finally, individuals and families with different ethnic or cultural backgrounds may also have needs and expectations that differ from those of the typical early-stage group participant. Clearly, more research is needed. But, in the interim, early-stage support groups offer hope to many participants and care partners. We have begun to define and objectively measure intervention benefits, and will undoubtedly learn much more about how these groups can best serve individuals and families in the future.

Cognitive Rehabilitation for People with Early-Stage Dementia

Cognitive rehabilitation (CR) involves the person with cognitive impairment, and where appropriate family members or other supporters, in working together with health professionals to develop ways of living with, managing, by-passing, reducing or coming to terms with difficulties resulting from damage or injury to the brain (Wilson 1997). CR builds on the person's strengths, aiming to harness personal resourcefulness to address the challenges of living with cognitive impairment.

The aim is to promote optimal management of the condition and reduce the level of functional disability. In terms of the (World Health Organization 1998) model of disability, cognitive rehabilitation focuses on reducing limitations on engaging in activity and restrictions on social participation, taking account of the individual's personal and social context.

Individualized rehabilitation approaches targeting relevant and personally meaningful aspects of everyday functioning have produced significant benefits in single-case and small-group intervention studies (Clare et al. 2000). This evidence has led to the development of a program of individual, goal-oriented cognitive rehabilitation for people with early-stage AD (Clare 2008). In this program, cognitive rehabilitation sessions take place for 60–90 min a week over 8 8 weeks. These 8 eight therapy sessions typically take place in the participant's own home, to facilitate implementation of strategies in the everyday setting. Participants are encouraged to work on goals and practice strategies between sessions. The intervention addresses five areas:

1. Rehabilitation goals. The aim is to identify and work on one or two personal rehabilitation goals relevant to the individual's daily life. A clinometric measure such as the Canadian Occupational Performance Measure provides a structured approach to eliciting goals and rating current performance and satisfaction with performance (Law et al. 2005). Rehabilitation goals relate to areas that are currently causing difficulty or concern, or reflect areas where the participant would like to see improvement. Goals might focus directly on the impact of cognitive difficulties in everyday life; for example, participants might aim to improve their ability to remember important events during the day or keep track of important personal belongings, or to absorb and retain important personally relevant information. However, some goals may have a broader focus; for example, the participant might express a wish to resume previously enjoyed activities, or to take up new activities so as to increase social contact. Once goals have been identified at the start of therapy, an individual approach to addressing these is designed, using evidence-based rehabilitation methods, and implemented over the course of the sessions. Work on personal goals forms the central element of the program and continues throughout all sessions. This effort to meet specific objectives is supported by the other components of the program.
2. Practical strategies. This component involves a review of the participant's current use of memory aids and practical coping strategies, explores whether it might be possible to build on these to promote more efficient use, and supports the introduction of new aids or strategies where appropriate.
3. Memory. The therapist introduces techniques for learning new associations and information, provides practice in these, identifies the person's preferred strategy, and encourages the wider application of this strategy in everyday life. The kinds of learning strategies presented include simple verbal and visual mnemonics, semantic elaboration, vanishing cues and forward cueing, and spaced retrieval. Face-name association learning is used as an example of the kind of new learning or relearning that is relevant for everyday life, with personally relevant stimuli such as photographs of family, friends or acquaintances selected for practice wherever possible.

4. Attention and concentration. Practice is provided for maintaining attention and concentration while processing information, drawing on rehabilitation methods devised for people with impairments of executive function.
5. Stress management. The person's current ways of coping with stress and anxiety are explored, suggestions are made to build on these strategies, and relevant practice is provided using simple stress management and relaxation techniques.
6. The participant's spouse or other family member or carer is invited to join the last 15 min of each session. This part of the session is devoted to reviewing the content of the session, agreeing on the home practice to be undertaken in preparation for the next session, and discussing ways of facilitating progress with the personal rehabilitation goals.

In a recently completed randomized controlled trial (RCT) in which CR was compared to Relaxation Therapy (RT) and a no-treatment control condition (NT) (Clare et al. submitted for publication), people in the CR group rated their performance, and satisfaction with performance, of personal rehabilitation goals significantly better following intervention, while the other two groups showed no change. For a sub-group of participants who underwent fMRI scanning, these significant gains were mirrored in changes in brain activation while carrying out a memory task. Similar effects were found in a single-case study of an individual with MCI who completed the CR program (Clare et al. 2009). This suggests that perceived improvements in behavioral functioning may reflect actual improvement in underlying neural plasticity. While this finding is tentative, it appears that CR may produce benefits at the neural as well as the behavioral level. As far as we can determine, this was the first RCT of individual, goal-oriented cognitive rehabilitation for people with dementia, and both behavioral and neuroimaging findings will need to be confirmed by future research. The results of the study suggest, however, that collaborative interventions of this kind can promote resilience through supporting attempts at problem solving and finding creative solutions to everyday difficulties.

Dyadic Interventions

Family members, as well as persons with MCI and early-stage dementia, face a host of threats and challenges related to caring for a relative with cognitive losses, and many intervention strategies have been documented that aim to help family members cope. However, intervention approaches targeting the caregiver/care-recipient dyad remain relatively rare. Yet dyadic interventions offer potential benefits to PWD and family caregivers by providing a structured environment within which the dyad is able to work together to maintain or develop resilience.

The Early Diagnosis Dyadic Intervention (EDDI) program was designed to respond to the growing and promising evidence that persons with mild to moderate cognitive impairment are able to communicate their preferences for care reliably, make informed decisions about their care (Clark et al. 2008), and choose a person (typically a family member) to make their decisions if they are no longer able to do so themselves (Feinberg and Whitlatch 2001; Logsdon et al. 1999). The goals of the EDDI program are to: (a) increase PWD and caregiver understanding of each other's care preferences and values; (b) learn and practice effective communication techniques; (c) understand discrepancies in care preferences and expectations; (d) increase the dyad's knowledge about available services; and (e) explore MCI-related relationship issues and emotional significance of the illness for both care partners (Whitlatch et al. 2006). The EDDI program evaluation found the intervention to be acceptable, feasible, and satisfactory to participants and EDDI Counselors (Whitlatch et al. 2006). Moreover, we found evidence indicating that PWD could voice care preferences and engage in discussions that helped them consider alternatives to care that did not rely solely on their family caregivers (Whitlatch et al. 2006). Unfortunately, these preliminary data did not provide clear evidence of the efficacy of EDDI for improving all well-being outcomes, or indication of whether the positive effects of EDDI can be maintained long term.

Based on the findings from the EDDI trial, a revised protocol has been developed that consists of seven sessions of structured counseling (see Table 16.1) conducted by a trained clinician with the critical goal of supporting the dyad "to work together to develop a mutual plan for coping with the disease over the long haul" (p. 689; Whitlatch et al. 2006). Sessions are designed so that the dyad meets with the EDDI Counselor for the entire session ("joint") or so that each care partner (caregiver and PWD) meets with the EDDI Counselor alone and with their care partner ("mixed"). A variety of EDDI materials and tools are used to enhance the learning and communication experience for both care partners. For example, caregivers and PWD have their own "EDDI Notebooks" that provides information about the program, appropriate worksheets, and notes from each session. Magnet boards with magnetic strips that correspond to a variety of EDDI procedures are used so that care partners can manipulate the strips as they make changes to their care plans. A variety of worksheets are filled out and revised over the course of the seven sessions as the dyad makes decisions about how to plan for the future. Together, these materials provide both the structure and flexibility to meet the diverse needs of care dyads as they work through the complex, demanding, and dynamic challenges associated with early-stage dementia.

The EDDI program offers hope and support for the growing number of persons with early-stage dementia and the family members who assist them. The program is one of a number of promising dyadic interventions (Logsdon et al. 2006; Zarit et al. 2004) that seek to decrease the stress experienced by early-stage families as they manage and adapt to their changing roles.

Resilience in a Period of Decline

Resilience is a quality expected in a healthy young person, and, as the other papers in this volume suggest, may increasingly be found among older people as well. More unexpectedly, the studies presented in this chapter demonstrate that there may be continued resilience even as cognitive function begins to decline. These findings

Table 16.1 Overview of EDDI sessions

Session	Time	Description
#1 Understanding memory loss (joint)	75 min	The EDDI Counselor creates an environment that is comfortable, safe, and friendly. The dyad meets jointly to address questions they have about dementia, learn about memory loss and other possible changes, discuss treatment options and begin addressing current needs for and ways of finding reliable information. Communication skills are introduced and will be practiced in subsequent sessions
#2 Care values & preferences (mixed)	90 min	CG and PWD meet separately to explore the PWD's care values and preferences for care tasks. Discussions provide the foundation for future sessions in working out a care plan
#3 Care preferences (joint)	75 min	The dyad engages in a care planning exercise that involves looking at the possible tasks that the PWD may need help with in the future and the preference for who would provide that help. Once the initial plan is constructed, the EDDI Counselor leads the dyad through steps in identifying ways of decreasing the load on the CG and encourages seeking help from other sources that would be acceptable to both
#4 Taking care of yourself – taking care of each other & barriers to receiving help (mixed)	90 min	Building on Sessions 2 and 3, the dyad is introduced to the concept of taking care of oneself as a way of managing the stresses of a chronic illness. The CG and PWD learn the concept of pleasant events and discuss strategies for building activities into their daily routines as a way of promoting health and well-being. PWD discuss how they can participate in activities on their own and together with others. Barriers to getting help are discussed
#5 Family and friends (joint)	75 min	Building on previous sessions, particularly the care plan exercise and pleasant activities strategy, the dyad explores the help and assistance that might be available from family in the future. They also explore effective ways to communicate with family about care-related concerns and changes associated with dementia
#6 Community resources (mixed)	75 min	This session continues the discussion of implementing the care plan, by supplementing the help provided by the CG and other family members with formal, paid help. The dyad will identify strategies for finding services and anticipate barriers. PWD discuss issues of independence and dependence and discuss when it might be appropriate for their caregiver to seek the help
#7 Looking to the future (joint)	75 min	Material will be covered from previous sessions and the plans participants have for the future. CGs and PWD review and follow-up on the issues that arose in previous sessions, and end with a discussion of how much they have accomplished since Session 1

combat the therapeutic nihilism that surrounds cognitive decline and dementia and the notion that only medication can make a difference. As the number of people with dementia in our population grows, it becomes increasingly important to identify strategies that may allow people with cognitive deficits to remain independent longer and function as well as possible. There has long been evidence that some people manage to maintain relatively good levels of functioning even though post-mortem examinations reveal extensive cognitive impairment (Katzman et al. 1988). A better understanding of mechanisms that lead to this kind of resilience in the face of a degenerative brain disease can be used to plan interventions that offer substantial improvements in functioning and in quality of life.

Compensation may be a major factor contributing to resilience in these studies. Compensatory processes have been hypothesized as a main component of successful aging (e.g. Baltes 1987, 1997; Carstensen et al. 2003; Riediger et al. 2006). From this perspective, people draw upon available cognitive and emotional resources to enhance those activities and relationships that are most important to them. This kind of compensation can be seen in the cognitive training and cognitive rehabilitation studies that we presented. People drew on remaining abilities to develop strategies to improve prospective memory or to achieve personally meaningful goals.

The finding that improvement in performance of a personally meaningful activity led to increased brain activity also raises the possibility of growth in cognitive ability. It would be overly optimistic to assume that these types of efforts might substantially alter the course of dementia, but some specific gains that have a reasonable duration may be possible. Teri et al. (2003) have shown that physical exercise can help people with dementia maintain performance of activities of daily living over a 2-year period. These effects are more substantial than found with any of the current medications for Alzheimer's disease. Comparable long-term benefits of cognitive interventions may be possible, especially when conducted while deficits are still mild.

The ESML and EDDI programs may operate in part through compensation and partly through a different mechanism. Resilience may emerge and be sustained through the support built with a care partner. The care partner will be able to provide compensation even when the person with dementia may no longer be able to do so. The care partner can draw upon earlier discussions with the person with dementia about his/her preferences and values. Dementia sufferers' improved understandings of their own emotional adjustments to cognitive and functional decline may also help care partners develop more personalized and effective strategies over the long haul. We now know that it is feasible to carry out frank discussions about the cognitive and emotional impact of dementia and the need to plan for future changes. It would be timely to test whether this type of planning has beneficial long-term effects.

We should note some potential sources of resilience in early dementia that have not been addressed. Technology may provide strategies that are useful for compensating for memory loss. These strategies, however, are likely to be more effective if they can be implemented at a time when the person with dementia can still learn to use them and incorporate them into everyday routines. Likewise, features of environmental design that may make it possible for people to live at home longer need to be implemented early on, rather than put in place as a last ditch effort when sustaining the person at home has become precarious.

Another issue is feelings of control. Blazer (2002) has argued that prevention programs in later life need to be built around a core component that helps increase feelings of self-efficacy. Studies have shown that greater feeling of being in control of one's life is related to continued independence in activities of daily living in very old populations (Fauth et al. 2007; Femia et al. 1997). The experience of cognitive decline is likely to precipitate feeling loss of control in one's life. Giving attention to increasing self-efficacy and to supporting the decisions made by people with dementia can be a critical aspect of interventions.

The resilience evidenced in the studies covered in this chapter provides affirmation of the humanity of those people affected by cognitive decline and dementia. Despite efforts to educate people about the "personhood" of those affected with dementia, it is easy to project our own fears onto the disease process, and to dismiss the requests and complaints made by people with dementia (Persson and Wästerfors 2009). The studies presented in this chapter demonstrate that people with MCI and dementia can actively engage in meaningful discussions about themselves, their goals, their emotions and their future. We need to take the opportunity to have these discussions while their memory loss is minimal and their ability to engage with us remains strong.

Acknowledgments Rebecca Logsdon's work is supported by grants from the National Alzheimer's Association (IIRG # 0306319) and the National Institute on Aging (R01AG23091–2). She would like to thank the Alzheimer's Association Western and Central Washington State Chapter, the Northwest Research Group on Aging staff, and the research study volunteers who made this investigation possible.

Linda Clare acknowledges support from the UK Alzheimer's Society. The trial described in this chapter was funded by the Alzheimer's Society through a grant to L. Clare (PI), D.E.J. Linden, R.T. Woods, and M.D. Rugg. She would like to thank the research participants and staff who contributed to the study, with particular thanks to Sue Evans and Caroline Parkinson.

Carol Whitlatch acknowledges the support of the Department of Health and Human Services, Administration on Aging grant number 90CG2566 (Zarit, PI) for her work on the Early Diagnosis Dyadic Intervention project.

Glynda Kinsella's research is supported by NHMRC, Australia through a grant to G. Kinsella (PI), D. Ames, E. Storey, B. Ong., M. Saling., E. Mullaly, E. Rand, and L. Clare. The study reported in this chapter was supported by Alzheimer's Australia Research, La Trobe University & Caulfield General Medical Centre. She would like to acknowledge her research collaborators and the support of the clinical staff in the memory clinics at Bundoora Extended Care Centre and Caulfield General Medical Centre, especially Margaret Winbolt and Luwene Heeney, and also thank the participants in the study.

References

Baltes, P.B. (1987) Theoretical propositions of life-span developmental psychology: On the dynamics between growth and decline. *Developmental Psychology, 23,* 611–626.
Baltes, P.B. (1997) On the incomplete architecture of human ontogeny: Selection, optimization, and compensation as foundation of developmental theory. *American Psychologist, 52,* 366–380.

Belleville, S. (2008) Cognitive training for persons with MCI. *International Psychogeriatrics, 20,* 57–66.

Blazer, D.G. (2002) Self-efficacy and depression in late life: A primary prevention proposal. *Aging and Mental Health, 6,* 315–324.

Carstensen, L.L., Fung, H.H., & Charles, S.T. (2003) Socioemotional selectivity theory and the regulation of emotion in the second half of life. *Motivation and Emotion, 27,* 103–123.

Clare, L. (2003) Managing threats to self: awareness in early-stage Alzheimer's disease. *Social Science and Medicine, 57,* 1017–1029.

Clare, L. (2008) *Neuropsychological Rehabilitation and People with Dementia.* Hove: Psychology Press.

Clare, L., Linden, D.E.J., Woods, R.T., Whitaker, R., Evans, S.J., Parkinson, C.H., van Paasschen, J., Nelis, S.M., Hoare, Z., Yuen, K.S.L. & Rugg, M.D. (submitted for publication) Goal-oriented cognitive rehabilitation for people with early-stage Alzheimer's disease: a single-blind randomized controlled trial of clinical efficacy.

Clare, L., van Paasschen, J., Evans, S.J., Parkinson, C., Woods, R.T., & Linden, D.E.J. (2009) Goal-oriented cognitive rehabilitation for an individual with Mild Cognitive Impairment: behavioural and neuroimaging outcomes. *Neurocase, 15,* 318–331.

Clare, L., Wilson, B.A., Carter, G., Gosses, A., Breen, K., & Hodges, J.R. (2000) Intervening with everyday memory problems in early Alzheimer's disease: an errorless learning approach. *Journal of Clinical and Experimental Neuropsychology, 22,* 132–146.

Clark, P.A., Whitlatch, C.J., & Tucke, S.S. (2008) Consistency of information from persons with dementia: An analysis of differences by question type. *Dementia: The International Journal of Social Research and Practice, 7,* 341–358.

Downs, M. (1997) Progress report: The emergence of the person in dementia research. *Aging and Society, 17,* 597–604.

Dresser, R., & Whitehouse, P.J. (1994) The incompetent patient on the slippery slope. *Hastings Center Report, 24(4),* 6–12.

Einstein, G.O., & McDaniel, M.A. (2005) *Memory fitness. A guide for successful aging.* New Haven: Yale University Press.

Einstein, G.O., Mc Daniel, M.A., Thoman, R., Mayfield, S., Shank, H., Morrisette, N., & Breneiser. J. (2005) Multiple processes in prospective memory retrieval: Factors determining monitoring versus spontaneous retrieval. *Journal of Experimental Psychology: General ,134,* 327–342.

Fauth, E. B., Zarit, S. H., Malmberg, B., & Johansson, B. (2007) Physical, cognitive, and psychosocial variables from the disablement process model predict patterns of independence and the transition into disability for the oldest old. *The Gerontologist, 47,* 613–624.

Feinberg, L.F. & Whitlatch, C.J. (2001) Are persons with cognitive impairment able to state consistent choices? *The Gerontologist, 41,* 374–382.

Femia, E.E., Zarit, S.H., & Johansson, B. (1997) Predicting change in activities of daily living: A longitudinal study of the oldest old. *Journals of Gerontology. Series B, Psychological Sciences and Social Sciences, 52,* P292–P304.

Fernández-Ballesteros, R., Zamarrón, M.D., Tàrraga, L., Moya, R., & Iniguez, J. (2003) Cognitive plasticity in healthy, MCI (MCI) subjects and Alzheimer's disease patients: A research project in Spain. *European Psychologist, 8,* 148–159.

Fratiglioni, L., Paillard-Borg, S., & Winblad, B. (2004) An active and socially integrated lifestyle in late life might protect against dementia. *Lancet Neurology, 3,* 343–353.

Gauthier, S. (2002) Advances in the pharmacotherapy of Alzheimer's disease. *Canadian Medical Association Journal, 166,* 616–623.

Johansson, B., Allen-Burge, R., & Zarit, S.H. (1997) Self reports on memory functioning in a longitudinal study of the oldest old: Relation to current, prospective, and retrospective performance. *Journals of Gerontology: Psychological Sciences, 52B,* P139-P146.

Katzman, R., Terry, R., DeTeresa, R., Brown, T., Davies, P., Fuld, P., Renbing, X., & Peck, A. (1988) Clinical, pathological, and neurochemical changes in dementia: A subgroup with preserved mental status and numerous neocortical plaques. *Annals of Neurology, 23(2),* 138–144.

Kinsella, G.J., Mullaly, E., Rand, E., Ong, B., Burton, C., Price, S., Phillips, M., & Storey, E. (2009) Early cognitive intervention for MCI: A randomized controlled trial. *Journal of Neurology, Neurosurgery and Psychiatry, 80*, 730–736.

Kitwood, T. (1997) *Dementia Reconsidered: the Person Comes First.* Buckingham: Open University Press.

Law, M., Baptiste, S., Carswell, A., McColl, M.A., Polatajko, H., & Pollock, N. (2005) Canadian Occupational Performance Measure (4th ed.). Ottawa, ON: CAOT Publications ACE.

Lingler, J.H., Nightingale, M.C., Erlen, J.A., Kane, A.L., Reynolds III, C.F., Schulz, R., & DeKosky, S.T. (2006) Making sense of MCI: A qualitative exploration of the patient's experience. *The Gerontologist, 46*, 791–800.

Logsdon R.G., Gibbons, L.E., McCurry, S.M., & Teri, L. (1999) Quality of life in Alzheimer's disease: Patient and caregiver reports. *Journal of Mental Health and Aging*, 5(1), 21–32.

Logsdon, R.G., McCurry, S.M., & Teri, L. (2006) Time-limited support groups for individuals with early stage dementia and their care partners: Preliminary outcomes from a controlled clinical trial. *Clinical Gerontologist, 30*, 5–19.

Persson, T., & Wästerfors, D. (2009) Such trivial matters: How staff account for restrictions of residents' influence in nursing homes. *Journal of Aging Studies, 23*, 1–11.

Petersen, R.C. (2004) MCI as a diagnostic entity. *Journal of Internal Medicine, 256*, 183–194.

Phinney, A. (2002) Living with the symptoms of Alzheimer's disease. In P. B. Harris (Ed.), *The Person with Alzheimer's Disease: Pathways to Understanding the Experience* (pp. 49–74). Baltimore: Johns Hopkins University Press.

Riediger, M., Li, S.-C., & Lindenberger, U. (2006) Selection, optimization, and compensation as developmental mechanisms of adaptive resource allocation: Review and preview. In J.E. Birren & K.W. Schaie (Eds.), *Handbook of the Psychology of Aging* (6th ed., pp. 289–313). San Diego, CA: Academic Press.

Robinson, L., Clare, L., & Evans, K. (2005) Making sense of dementia and adjusting to loss: Psychological reactions to a diagnosis of dementia in couples. *Aging and Mental Health, 9*, 337–347.

Snyder, L., Bower, D., Arneson, S., Sheperd, S., & Quayhagen, M. (1994) *Coping with Alzheimer's disease and related disorders: An educational support group for early stage individuals and their families.* San Diego: UCSD Alzheimer's Disease Research Center.

Stern, Y., Zarahn, E., Hilton, H.J., Flynn, J., De La Paz, R., & Rakitin, B. (2003) Exploring the neural basis of cognitive reserve. *Journal of Clinical and Experimental Neuropsychology, 25*, 691–701.

Teri, L., Gibbons, L.E., McCurry, S.M., Logsdon, R.G., Buchner, D.M., Barlow, W.E., Kukull, W.A., LaCroix, A.Z., McCormick, W. & Larson E.B. (2003) Exercise plus behavioral management in patients with Alzheimer's disease: A randomized controlled trial. *Journal of the American Medical Association, 290*(15), 2015–2022.

Troyer, A.K., Murphy, K.J., Anderson, N.D., Moscovitch, M., & Craik, F.I.M. (2008) Changing everyday memory behaviour in amnestic MCI: A randomised controlled trial. *Neuropsychological Rehabilitation, 18*, 65–88.

Troyer, A.K. & Rich, J.B. (2002) Psychometric properties of a new metamemory questionnaire for older adults. *Journal of Gerontology, 57B*, 19–27.

Whitlatch, C.J., & Feinberg, L.F. (2003) Planning for the future together in culturally diverse families: Making everyday care decisions. *Alzheimer's Care Quarterly, 4*, 50–61.

Whitlatch, C.J., Feinberg, L.F., Tucke, S.T. (2005) Measuring the values and preferences for everyday care of persons with cognitive impairment and their family caregivers. *The Gerontologist, 45*, 370–380.

Whitlatch, C.J., Judge, K., Zarit, S.H., & Femia, E. (2006) Dyadic intervention for family caregivers and care receivers in early-stage dementia. *The Gerontologist, 46*, 688–694.

Willis, S.L., Tennstedt, S.L., Marsiske, M., Ball, K., Elias, J., Koepke, K.M., Morris, J.N., Rebok, G.W., Unverzagt, F.W., Stoddard, A.M. & Wright, E. for the ACTIVE Study Group. (2006) Long-term effects of cognitive training on everyday functional outcomes in older adults. *Journal of the Medical Association of America, 296*, 2805–2814.

Wilson, B.A. (1997) Cognitive rehabilitation: How it is and how it might be. *Journal of the International Neuropsychological Society*, *3*, 487–496.

Wilson, R.S., Bennett, D.A., Bienias, J.L., Aggarwal, N.T., de Leon, C.F.M., Morris, M.C., Schneider, J.A., & Evans, D.A. (2002) Cognitive activity and incident AD in a population-based sample of older persons. *Neurology*, *59*, 1910–1914.

World Health Organization. (1998) *International Classification of Impairments, Disabilities and Handicaps*. 2nd Edition. www.who.int/msa/mnh/ems/icidh/introduction.htm

Yale, R. (1995) *Developing support groups for individuals with early-stage Alzheimer's disease.* Baltimore: Health Professions Press.

Zarit, S.H., Femia, E.E., Watson, J., Rice-Oeschger, L., & Kakos, B. (2004) Memory Club: A group intervention for people with early-stage dementia and their care partners. *The Gerontologist*, *44*, 262–269.

Chapter 17
African American Caregivers Finding Resilience Through Faith

Joseph G. Pickard and M. Denise King

The field of gerontology takes a multidisciplinary approach to the study of aging and issues related to older adults by combining knowledge from the fields of biology, medicine, political science, psychology, sociology, social work, and other disciplines. The study of religion and spirituality in each of these fields has increased dramatically as evidenced by the explosion of high-quality, peer-reviewed articles that have been produced within each of these sub-disciplines in the past several years.

Koenig et al. (2001) suggest three reasons for the sudden increase in academic interest in this area. First, though science and psychology have made great advances, religion continues to play a large role in the lives of many people, and the social sciences are just now beginning to recognize their reticence to address such an important source of strength and resilience in people's lives. Second, due to the burgeoning cost of health care, alternatives must be found to fill the gaps in what treatments are actually available to people and to complement existing treatments. Third, the face of medicine as a cold, uncaring science based on remediation of symptoms is changing to a field in which medical professionals actively encourage people to change their lifestyles to include more healthy behaviors. The increase in scholarly attention to religion and spirituality is also due to the revival of religion as a legitimate political issue, the increase in policies concerning faith-based initiatives, the realization among researchers and providers that many positive associations exist between religiosity and health and mental health outcomes, and a growing awareness that religiosity, though difficult to clearly define in a manner that all would find acceptable, still can be studied scientifically.

Defining Spiritually and Religion

The two terms, spirituality and religion, are often used interchangeably and, indeed, difficulty exists in distinguishing strongly between the two. Spirituality can be thought of as a relationship with a transcendent being – God – and refers to the quest

J.G. Pickard (✉)
University of Missouri, St Louis, MO, USA
e-mail: pickardj@umsl.edu

B. Resnick et al. (eds.), *Resilience in Aging: Concepts, Research, and Outcomes*,
DOI 10.1007/978-1-4419-0232-0_17, © Springer Science+Business Media, LLC 2011

to deepen that relationship, to find meaning and purpose, and to make sense of complex life experiences. It is usually informed by a historical religious tradition. The utility of characterizing spirituality this way is twofold: this conceptualization identifies the importance of spirituality in its own right, and also ties spiritual development to cultural influences without directly connecting spirituality to any specific religious affiliation. This definition recognizes that individuals do not develop spirituality in a vacuum. Instead, spirituality is based on cultural influences that run deeply in individuals, families, and societies.

The term religion can include beliefs, attitudes, knowledge, rituals, personal and public behaviors, laws, and social organization. Religion can be understood best, however, from a multidimensional point of view than as a single, all-encompassing term, because religion is so complex and wide ranging in its manifestations and effects. Religion includes patterns of behaviors, ritual practices, membership in some form of community, sacred texts, beliefs, values, and attitudes. A review of Hill and Hood's (1999) book, *Measures of Religiosity*, reveals that the majority of scales developed to quantify and compare levels of religiosity include items that address behavioral, emotional, and experiential aspects of faith. Furthermore, this occurs in the context of social, emotional, and metaphysical experiences. Religion can be considered to be very personal or it can be public; it can be a source of strength and resilience to individuals, groups, families, or communities.

For the purposes of this chapter, the term religion is defined as an institutionalized set of beliefs and behaviors, involving a sense of spirituality that provides meaning, direction, values, and support. Religiosity, then, refers to the practice of religion and the salience of respondents' spiritual and religious beliefs in their lives. The term religion includes spirituality, unless a specific distinction is needed for clarity.

An Aging America

The remarkable increase in academic literature addressing the relationship between religion and aging is not surprising when one considers the current and impending growth of the population of older adults in the United States and, indeed, the world. For example, in 1900 approximately 4% of Americans were over age 65, yet the proportion of adults over the age of 65 is currently about 12.3%; by the year 2030 the proportion of the US population over age 65 is expected to approach 20% (Administration on Aging 2006). African Americans, like other groups, are living longer than ever before, and African Americans and Caribbean and African immigrants make up the largest group of elders of color in the United States. At the same time, the growth of the population of African Americans over the age of 65 during the next half century has a remarkable trajectory when contrasted with the change in the population of non-Hispanic Whites (Administration on Aging 2009). In 2004, the proportion of African Americans among the population of those aged 65 and older was 8%. This percentage is projected to increase to 12% by 2050. By comparison, the proportion of non-Hispanic White Americans will decrease from 82% to 61% during the same time period.

Importance of Religion and Spirituality to Older Adults

Religion appears to have a greater presence and influence in the lives of the current cohort of older adults than in the population in general. In one study of religious congregations in the United States, researchers found that 24% of all congregants were age 65 or older (Cnaan et al. 2002). Another study that estimated membership in mainline Protestant churches found that about 50% of members in these congregations are over age 60 (Brat 2002).

Overall, older people appear more religious than younger people, a trend that is true for both Caucasian–Americans and African Americans. The ongoing importance of religiosity in the lives of older Americans is illustrated by Cutler's (1976) findings based on the General Social Surveys of 1974 and 1975. Cutler found that among older adults belonging to voluntary associations, 49% belonged to groups affiliated with churches. The next most commonly reported associations were fraternal groups, which only claimed volunteer participation by 18% of older adults. More recently, the most common form of volunteering by older adults was found to be in synagogues and churches, where 53% of those aged 65 and over attended weekly (Koenig 1992). Increased health in late life is associated with older adults helping others within their religious congregations, but the association appears strongest when the people are committed more deeply to their faith (Krause 2009).

Nationally, 59% of Americans over age 18 say that religion is "very important" in their daily lives (Carroll 2004), but a breakdown by age group highlights differences among age cohorts. Only 46% of younger adults aged 18–29 and 65% of older adults aged 50–64 rate religion as "very important," while 73% of those over age 65 view religion as "very important" (Gallup and Lindsay 1999; Newport 2004). Further accentuating the importance of religion for seniors as a socializing factor, more than half of the respondents among patients being seen at a geriatric assessment clinic reported that at least four out of five of their friendships were with people within their religious organizations (Koenig et al. 1988).

While it is unclear if the greater religiosity of older people as compared to younger people is a developmental or a cohort effect, Glamser (1988) found support for the "stability hypothesis" in a 6-year longitudinal study that indicated little change in church activity during the early retirement years. However, those who attended church regularly at a younger age seemed to attended church even more after retirement. It seems that the more religiosity one displays in early and middle adulthood, the more religiosity one will display when older. Though older adults are known to attend religious services more frequently than their younger counterparts, their attendance tends to decline with the onset of age-related disabilities, loss of ability to complete activities of daily living independently, reduction in mobility, and loss of driving privileges.

African American Elders, Religion, and Spirituality

In a review of the literature, Taylor et al. (2004) conclude that African Americans display certain general religious characteristics. They suggest most African Americans feel the church is a valuable institution, are Protestant Christians (over half report that they are Baptist), tend not to participate in denominational switching, and have high levels of religious participation that often includes attendance at religious services and daily prayer. They also found that gender was the most influential factor in determining who among the elderly would actively engage in religious attendance. In fact, in Western societies, at all ages, females tend to be more religious than males on almost every measure of religiosity. In the United States, religion is ranked as "very important" in the lives of women 67% of the time and 53% of the time for men (Gallup and Lindsay 1999). Perhaps, one of the reasons that older adults appear more religious than younger adults has to do with the fact that so many more women than men live into late life. This is particularly true for African Americans. In 2002, if African American men lived to be 65, their life expectancy would become 79.6 years; for African American women who reached age 65, life expectancy was 83.0 years (Administration on Aging 2006).

African Americans tend to report being more religious/spiritual than Whites, and this is even more pronounced for older adults (Taylor et al. 2004). Regardless of age, over 90% of Blacks report that they have attended church services as an adult for services other than weddings or funerals, and about 70% report regular attendance at church services at least a few times per month with close to two-thirds reporting that membership in a church. Neighbors et al. (1998) assert that the African American minister serves as a primary mental health service provider and gatekeeper to other mental health resources; however, they caution that little research has been done that would validate the efficacy of the services they provide.

Caregiver Strain and Religious Coping

Religious coping has consistently emerged among African American caregivers as an important strategy for adapting to the challenges of providing care. It has been conceptualized as a resource called upon in times of stress to help people cope with and adapt to changing life circumstances. Moreover, religious involvement can be a determinant of well-being among African Americans; religiosity has positive associations with life satisfaction, happiness, and congruence, and negative associations with distress. Clearly, religious participation is vital to the lives of Black Americans, particularly those in older cohorts (Taylor et al. 2004). Indeed, historical and present-day scholarship unmistakably documents the pivotal role of religion and religious institutions in the development of Black communities in America and their promotion of individual well-being.

The burdens of caregiving, both physical and emotional, have been studied extensively and are well documented. The negative effects of caregiving are of particular concern to African American women, as they are more likely than their Caucasian counterparts to become caregivers for older adults. According to the National Alliance for Caregiving and American Association of Retired Persons (2004), African American caregivers usually need to manage multiple tasks and are more likely to face financial difficulties.

The experience of caregiving strain varies greatly from one individual to the next, and the reasons for strain are many. Although multiple sources of stress exist, caregiver burden may be based more on the amount of time spent thinking about caregiving tasks and responsibilities than on actual time spent managing the elder's symptoms and providing direct care. This stems from the fact that mental stress is often conceptualized as worry, and time spent thinking about caregiving is, in effect, worry. Further, it is a self-perpetuating cycle in which excessive thinking about a thing becomes difficult to stop. Stress causes worry, which, in turn, leads to more stress. When thoughts become overwhelming, these thoughts can be disruptive to an individual's ability to function effectively and live with serenity.

The National Survey of American Life included a nationally representative sample of approximately 4,000 African Americans, 1,500 Black Americans of Caribbean descent, and 1,500 non-Hispanic Whites (Taylor et al. 2004). Surprisingly, lifetime prevalence rates of dysthymia, major depression, agoraphobia, social phobia, panic disorders, and generalized anxiety disorder were found to be lowest for African Americans despite the fact that they also scored lowest on most other indicators of positive social status and health (Sue and Chu 2003). The source of this resilience can be found in the coping styles that are often employed by African Americans – namely religious coping. Coping refers to the manner in which a person makes sense of or masters stressful life events. Religious coping refers to coping methods that are specifically oriented toward the use of religious/spiritual-based methods such as prayer or talking to a clergy member. Religious coping is not the same as other forms of coping in that it is specifically of a religious or spiritual nature (Fetzer Institute 1999).

When stress is present, people consciously and unconsciously mobilize their coping strategies. Most – though clearly not all – older African Americans look to their faith and images of God for comfort as a primary way of coping with the stress of caregiving. Cognitive appraisal is, in turn, affected by one's sense of spirituality or one's relationship with God. People commonly say such things as, "God will not give you more than you can handle," or "God has a plan." When approached from this world view, outside stressors are buffered, and the negative effects of life events are dampened.

Research suggests that African Americans underutilize psychotherapeutic services as a way to cope with emotional problems, and, when compared with Whites, they seem less willing to visit community mental health centers, a reluctance stemming from a distrust of the medical and scientific system in general, as well as a distrust of the White population (Kennedy et al. 2007). Instead, many African American caregivers turn to clergy in times of distress, and there they find strength and resilience.

The Role of the Church in African American Communities

The church is known to be a central institution in African American communities that generates positive community outcomes on a variety of measures and provides many types of support. In African American communities, the church occupies a special place that provides spiritual guidance, fellowship, a sense of shared purpose, and a political voice. While church attendance among mainstream White American churches has declined, membership in African American churches has remained steady. Historically, African Americans have been denied access to political participation and many of the social services that Caucasian Americans have had. For this reason, the church developed as a force for political activism and a voice of political change, an important provider of human services that might otherwise not be provided, and an institution that offered stability in often turbulent times. African American churches in inner cities have remained a source of shared community for parishioners and continue to provide support to those lacking in influence and affluence.

Dating back to slavery, the supportive efforts of churches spurring social, political, and economic self-help among congregants have been beneficial to individuals and benefits have often expanded into communities. The church was perceived as an institution that helped communities to survive, helped to organize resistance and promoted social change, and provided a sense of communal identity. In addition, when formalized social services were not available, the church often functioned as a surrogate family and support system for African Americans by providing concrete assistance (e.g. food, clothing, money, education, and job opportunities) and psychosocial assurance, especially to older adults.

Help Seeking from Clergy

In the United States, clergy of all races are important in the provision of mental health services; they serve as gatekeepers as well as providers. Generally, clergy are considered to be any religious leaders who are ordained and/or have the mandate of those they serve to provide religious/spiritual guidance. Clergy often are congregational ministers who provide pastoral counseling, though they are not necessarily trained specifically as counselors or therapists. By contrast, pastoral counselors and chaplains have in-depth training similar to that of clinical social workers. In general, clergy are neither certified nor licensed as mental health providers and do not normally charge a fee for their counseling services. The training they receive in counseling is usually a minor part of their overall training, with the bulk of their training focusing on theological issues. Counseling is considered only one element, albeit a large one in practice, of the ministry for which they are responsible.

Individuals with serious mental health problems, such as antisocial personality disorder, bipolar disorder, major depression, and obsessive compulsive disorder, are just as likely to seek help from religious leaders as they are from other mental health professionals; the only problems for which they are significantly more likely to seek help from mental health professionals are alcohol abuse, drug abuse, and panic disorder (Hohmann and Larson 1993). A 20-year study indicated that about 40% of Americans sought help from a religious leader when dealing with personal problems (Veroff et al. 1981), and of those attending religious services weekly, more than 50% considered their primary mental health service provider to be their religious leader (Larson et al. 2000). Among 1,200 randomly sampled adults (600 White and 600 Black) in the Nashville area, 36.9% of African Americans and 24.2% of Whites used clergy for assistance with emotional problems (Husaini et al. 1994). Older adults are generally more likely to seek help from a member of the clergy than from another source of help (Pickard 2006; Pickard and Guo 2008). Furthermore, people who have less support are even more likely to turn to clergy for help than those who have other people in their lives to whom they can turn.

The National Survey of Black Americans (NSBA) was a cross-sectional, nationally representative survey of 2,107 adults who identified themselves as Black Americans. The original interviews were conducted in 1979–1980, followed by three waves of interviews conducted by phone in 1987–1988, 1988–1989, and 1992. Using NSBA data, Neighbors et al. (1998) found that of all 612 respondents seeking help, 29.46% turned first to their church. People who first sought help from their churches were less likely to continue seeking help elsewhere than those who first sought help from a secular source. Among those who sought assistance from a church first, only 29.5% went elsewhere to seek further help. In contrast, 46.4% of those first seeking help from a secular source continued to seek help from another source. These statistically significant findings suggest that people who initially seek help from a church are not likely to continue seeking help elsewhere. They also found that among people who sought help from only one source, those who relied on clergy were significantly more satisfied with the services they received than those who sought help from other sources. Additionally, among people who sought help from more than one source, those who sought help from clergy first were significantly more satisfied with the services they received than those who sought help from another source first. Moreover, people who sought help from clergy were significantly more likely to refer someone else to the same source than were those who had sought help elsewhere.

Preparation of Clergy for Counseling Older Adults

Clergy often come from theological perspectives that are antithetical to science, and social science researchers come from scientific perspectives that insist on carefully and thoroughly examining the specifics of clergy-provided mental health services. Furthermore, clergy provide their services outside the purview of professional organizations such as the National Association of Social Workers or the American Psychological Association, and they are likely to resist any type of governmental oversight or mandated regulation as a result of secular examination. It is important to note, however, that many African American clergy are not full-time paid representatives of their religious bodies. African American clergy are more likely than clergy members from other racial and ethnic groups to have other full-time employment outside their religious roles. Therefore, they often have less opportunity for training and career preparation specific to counseling or working with older adults. While outcome studies are scarce, in 11 different studies conducted from 1976 to 1989, United States' and Canadian Jewish, Protestant, and Catholic clergy all reported that they needed more training in the skills of counseling, and 50–80% of them indicated that their seminary training in pastoral counseling did little to prepare them for the demands of providing mental health services to their congregations (Weaver 1995).

The results of a small study by Domino (1990) indicated that American Jewish, Protestant, and Catholic clergy ($N = 157$) had about the same level of knowledge of the symptoms of psychological distress as a group of college undergraduates in an introductory psychology class. Similar findings have been reported by other researchers. One study found that clergy scored significantly lower than professionally trained mental health service providers on their ability to assess for suicidal ideation (Larson et al. 2000). Through his review of 11 different studies, Weaver (1995) highlights the marked lack of counseling skills provided to clergy in their typical professional training:

- 50–80% of clergy considered their seminary training insufficient preparation for actual practice in their ministries for either identification of parishioner needs or the types of services being requested (e.g. marital counseling, assisting severely mentally ill parishioners).
- In a review of studies between 1976 and 1989, the majority of clergy reported a significant need for more training in counseling skills.
- As recently as 1981, approximately one half of Protestant seminaries in the United States had no course requirement for counseling.
- In a survey of 1,927 United Methodist ministers, one in four reported that they felt the overall quality of mental health services provided by clergy was poor.

Assisting Clergy in Their Efforts

Collaboration between clergy and mental health professionals is needed to optimize provision of mental health assistance. Clergy often have long-term relationships with older adults and their families. Relationships are at the heart of the helping professions, and these particular relationships provide clergy with unique opportunities to detect changes that may hint at the presence of emotional problems. In turn, this may increase the likelihood that clergy will be able to connect those in need with the most helpful services available. If mental health professionals increase their collaborative efforts with clergy, clergy are likely to respond in kind, thus leading to better overall care for older adults in need of mental health services. This is particularly important considering the impending rise in the numbers of older adults and the lack of qualified mental health professionals trained and available to work with them, a problem that is particularly pronounced in rural areas and with respect to African American caregivers. Mental health professionals should be made aware of the high frequency of requests for assistance with emotional and behavioral concerns encountered by clergy and remember to include questions regarding the use of clergy in their assessments of client resources.

If social workers, mental health workers, and other geriatric helping professionals know that caregivers are turning to clergy for help with emotional problems, it seems a worthwhile endeavor to assist clergy and promote collaboration between religious and secular service providers. Outreach efforts aimed at African American clergy would have a positive, though indirect, impact on the well being of African American caregivers. While actively engaging with clergy would not be a small task, there are some things that can certainly be accomplished. For example, in recognition of the reality that African American caregivers are seeking help from clergy, training programs for mental health professionals should include instruction regarding working with clergy. Such instruction has been used in the past, and it effectively increased the self-report of psychologists in training that they would likely work more closely with clergy in the future (Meylink 1988), particularly for co-treatment of clients, rather than a more traditional refer and release model.

Conclusions

As the baby boom generation ages, a corresponding need for people in the helping professions trained to work with older adults will arise. Unfortunately, the United States currently faces an apparent shortage of professionals who are specifically trained to work with older adults, and help will probably not be available for everyone in need. This circumstance is magnified for African American caregivers, a group who are more likely to be negatively impacted by their caregiving roles and less likely to seek help from professional sources. One way to support these caregivers and enable them better to care for their loved ones is to provide appropriate aging and counseling education to the clergy who serve them. In African American communities, churches in general and clergy in particular represent a prominent and trusted resource for people in need of assistance with many types of problems. Providing greater clergy preparation for counseling older adults could very likely become a factor that contributes to greater resilience and, thus, more positive outcomes for African American caregivers.

References

Administration on Aging (2006) *A statistical profile of Black older Americans aged 65+.*
Administration on Aging (2009) *Statistics on the aging population.* Retrieved August 31, 2009, from http://www.aoa.gov/AoARoot/Products_Materials/fact/pdf/Black_Americans_Aged_65 plus_statistics.pdf.

Brat, P. (2002) Aging, mental health and the faith community. *Journal of Religious Gerontology*, *13*, 45–54.

Carroll, J. (2004) Religion is "very important" to 6 in 10 Americans. *The Gallup Poll: Tuesday Briefing*, 24.

Cnaan, R., Boddie, S., Handy, F., Yancey, G., & Schneider, R. (2002) *The invisible caring hand: American congregations and the provision of welfare*. New York: New York University Press.

Cutler, S.J. (1976) Membership in different types of voluntary associations and psychological well-being. *Gerontologist*, *16*, 335–339.

Domino, G. (1990) Clergy's knowledge of psychopathology. *Journal of Psychology and Theology*, *18*, 32–39.

Fetzer Institute (1999) *Multidimensional measurement of religiousness/spirituality for use in health research*. Kalamazoo: The Fetzer Institute.

Gallup, G. & Lindsay, D.M. (1999) *Surveying the religious landscape: Trends in U.S. beliefs*. Harrisburg: Morehouse Publishing.

Glamser, F.D. (1988) The impact of retirement upon religiosity. *Journal of Religion and Aging* *5*(1), 27–37.

Hill, P. & Hood, R. (1999) *Measures of religiosity*. Birmingham: Religious Education Press.

Hohmann, A.A. & Larson, D.B. (1993) Psychiatric factors predicting use of clergy. In E.L. Worthington (Ed.), *Psychotherapy and religious values* (pp. 71–84). Grand Rapids: Baker Book House.

Husaini, B.A., Moore, S.T., & Cain, V.A. (1994) Psychiatric symptoms and help seeking behavior among the elderly: An analysis of racial and gender differences. *Journal of Gerontological Social Work*, *21*, 177–195.

Kennedy, B.R., Mathis, C.C., & Woods, A.K. (2007) African Americans and their distrust of the health care system: Healthcare for diverse populations. *Journal of Cultural Diversity*, *14*(2), 56–60.

Koenig, H.G. (1992) Religion and mental health in later life. In J. Schumaker (Ed.), *Religion and mental health* (pp. 177–188). New York: Oxford University Press.

Koenig, H.G., Moberg, D.O., & Kvale, J.N. (1988) Religious activities and attitudes of older adults in a geriatric assessment clinic. *Journal of the American Geriatrics Society*, *36*, 362–374.

Koenig, H.G., McCullough, M.E., & Larson, D.B. (2001) *Handbook of religion and health*. New York: Oxford University Press.

Krause, N. (2009) Church-based volunteering, providing informal support at church, and self-rated health in late life. *Journal of Aging and Health*, *21*(1), 63–84.

Larson, D.B., Milano, M.G., Weaver, A.J., & McCullough, M.E. (2000) The role of clergy in mental health care. In J.K. Boehlein (Ed.), *Psychiatry and religion*: The convergence of mind and spirit, (pp. 125–142). Washington DC: American Psychiatric Press.

Meylink, W.D. (1988) Impact of referral training of psychologists on the clergy-psychologist interaction. *Journal of Psychology and Christianity*, *7*(3), 55–64.

National Alliance for Caregiving & American Association of Retired Persons (2004) *Caregiving in the U.S.* Retrieved June 15, 2007 from http://www.caregiving.org/data/04finalreport.pdf.

Neighbors, H.W., Musick, M., & Williams, D.R. (1998) The African American minister as a source of help for serious personal crisis: Bridge or barrier to mental health care? *Health Education & Behavior*, *25*, 759–777.

Newport, F. (2004) A look at Americans and religion today. *The Gallup Poll: Tuesday Briefing*, 23.

Pickard, J.G. (2006) The relationship of religiosity to older adults' mental health service use. *Aging and Mental Health*, *10*(3), 290–297.

Pickard, J.G. & Guo, B. (2008) Clergy as mental health service providers to older adults. *Aging and Mental Health*, *12*(5), 615–624.

Sue, S. & Chu, J. (2003) The mental health of ethnic minority groups: Challenges posed by the supplement to the surgeon general's report on mental health. *Culture, Medicine and Psychiatry*, *27*, 447–465.

Taylor, R.J., Chatters, L.M., and Levin, J. (2004) *Religion in the lives of African Americans: social, psychological, and health perspectives*. Thousand Oaks: Sage Publications.

Veroff, J., Kulka, R.A., & Douvan, E. (1981) *Mental health in America: Patterns of help-seeking from 1957 to 1976*. New York: Basic Books, Inc.

Weaver, A.J. (1995) Has there been a failure to prepare and support parish-based clergy in their role as frontline community mental health workers: A review. *The Journal of Pastoral Care*, *49*, 129–147.

Chapter 18
The Age-Friendly New York City Project: An Environmental Intervention to Increase Aging Resilience

Julie Netherland, Ruth Finkelstein, and Paula Gardner

As the growing body of research affirms, resilience in aging is a multidimensional concept influenced by demographics, social support and connectedness, health status, psychological factors, and material resources. Most, if not all, of these factors are profoundly shaped by the social, cultural, and physical environments in which older adults live. Increasingly these environments are cities. In 2008, for the first time in human history, more than half of the world's population was living in cities and towns (UNFPA, undated). In the U.S., 73% of older men and 77% of older women live in metropolitan areas (Fried and Barron 2005). These urban environments have the potential to promote or inhibit aging resilience among millions of older adult residents. This chapter describes the conceptual framework that underlies the Age-friendly New York City (AF NYC) initiative – a project that seeks to change the urban environment in ways that enhance aging resilience for older New Yorkers – and summarizes findings from a year-long assessment about the age-friendliness of New York City (NYC), including features of the urban environment that promote and restrict aging resilience. We conclude with a discussion on how these findings are being used to shape the urban environment in ways that can improve the social resilience and active engagement of older adults in NYC.

Background & Conceptual Framework

Since the 1980s, the field of environmental gerontology has emphasized the influence of environment on aging and the importance of the relationship between the person and his or her physical, social and cultural environment (Wahl and Weisman 2003). As Phillipson (2007, p.330) explains: "The experience of being old... varies according to one's environment. Situation can thus affect aging." While some have argued that environmental gerontology has languished (Wahl and Weisman 2003),

R. Finkelstein (✉)
The New York Academy of Medicine, New York, NY, USA
e-mail: rfinkelstein@nyam.org

B. Resnick et al. (eds.), *Resilience in Aging: Concepts, Research, and Outcomes*,
DOI 10.1007/978-1-4419-0232-0_18, © Springer Science+Business Media, LLC 2011

most agree that globalization has led to greater variation in the communities and environments in which older people live, increasing the importance of environmental perspectives for understanding aging resilience (Phillipson 2007). In general, cities have not been viewed as environments that cultivate aging resilience. Rather, much of the scholarship on urban aging has focused on the risks of urban environments to older people, especially those living in impoverished inner-cities (see for example, Klinenberg 2002; Newman 2006; Rodwin and Gusmano 2006; Smith et al. 2004). Much less attention has been paid to the ways in which cities might foster aging resilience and promote healthy aging. Some notable exceptions are Rodwin and Gusmano's (2006) *Growing Old in World Cities*, which describes the paradox of cities as places of both tremendous potential and peril for older people, and Fried and Barron's chapter (2005), which discusses the positive and negative health effects of cities on older adults. The AF NYC project is concerned with how we can intervene in urban environments to foster and strengthen the resilience of older residents, regardless of their income or the neighborhood in which they live. Understanding how urban environments, like NYC, might enhance aging resilience is more important than ever as the trends of urbanization, population aging and globalization converge to produce complex, cosmopolitan cities that are home to millions of older adults.

More than 8.2 million people live in NYC (NYC DOHMH: Bureau of Vital Statistics 2007). The number of people over the age of 65 in NYC is projected to reach 1.35 million by 2030. By 2030, older people will outnumber school aged children in NYC (NYC Department of City Planning 2006). The diversity of New York's older population is also expected to grow as immigrants of all ages continue to move into the city (NYC Department of City Planning 2004). New Yorkers come from all corners of the globe and speak more than 174 languages. According to figures from the 2000 census, 44% (2.9 million) of the adult population is foreign-born and 46% of the population speaks a language other than English at home (NYC Department of City Planning 2004). These trends have placed unprecedented demands on the city's infrastructure and need for planning.

Traditionally in the United States, planning efforts have addressed the challenges of urban aging by implementing a set of "aging services" targeted to the old and infirm – an approach that fails to maximize either the potential of older adults or the strengths of the urban environment. The age-friendly cities model, in contrast to previous planning approaches, is rooted in the belief that the urban environment is a key determinant of *active aging*. This model challenges planners, policy makers, researchers, and residents to view *all* aspects of urban life through the lens of aging and to imagine a city that fosters active aging. Active aging, a concept developed by the World Health Organization (WHO) Ageing and Lifecourse Programme (WHO 2007, p.5), is "the process of optimizing opportunities for health, participation and security in order to enhance quality of life as people age." As shown in Fig. 18.1, the ability of individuals to remain active and engaged depends in part on their health status and level of functionality. However, external social, environmental, and economic factors also influence whether or not older people are able to remain independent. For example, barrier-free buildings, streets, and transportation systems increase the capacity of people with limited mobility to continue to live independently, participate in meaningful activities, and maintain important social

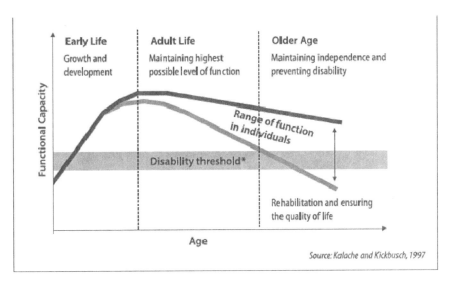

*Changes in the environment can lower the disability threshold, thus decreasing the number of disabled people in a given community.

Fig. 18.1   Health status and level of functionality

ties and connections. The goal of the AF NYC project is to transform the urban environment in ways that promote active aging, thus fostering social connection, social engagement, and participation; all key factors associated with aging resilience.

The Age-Friendly New York City Project

The AF NYC project is a direct outgrowth of the WHO's global age-friendly cities program, which produced a Global Age-friendly Cities Guide offering age-friendly indicators for eight domains: access to outdoor spaces and buildings, transportation, housing, respect and social inclusion, social participation, communication and information, civic participation and employment, and community support and health services (World Health Organization 2007).

The AF NYC project, which is housed at and staffed by The New York Academy of Medicine (NYAM), adopted the Global Age-friendly Cities project as its starting place and then adapted it to meet the unique political and social environment of NYC. Recognizing that key decisions about the urban environment are made at the municipal level and to avoid producing another report that would sit idle on the shelves of policymakers, the NYAM's first step was for staff to meet with the city' political leaders. NYAM approached the NYC departments of aging and health, the leadership of the city Council, and the Mayor's Office knowing that to shift the planning paradigm for older residents, most, if not all, city agencies would need to be engaged.

To acquire a solid commitment from these government leaders, NYAM educated them about the new approach and assured them that the project would be a true partnership between the public and private sectors. Elected leaders were already grappling with how to meet the demands of the city's growing population of older adults, and they recognized that older adults are among their most politically active and engaged constituents. The city's executive branch, on the other hand, understood that older residents are high users of city services. The age-friendly cities approach appeals to political leaders because it addresses a real key constituent group need in a way that optimizes the strengths of the city. Moreover, this paradigm generates recommendations for change that may be no-cost or low-cost and can be implemented by a wide range of city constituents including businesses, cultural institutions, religious groups, and non-governmental agencies. One guiding principle of the AF NYC project is the belief that creating an age-friendly city requires the involvement of all sectors – not just government.

Assessing New York's Age-Friendliness

NYAM undertook a year-long process to assess the current age-friendliness of New York with the goal of identifying which features of the urban environment fostered active aging and what impeded it. Because NYC is such a large, diverse and complex city, NYAM used a number of assessment activities and methods to collect the views of aging experts and older New Yorkers. These included:

- Five expert roundtables to discuss current practices and innovative ideas in the areas of business, housing development, civic engagement, transportation and outdoor spaces, tenants rights, social services, and health.
- Fourteen community forums to gather the experiences, ideas and opinions of older adults and service providers.
- A widely disseminated request for information soliciting policy and programmatic ideas.
- Focus groups and interviews with under-represented older New Yorkers (e.g. low income, formerly homeless, and immigrant).
- Comprehensive review of the literature.
- Geographical Information System analysis to map key indicators of age friendliness/unfriendliness in relation to where older adults live.

In total, NYAM consulted with more than 1,500 older adults and dozens of policy makers, service providers, and researchers. In keeping with the public-private framework of the project, each community forum was co-sponsored by one or more City Council member(s), and staff representatives from the City Council were active partners throughout the assessment. Data from these activities were analyzed and published Fall 2008 in *Toward and Age-friendly New York City: A Findings Report* (Finkelstein et al. 2008).

While NYAM was leading an assessment of the NYC community, the Mayor's Office asked city agencies to assess the "age-friendliness" of each agency and what could be done to improve the way they addressed the needs of older residents. This marked a breakthrough in conventional thinking as agencies that normally did not focus on aging issues examined their services through the lens of aging. After this process, each agency generated a list of activities and policy changes that it could implement to make NYC more age-friendly.

Overview of Findings

Importance of Place

As Shaw (2004) explains: "People do not just live in houses: They live in and experience neighborhoods (p. 412)." The meaningfulness of place, including a sense of attachment, familiarity and satisfaction, can be an importance source of resilience, providing a sense of comfort, belonging and control over one's space (AARP 2005; Oswald and Wahl 2004). One of the central findings of the AF NYC assessment involved identification of a prevalent, deep and abiding love for and attachment to NYC. Many people reported having lived happily in their neighborhoods and even their apartments for 30, 40, 50 years, or even longer. As one focus group participant explained about her neighborhood, "I was born here. To me, it's the center of the Earth and to go anywhere else is a step down. Anywhere else I'd be a fish out of water." Attachment to the city was a widely shared experience, but in many ways the rich diversity of NYC neighborhoods means that it is a very different city for each person. Residents on the Upper West Side spoke enthusiastically about their proximity to cultural institutions. Older immigrants in Jackson Heights said they liked living among the hustle and bustle of younger immigrant families. Staten Island residents appreciated owning their own homes. Residents of Jamaica, Queens, said they appreciate the calmness of their area and rarely travel into the noise and traffic of Manhattan.

Older New Yorkers also recognized that NYC offers particular advantages as they age. Many cited the easy access to public transit, the convenience of having stores and other amenities in close proximity, the many events, activities and institutions to enjoy in retirement, and availability of high-quality health care facilities as advantages of aging in an urban environment. Several noted that the city allowed them to remain independent in ways they could not in other settings. For example, some older New Yorkers had moved to the suburbs to live with their grown children but disliked having to rely on others to drive them everywhere. In the city, by contrast, they were able to walk to business, services, and social activities or take the bus and subway to just about anywhere in the five boroughs. The attachment to NYC, however, was not just grounded in these practical advantages. Phillipson (2007) argues: "some people select locations as a means of 'announcing' or 'reaffirming' their identities (p.329)." Indeed, many who participated in the AF NYC assessment made clear that living in NYC and being a New Yorker was absolutely central to their sense of self.

Social Connectedness

Social connectedness and social support have emerged as key predictors of aging resilience (Fuller-Iglesias et al. 2008; Hildon et al. 2008; Kinsel 2005). Fuller-Iglesias et al. (2008) suggest that social relations may be especially important for older people as they have fewer resources available to them as they age. According to the WHO, inadequate social support is associated with increased mortality, morbidity, and psychological distress and decreased overall health and well being (Marmot and Wilkinson 1999; World Health Organization 2003). Belonging to a supportive social network makes people feel cared for, loved, esteemed and valued – all of which have a powerful protective effect on health (World Health Organization 2003). The social networks older adults develop, as well as their ability to sustain these relationships, are central to their ability to live independently and their continued integration into the life of the City. The AF NYC assessment uncovered several ways in which urban environments challenge some forms of social connection but foster others.

The older New Yorkers in the AF NYC assessment recognized the centrality of their social networks but acknowledged that they had commonly diminished with age. Many indicated that few or none of their children lived nearby. A woman from the East Harlem forum noted: "Once children get married, they leave the community because they want a better life, and there's nothing for them here." Several participants described watching their social networks disappear as they lost partners, friends, and peers. One focus group member said "That's the bad part of longevity: everybody goes away. It has been very hard watching everyone die." Researchers concur that social networks often decline with age (Moen et al. 1992), with both the amount and variety of social interactions decreasing over time (Sauer and Coward 1985).

However, not all kinship networks diminish with age, especially in urban environments. The AF NYC assessment confirmed previous research findings that large numbers of older New Yorkers are the primary caregivers for grandchildren. As Newman (2006) points out in her study of African American and Latino older New Yorkers, many older adults, especially those living in inner cities, are caring for children in their communities. She notes that many of those growing older in New York's poorer neighborhoods today are dealing with the consequences of the extreme poverty, infrastructure decline, high rates of crime, and the HIV and crack epidemic of the 1970s and 1980s that left many of their children unable to raise the next generation. In the AF NYC assessment, many older women, despite health conditions, and extreme financial hardship, had taken on primary caretaking responsibilities when their children could no longer act as parents for their grandchildren. "If it wasn't for the older people, the younger people wouldn't have a place to stay," said one resident of Queens. Another woman put it simply: "Older people are the ones who bear the burden. They take care of kids left behind." Unfortunately, this role is not well-acknowledged by social service systems, and grandparents often have difficulty accessing benefits and obtaining the legal services needed to secure guardianship. While many older adults derive meaning and satisfaction from their social connections and caregiving role (Waldrop and Weber 2001), they also associate caregiving with increased stress, depression, and financial strain (Sands and Goldberg-Glen 2000).

The AF NYC assessment suggests that the city's booming housing market of the 1990s and early 2000s also played a role in changing and disrupting the social networks of some older people. Participants expressed alarm at the rise of luxury apartment buildings and loss of affordable housing. A community leader in Harlem voiced a common frustration: "poor and working-poor people who have been in this community for generations are being marginalized. They are tearing down their buildings and putting up new apartment complexes that they cannot afford." Some older people felt they could not afford to move away from their subsidized apartments to areas where children or relatives might be living, and grown children and relatives could not afford to move into (or back to) the neighborhood to be near them. Similarly, some older adults were separated from long-time friends and neighbors when they were forced out of a neighborhood by high rents. These changes directly impacted people's feelings of security and neighborhood cohesion. A participant at a forum in the South Bronx noted that when she sees strangers in the hall she "just hopes they live here" because she's no longer sure who her neighbors are.

The reality of losing friends, family, and neighbors combined with declining functionality led some older people to describe fears of being alone, especially in a crisis. Many, like this woman from a Chinese-language focus group in Queens, expressed feelings of vulnerability: "My biggest fear in life is that I would come down with some incurable disease or some crippling disease and I would have to fend for myself with no family and just a handful of friends." Older New Yorkers confirm what other researchers, like Klinenberg (2002) have found: social isolation is a serious problem and major concern. One woman said, "I know a blind woman whose aide leaves at noon, and she's alone all day and all night." Several others told stories of people dying alone in apartments, people who lived alone, or of older adults who were unable to get help for themselves when they fell down. This story told by a focus group member was typical: "A friend of mine fell out of bed and it took two days for her to get to the phone."

Despite these stories of social isolation and the acknowledgement that traditional social networks were diminishing, older New Yorkers reported important and varied forms of social connectedness that were facilitated by living in a densely populated City. The social networks of older New Yorkers are as varied as any other cross-section of New Yorkers – they are opera goers to mahjong players, bingo enthusiasts, historians, and activists. Many people, like participants in a forum for lesbian, gay, bisexual and transgender (LGBT) older adults, noted that their primary identification was not as an older adult; they wanted their social interaction to center on their existing communities of affiliation within the LGBT community. Several members of the United Hindu Cultural Council Senior Center in Queens described how important it was for them to have a designated place where their culture and beliefs were specifically supported and recognized. Some older adults found connection through religious institutions. One focus group participant put it succinctly: "No children and no family. My friends and my synagogue are my sup-port." Others described primary social and support networks based on profession or shared interests. A recent report by Columbia University (Jeffri 2007) asserts that older artists' strong relationships with other artists trump their communication with partners, family, and children. These finding are consistent with the idea of the "changing face of social networks" as non-family become increasingly important to aging individuals (Walker and Hiller 2007).

Although changes in some areas have disrupted neighborhood social networks, neighbors remain an important source of social connection for many. In fact, some housing policies and configurations seemed to nurture important pockets of social cohesion. Whether living in public housing, privately owned co-ops, or condo-minium high-rise buildings, people appreciated and benefited from living in close-knit, micro-communities. For example, residents in some public housing complexes explained that affordable rents or subsidized housing had kept them in the same place for decades and allowed them to form close relationships with their neigh-bors. Many described informal networks of neighbors who regularly checked up on and assist older residents. One focus group participant from the Bronx said "When I got cancer, my neighbor always checked on me. I loved that. That's beautiful."

Housing arrangements as well as the density and diversity of urban populations in cities like NYC produce settings with the potential to support and enhance forms of social connectedness and resilience even as an individual's traditional kinship networks diminish. This finding is consistent with that of Newman's (2006) study of older African American and Latinos in New York who reported significantly higher levels of social integration than a national sample of older adults. Whether through shared attachment to place, tight neighborhood networks, or groups based on affiliations and interests, older adults living in cities have opportunities to form the social connections that are important to aging resilience. As discussed below, cities can do much to improve the quality of life of older residents by removing the barriers that prevent these connections from flourishing.

Social Engagement & Participation

Social connection is fostered in part by the ability of individuals to engage with and actively participate in the life of the city. Most models and theories of successful or healthy aging (e.g. Rowe and Kahn 1997, 1998) include engagement in life as a key component. Moreover, research has consistently reported a positive relationship between activity and life satisfaction (Menec and Chipperfield 1997) and between social participation and quality of life (World Health Organization 2007). Increasingly, evidence suggests that higher rates of participation in leisure and productive activi-ties are also associated with good health and that older adults in cities have more opportunities for socializing and participation than those in the suburbs (Fried and Barron 2005). One important arena of engagement for older adults is civic participa-tion and volunteerism. Civic participation has been positively associated with better physical and mental health in older adults (Fried et al. 2004; Kaskie et al. 2008), and engagement in volunteering has been linked to reduced mortality (Musick et al. 1999) and higher levels of well-being (Morrow-Howell et al. 2003).

Putnam (2000) has called this generation of older adults "the long civic generation," and in the AF NYC assessment, many people had a rich history of giving to the City. Many older adults continued to play critical civic roles – leading campaigns and serving on advisory councils, tenant associations, and non-profit boards. "Older people carry the community around here. We go to the tenant meetings, the PTA, all the meetings," said one participant. Older New Yorkers recognized that staying involved enriched both their communities and their own lives. One older person explained: "I'd like to do something that I can be proud of. I don't mind getting old. I just want to be doing something." Engagement must be meaningful, and for older New Yorkers, one clearly meaningful role is participating in activities that influence the future of their City. Older adults asked for opportunities to be included in all levels of decision-making about their own futures, including continued involvement in the AF NYC initiative. Some identified political activism as an important social role they discovered late in life. At the forum in the East Tremont section of the Bronx, an older woman in a wheelchair said, "two to three years ago I took a class at JPAC [the Joint Public Affairs Committee of the Jewish Association of Services for the Aged] and it opened up my life. I'm never home now. I'm more active than I've been in 50 years. I'm an activist." For others, activism has been a life-long commitment. A focus group participant in Harlem said, "Every time we think we can relax it never lasts. It's here we go again!"

Older adults in the AF NYC assessment were also clear that their continued civic engagement and participation were made possible by the City's infrastructure. Without the superior transportation system, older adults would have a much more difficult time getting to meetings and events, volunteering, or handling their care-giving responsibilities. At a community forum on the Upper East Side, audience members applauded when a participant declared, "This city has the best transportation system in the country!" Some people explained that they moved back to New York from the suburbs and other parts of the country specifically for the public transportation because it allowed them to continue to engage in the activities that were important to them. The City's parks, libraries, senior and community centers, and cultural institutions also clearly play an important role in helping older New Yorkers stay engaged and connected to one another and the life of the City.

Barriers

The AF NYC assessment demonstrates the complex ways which the urban environment impacts aging resilience by fostering a meaningful sense of place and familiarity and providing opportunities for social connection, engagement, and participation. Unfortunately, the urban environment also creates a number of challenges that make it difficult for aging resilience to fully flourish. In fact, several researchers have suggested the urban environment dampens resilience because of the concentration of poverty, poor housing, and crime in cities (Klinenberg 2002; Newman

2006; Phillipson 2007; Sanders et al. 2008). While the AF NYC assessment found a number of features of the urban environment that foster resilience, it also found that poverty, linguistic isolation, lack of information, and impediments in the built environment hinder aging resilience.

New York is ranked the fifth most expensive city in the world in which to live (Employment Cities Abroad (ECA) International 2008). The high cost of living in NYC is a financial burden for many residents and can increase their risk of living in poverty. In 2005, the poverty rate among older New Yorkers was twice the national average: 20.3% vs. 9.9% (*American Community Survey*). However, when the definition of poverty is tailored to acknowledge the high cost of living in NYC, that figure grows to one in three older New Yorkers (Finkelstein et al. 2008). Older adults with incomes below the poverty line can be found in most neighborhoods across the five boroughs. In the AF NYC assessment, older New Yorkers cited poverty and affordability as the primary challenges to staying in the City as they age and to being socially connected and engaged in what the City has to offer. Poverty – with its attendant fear of crime, stress, and strains on time – undermines connectedness (Phillipson 2007). Moreover, as Klinenberg's landmark work *Heat Wave* (2002) vividly illustrates, obstacles to social connectedness, including poverty, can lead to social isolation with deadly consequences.

The AF NYC assessment also revealed that linguistic isolation is a barrier to social connectedness and participation for many older immigrants, which may diminish their aging resilience. In NYC, approximately 27% of older adults speak English "less than very well" (Walker and Herbitter 2005). In some neighborhoods, linguistic isolation is particularly concentrated. For example, in one census tract of Manhattan's Chinatown, two-thirds of persons age 65 and older are linguistically isolated (Gusmano et al. 2008). In cities like New York, immigrant networks and enclaves can be important sources of connection and material assistance, and many established immigrant communities have ethnic and linguistically appropriate service agencies to support older adults. For some, however, linguistic barriers still pose an obstacle to accessing critical information and engaging fully in life of the city. At a forum in Chinatown, an older woman who speaks only Chinese said: "I'm blind because I cannot read documents written in English. I'm deaf because people speak to me in English and I don't understand. And I'm mute because I cannot communicate with anyone who does not know my language."

Barriers to accessing information emerged in the AF NYC assessment as a problem that extended to adults from all ethnic and linguistic backgrounds. With information increasingly dispersed through electronic means, many older adults felt left behind, indicating they could not access critical information that would allow them to get government benefits, participate in activities, and stay connected to others. Some elders expressed anger and frustration at the increasing expectation that everyone access information online: "You know what burns me up? When people say that they will e-mail me. I don't have e-mail. I can't afford a computer." Barriers to computer access include affordability (purchasing a computer, paying fees associated with computer training, and costs of ongoing internet service) and lack of skills and knowledge. Increasingly, email and online forums, such as *Facebook* and

MySpace, are becoming important sites for social connection and have tremendous potential to help older adults stay in touch with families and friends, to engage in social and civic activities, and to access needed information (Jones 2009; U.S. Department of Commerce 2002). However, many older adults have yet to realize this potential. In addition, many older adults are not getting the information they need to foster connection, stay engaged, and sustain and build resilience.

The AF NYC assessment also revealed how impediments in the built environment and inadequacies in transportation can negatively influence aging resilience. Social connection and social participation are core features of aging resilience that are undermined when older adults cannot negotiate their neighborhoods or the City. As mentioned above, in general participants had high praise for the City's transportation system and saw it as essential to their ability to remain independent, stay connected to others, and participate in activities and services. However, they also identified many inaccessible subway stops, gaps in bus service in particular neighborhoods, and the increasing cost of public transit. In addition, many older New Yorkers are in difficult housing situations (e.g. walk-ups or over-crowded apartments), struggle to negotiate cluttered and broken sidewalks, and cannot safely cross busy intersections.

Intervening in Urban Environments to Build Aging Resilience

In contrast to much of the work that focuses on the risks city life poses to resilience among urban elders, the AF NYC project is aimed at building upon the unique features of urban life that promote aging resilience. In many ways, NYC is an optimal place in which to grow old. In addition to its fine social and health services, public transportation system, and array of cultural institutions, NYC harbors tremendous potential to enhance aging resilience by providing older adults with a sense of place and identity, facilitating a wide array of social connections and networks, and providing opportunities for meaningful engagement. However, a number of barriers prevent many older New Yorkers from accessing all that the City has to offer. A central challenge of environmental interventions, like the AF NYC project, is to bring the urban advantages of the city to *all* neighborhoods and *all* residents. It is the work of the AF NYC project to spread the urban advantages that foster aging resilience by ameliorating barriers and enhancing the capacity of all New Yorkers – regardless of age, national origin, income, or physical ability – to live and thrive in the City.

This work has already begun. Following the assessment and the publication of the findings, NYAM convened work groups from different sectors to develop concrete recommendations for moving forward. These included leaders from civil society, health and social services, business, academia and research. Each sector is being asked to make specific commitments regarding how their participation will make NYC more age-friendly. In August 2009, the Mayor and Speaker of the City Council announced the City's response to the AF NYC findings, which included 59 new initiatives to make NTC a better place to grow old and the formation of an

AF NYC Commission. The Commission is charged with developing a *Blueprint for an AF NYC* and overseeing its implementation. The Commission will include high-level representatives who have an understanding of the structures, systems, and programs that affect the lives of older adults and who can provide leverage for meaningful action. The Commission will convene work groups to synthesize evidence, design policies and programs, develop indicators of success, engage additional part-ners, build private/public partnerships, and conduct additional research as needed. The AF NYC Commission is conceived as a public-private partnership that will meet regularly for four years and will release an annual progress report on what concrete steps that have been made towards improving the age-friendliness of New York.

At the same time that progress is being made on city-wide recommendations and policy initiatives, local communities will work to transform their neighborhoods. Many of the improvements to New York's age-friendliness will be neighborhood changes in the built environment, a re-visioning of neighborhood services, and/or community outreach and education campaigns. Community boards, local planning groups, business improvement districts, and borough-level decision makers will be convened and trained on how to incorporate the perspectives and needs of older people in their planning and decision-making. These local community efforts have been conceptualized as "Aging Improvement Districts," where businesses, service providers, academic and cultural institutions will join with older residents to iden-tify the specific issues in their neighborhoods that diminish aging resilience and work together to resolve them.

Conclusions

Globalization, urbanization, and population aging are converging trends that have ever increasing numbers of older adults living in large, global cities like New York. Fortunately, cities can be sources of the social connection and social engagement that are vital to aging resilience. For most of the more 1,500 older New Yorkers who participated in the AF NYC assessment, NYC is not only home; it is an impor-tant source of identity and meaning in their lives. It is in and through their connec-tion to neighborhoods, affinity groups, and the City that they feel better able to face the joys and challenges of growing old. Even as their traditional social networks shrink, the City provides them rich opportunities for connection with people of all ages along a wide array of interests and affiliations. The neighborhood bonds that have formed over decades of living in proximity offer the security as well as mate-rial and emotional support they need in times of trouble. The City has a multitude of activities, projects, institutions, and problems that need the experience, skill and time older New Yorkers have to offer, and many older New Yorkers want opportuni-ties to give back to their families, neighborhoods, and city. These exchanges between older people and their environment have tremendous potential to build connection and engagement in ways that promote aging resilience and active aging, while making the City a better place for people of all ages. However, to take advan-tage of these urban assets that promote aging resilience, cities must make them affordable, accessible, and visible. Most importantly, the urban advantages for active aging must be extended to even the most disadvantaged neighborhoods and individuals. Rather than starting from scratch to build new models and programs, urban environments like New York can be modified to foster aging resilience by:

- Helping neighbors connect with and support one another as they age.
- Creating opportunities for older adults to stay engaged in their communities of affiliation.
- Supporting ongoing opportunities for older adults to be engaged in civic city life, particularly to plan for their own needs and communities.
- Expanding access to material and emotional support for older adults who are caregivers.
- Developing meaningful jobs and opportunities for older adults who want to work or volunteer.
- Insuring that housing and the cost of living remain affordable for older adults.
- Devising new ways of centralizing and disseminating information to older adults from all cultural and linguistic backgrounds.
- Helping older adults obtain the skills and tools needed to connect to people and information online.
- Fostering strong a city infrastructure to keep neighborhoods free of crime, streets and sidewalks accessible and safe, and transportation systems affordable and easy to access.

Cities, such as New York, are not currently doing all that they can to promote the resilience of their aging populations. Moreover, there remain profound inequities regarding who is able to take advantage of the best that cities have to offer. Urban areas have some unique environmental advantages they can exploit to confront the pressing demographic challenges before them. Mass transit, population density and diversity, existing social networks and affiliations, and access to health care, services, and activities promote connection, engagement, and health among older adults. Thoughtful and creative planning can transform these urban assets into environments that support resilient, active, and healthy aging for *all* city dwellers.

References

AARP. (2005) *Livable communities: An evaluation guide.* Washington, DC: AARP Public Policy Institute.

City Mayors. (2009). *The most expensive cities in the world. http://www.citymayors.com/economics/expensive_cities2.html.* Accessed 2 September 2010.

Finkelstein, R., Garcia, A., Netherland, J., & Walker, J. (2008) *Toward and age-friendly New York City: A findings report.* New York: The New York Academy of Medicine.

Fried, L., & Barron, J. (2005) Older adults. In S. Galea, & D. Vlahov (Eds.), *Handbook of urban health: Populations, methods, and practice.* New York, NY: Springer.

Fried, L., Carlson, M., Freedman, M., Frick, K., & Glass, T. (2004) A social model for health promotion for an aging population: Initial evidence on the experience corps model. *Journal of Urban Health, 81*(1), 64.

Fuller-Iglesias, H., Sellars, B., & Antonucci, T. (2008) Resilience in old age: Social relations as a protective factor. *Research in Human Development, 5*(3), 181–193.

Gusmano, M., Rodwin, V., & Schwartz, H. (2008) Vulnerable older people in Chinatown: report on a neighborhood workshop. Unpublished report from the authors.

Hildon, Z., Smith, G., Netuveli, G., & Blane, D. (2008) Understanding adversity and resilience at older ages. *Sociology of Health & Illness, 30*(5), 726–740.

Jeffri, J. (2007) *Above ground: Information on artists III: Special focus new york city aging artists.* New York, NY: Research Center for Arts and Culture.

Jones, S. F. S. (2009) *Generations online in 2009* Pew Internet & American Life Project.

Kaskie, B., Imhof, S., Cavanaugh, J., & Culp, K. (2008) Civic engagement as a retirement role for aging Americans. *Gerontologist, 48*(3), 368–377.

Kinsel, B. (2005) Resilience as adaptation in older women. *Journal of Women & Aging, 17*(3), 23–39.

Klinenberg, E. (2002) *Heat wave: A social autopsy of disaster in Chicago.* Chicago: University of Chicago Press.

Marmot, M., & Wilkinson, R. (1999) *Social determinants of health.* Oxford: Oxford University Press.

Menec, V. H., & Chipperfield, J. G. (1997) Remaining active in later life – the role of locus of control in seniors' leisure activity participation, health, and life satisfaction. *Journal of Aging and Health, 9*(1), 105–125.

Moen, P., Dempster-McClain, D., & Williams, R. M. (1992) Successful aging: A life-course perspective on women's multiple roles and health. *American Journal of Sociology, 97*(6), 1612–1638.

Morrow-Howell, N., Hinterlong, J., Rozario, P., & Tang, F. (2003) Effects of volunteering on the well-being of older adults. *Journals of Gerontology Series B: Psychological Sciences and Social Sciences, 58*(3), 137–145.

Musick, M. A., Herzog, A. R., & House, J. S. (1999) Volunteering and mortality among older adults: Findings from a national sample. *Journals of Gerontology Series B: Psychological Sciences and Social Sciences, 54*(3), S173–S180.

Newman, K. (2006) *A different shade of gray: Midlife and beyond in the city.* New York: New Press.

NYC Department of City Planning. (2004) *The newest New Yorkers: Immigrant New York in the new millennium.* NYC Department of City Planning Population Division.

NYC Department of City Planning. (2006) *New york city population projections by Age/Sex & borough, 2000–2030* NYC Department of City Planning Population Division.

NYC DOHMH: Bureau of Vital Statistics. (2007) *Summary of vital statistics 2006: The City of New York.* http://www.nyc.gov/html/doh/html/vs/vs.shtml.

Oswald, F., & Wahl, H. W. (2004) Housing and health in later life. *Reviews on Environmental Health, 19*(3–4), 223–252.

Phillipson, C. (2007) The 'elected' and the 'excluded': Sociological perspectives on the experience of place and community in old age. *Ageing and Society, 27*(3), 321.

Putnam, R. (2000) *Bowling alone: The collapse and revival of American community.* New York, NY: Simon & Schuster.

Rodwin, V., & Gusmano, M. (2006) *Growing older in world cities: New York, London, Paris, and Tokyo.* Nashville, TN: Vanderbilt University Press.

Rowe, J., & Kahn, R. (1997) Successful aging. *Gerontologist, 37*(4), 433–440.

Rowe, J., & Kahn, R. (1998) *Successful aging.* New York, NY: Pantheon.

Sanders, A. E., Lim, S., & Sohn, W. (2008) Resilience to urban poverty: Theoretical and empirical considerations for population health. *American Journal of Public Health, 98*(6), 1101–1106.

Sands, R., & Goldberg-Glen, R. (2000) Factors associated with stress among grandparents raising their grandchildren. *Family Relations, 49*, 97.

Sauer, W., & Coward, R. (1985) *Social support networks and the care of the elderly: Theory, research, and practice.* New York: Springer.

Shaw, M. (2004) Housing and public health. *Annu Rev Public Health, 25*, 397.

Smith, A., Sim, J., Scharf, T., & Phillipson, C. (2004) Determinants of quality of life amongst older people in deprived neighbourhoods. *Ageing and Society*, *24*(5), 793.

U.S. Census Bureau. (2005) *American Community Survey*, Poverty Status in the Last 12 Months by Sex by Age, Table C17001, New York City.

U.S. Department of Commerce. (2002) *A nation online: How Americans are expanding their use of the internet*. Washington, DC: U.S. Government Printing Office.

UNFPA. (undated) *Urbanization: A majority in cities: Population & development*. http://www. unfpa.org/pds/urbanization.htm. Accessed 30 July 2009.

Wahl, H., & Weisman, G. (2003) *Environmental gerontology at the beginning of the new millennium: Reflections on its ... The Gerontologist*. *43*(5), 616–627.

Waldrop, D., & Weber, J. (2001) From grandparent to caregiver: The stress and satisfaction of raising grandchildren. *Families in Society*, *82*, 461.

Walker, J., & Herbitter, C. (2005) *Aging in the shadows: Social isolation among seniors in new york city*. New York: United Neighborhood Houses of New York.

Walker, R. B., & Hiller, J. E. (2007) Places and health: A qualitative study to explore how older women living alone perceive the social and physical dimensions of their neighbourhoods. *Social Science & Medicine. Soc Sci Med*, *65*(6),1154–65.

World Health Organisation. (2003) *Social determinants of health: The solid facts*. Copenhagen, Denmark: Word Health Organisation.

World Health Organisation. (2007) *Global age-friendly cities: A guide*. Geneva: World Health Organisation Press.

Chapter 19
Promoting Resilience in Small-Scale, Homelike Residential Care Settings for Older People with Dementia: Experiences from the Netherlands and the United States

Hilde Verbeek, Rosalie A. Kane, Erik van Rossum, and Jan P.H. Hamers

Supported by a cultural change movement, resilience in long-term dementia care has become increasingly relevant and important. The process of cultural change promotes resident-directed care and quality of life, with the care-based relationship between the resident and direct care workers emphasized (Foy Whithe-Chu et al. 2009). Examples of this cultural change include care settings in a homelike environment focusing on residents' autonomy, opportunity for choice, and sustaining a sense of self and control. This chapter illustrates characteristics and experiences with homelike dementia care setting in the Netherlands and United States.

Although the majority of people with dementia live at home, long-term institutional care is often inevitable as the disease progresses, and is especially likely for those without family members available to provide care. Traditionally, long-term care for people with dementia was based on a medical-somatic model of care, emphasizing illness and treatment of underlying pathology. Basic nursing and medical care services were emphasized in a protected setting where the resident would be safe. Physically long-term care facilities often resemble hospitals, with long double-loaded corridors, a nurses' station and staff uniforms. Their rules and routines governing daily life permit little individualization. Currently, there is a shift toward strength-based and person-centered care for people with dementia living in care facilities: care aimed at building on a patient's personal strengths and supporting the overall well-being of the individual (e.g. Foy White-Chu et al. 2009).

Implementation of person-centered care required changes in environmental design practices to promote greater autonomy, privacy, personal identity and personhood, and socialization (Calkins 2001; Cutler et al. 2007; Zeisel et al. 2003). Guiding principles for these environmental changes can be traced back to Lawton's ecological model of a supportive and stimulating care environment (Lawton and Nahemow 1973). Additionally, it was suggested that people with dementia thrive best in small settings that are similar to homes where they have lived during their

H. Verbeek (✉)
CAPHRI School for Public Health and Primary Care,
Maastricht University, Maastricht, The Netherlands
e-mail: H.Verbeek@ZW.unimaas.nl

B. Resnick et al. (eds.), *Resilience in Aging: Concepts, Research, and Outcomes*,
DOI 10.1007/978-1-4419-0232-0_19, © Springer Science+Business Media, LLC 2011

lives rather than in complex organizations that are hotel-like or hospital-like, and therefore, hard to navigate.

Together, conceptual and environmental design changes have resulted in the development of new long-term care settings for older people with dementia: small-scale, homelike settings, in which normal daily life is emphasized. These facilities correspond with a common and desirable policy trend in many countries towards making institutional dementia care as homelike as possible and enabling residents as much as control over their lives as possible (Moise et al. 2004). Internationally, various small-scale, homelike dementia care settings have been established (Verbeek et al. 2009a). Examples include small-scale living in the Netherlands (te Boekhorst et al. 2009; Verbeek et al. 2009a), Green Houses® in the United States (Kane et al. 2007), group living in Sweden (Annerstedt 1993), residential groups in Germany (Dettbarn-Reggentin 2005) and group homes in Japan (Funaki et al. 2005).

In this chapter, we discuss types of small-scale, homelike nursing-home settings in two countries: the Netherlands and the United States. In the latter, small-house nursing homes are emphasized, some of which are known as Green House® settings. After presenting descriptive information and research findings about programs, physical environments, staffing, and family involvement, we conclude the chapter with some general implications for further research, practice, and policy development.

Experiences from the Netherlands

Dutch Nursing Home Care

Dutch nursing home care is delivered mainly through the non-profit sector and covered by insurance mandated by the Exceptional Medical Expenses Act. Nursing home care is primarily provided for people with chronic somatic (i.e. physical) diseases or with progressive dementia; they are cared for within specialized somatic or psychgeriatric wards (Schols et al. 2004). Residents in psychogeriatric wards, also known as dementia care units, usually live in the nursing home until death.

The majority of nursing home care for people with dementia is provided in psychogeriatric wards located within traditional nursing homes. These wards can be compared with specialized Alzheimer units in the United States (Schols et al. 2004) and normally house around 20–30 residents. Although the environment is adapted for people with dementia, the wards often have an institutional character (Verbeek et al. 2009b). Institutional features may include long corridors, staff wearing uniforms, the nurses' station, and daily life organized by routines of the nursing home.

Long-term care for older people with dementia is currently in a transformation phase in the Netherlands (Schols 2008). Socialization of care has resulted in deinstitutionalization and normalization of long-term dementia care. Values such as preserving residents' autonomy, offering a familiar and homelike environment, enabling residents to continue their own lifestyles and promoting overall well-being hold a prominent place in long-term care. Therefore, dementia care is increasingly organized in small-scale and homelike settings, also referred to as small-scale living or group living (te Boekhorst et al. 2007; Verbeek et al. 2009a). It is estimated that by 2010, about one-fourth of all psychogeriatric nursing home care will be organized in these small-scale settings. The Dutch government stimulates the development of these care settings by adjusting policies and financial support.

Small-Scale Living in the Netherlands

Small-scale living promotes domesticity, familiarity, sense of belonging, trust, and normality. These values should be equally reflected in both the physical environment and care giving philosophy. Residents are offered opportunities to perform tasks for themselves (increasing autonomy) and have as much control over their own lives as possible (increasing empowerment) (Van Audenhove et al. 2003).

Definition of Small-Scale Living. Although small-scale living is rapidly expanding, there is debate about its precise definition. Te Boekhorst et al. (2007) used Concept Mapping analysis to define small-scale living. Their analyses resulted in six clusters, which reflect the essential elements of small-scale living: (1) a home for life; (2) normalization of daily life (activities are centered within household daily life); (3) resident autonomy and choice; (4) nursing staff as members of the household; (5) the social environment resembles a family; and (6) small-scale living is situated in an archetypical house. The emphasis in all clusters is to provide opportunity for residents and their family members to sustain a sense of self, preserve identity, and exert control over daily life. Normalizing activities of daily life, engaging in meaningful activities, and including nursing staff as members of the household all contribute to the resilience of the residents.

In everyday practice, daily routine in small-scale settings is mainly determined by household chores, in which residents are encouraged to participate. In general, domestic features such as a kitchen, dining area, bathing room and laundry area are present in all small-scale living settings. However, there is a large variety in scale, location, and other physical features of small-scale living in the Netherlands.n investigation of physical characteristics, of small-scale living in the southern part of the Netherlands (Verbeek et al. 2008a) revealed that the majority of small-scale living settings served a small number of residents ($M = 32$ residents). Most small-scale living settings included a clustering of units, ranging from three to eight per location, situated within the community or as part of a larger service facility. A broader service facility might offer, in addition to these specialized dementia care units, a home for frail elders, or assisted living care for people with psychiatric problems or intellectual disabilities. The majority of all care settings are purpose-built. Although stand-alone settings reduce the institutional look of the care setting, they often are difficult to maintain due to financial and organizational constraints. All small-scale living care settings used technology support – in the Netherlands referred to as "domotica." The main goals of domotica are mobile communication among staff (nursing staff as well as other staff), safety, and increasing resident's well-being, comfort, and ease.

Nursing staff consist of nursing assistants (NAs), certified nursing assistants (CNAs), and registered nurses (RNs). Staff members may also include specialists other than nurses, such as social work, and may receive extra trainings such as in medication administration. To ensure that daily life is as normal as possible, personal care is integrated in daily routines. Nursing staff are responsible for personal and medical care and performing domestic chores (i.e. cooking, cleaning) and organize recreational activities (te Boekhorst et al. 2008b). In small-scale living only one or two nurses are usually present during the day to manage all tasks. A traditional psychogeriatric ward requires many more staff members.

The nursing home physician, an officially recognized medical discipline in the Netherlands, supports the nursing staff. Consultation is also provided by psychologists, physiotherapists, dieticians, occupational therapists, and recreational therapists. While physicians are considered central employees of regular psychogeriatric wards, all supplemental medical specialists are regarded as visitors to the small-scale care setting.

Residents

Small-scale living is regarded as an alternative care setting for regular psychogeriatric wards in a traditional nursing home, and therefore does not require additional admission criteria. All residents require a nursing home level of care, although residents' level of cognitive and functional performance may be higher in small-scale living (te Boekhorst et al. 2009; Verbeek et al., 2010).

Van Audenhove et al. (2003) argue that small-scale living settings may not be appropriate for all residents. Relationships with others (residents, family, and nursing staff) are very personal and intimate. Residents who prefer to be alone, or who are sensitive about privacy, may not find small-scale living appropriate. In addition, it might not be suitable for residents who have extreme behavioral problems (Verbeek et al. 2008a) or need to walk around a lot or need a lot of space. Admission decisions need to be made very carefully and require experience and knowledge from staff and management.

Findings from the few studies that have assessed the effects of small-scale living suggest several resilience-promoting outcomes for residents (de Rooij et al. 2009). For example, residents of small-scale living were more socially engaged, have more things to do, and enjoy more aspects of the environment than residents living in regular psychogeriatric wards (te Boekhorst et al. 2009). In addition, physical restraints were used less with residents in small-scale living than with residents of psychogeriatric facilities. Declercq (2009) found that residents in small-scale living compared to those residing in traditional psychogeriatric wards interacted more with nursing staff and residents in advanced stages of dementia and initiated more frequent non-verbal communication. However, most studies suffer from methodological limitations such as a small sample size and base-line differences between residents. Verbeek et al. (2009b) have designed a study to tackle these issues and investigate effects on residents, family caregivers and nursing staff.

Family Caregivers

In small-scale living, family caregivers are a part of the household. They can visit at any time, help with daily activities and household chores, join residents for dinner, and are actively involved with all residents. To investigate the experiences of family caregivers with respect to small-scale living settings, Verbeek et al. (2008a) conducted interviews with family members of residents. Almost all family members were very positive about small-scale living. They felt the needs, wishes, and beliefs of their residents were very well respected and residents were encouraged to live their lives as they were accustomed. Staff members were very involved with both residents and family members. This personal attention and compassion was highly appreciated. Additionally, family members appreciated their involvement with care and the household in the small-scale care setting. All settings were perceived as very homelike; the atmosphere and ambience played a crucial role. Collective meal preparation was highlighted as a crucial component of this special, homelike environment. Other daily activities such as reading the newspaper and playing games increased the feeling of being at home. Family members also valued physical characteristics of living rooms, kitchens, and the residents' private rooms. They also appreciated residents being allowed to bring their own furniture and other personal belongings into the house. Finally, families found it very important that small-scale living had a home-for-life principle. Once admitted, residents should not be transferred to another care setting, even when the disease progresses because of the potential stress and negative outcomes for the residents.

Family caregivers of people with dementia often experience high level of stress. Te Boekhorst et al. (2008a) investigated the effects of small-scale living settings on three aspects of family caregivers' psychological distress: burden, psychopathology, and competence. No location effects were found: family caregivers in small-scale living did not experience less psychological distress compared with those in traditional nursing homes. These findings conflict with previous research which reported group-living care to be more effective in reducing caregiver burden compared with other types of nursing home care (Colvez et al. 2002). However, differences were identified in how caregivers in small-scale living and traditional nursing homes experienced the care delivered and contact with nursing staff (te Boekhorst et al. 2009). Family in small-scale living felt that nursing staff had more respect for a residents' perception of the environment, asked more frequently for former habits, and appeared less hurried. Additionally, they perceived more personal attention from staff as family caregivers.

Staff's Perspective

Working in a small-scale living setting is very different from employment in a regular psychogeriatric ward. Small-scale living resembles family life and only 1–2 nurses manage the household each day. What does this mean for the nursing staff?

To investigate this, we interviewed nursing staff and managers working in four small-scale living settings in the southern part of the Netherlands (Verbeek et al. 2008a). Most staff members had deliberately chosen to work in a small-scale living setting. Personal contact with residents was the main reason for making this choice. They had more time for personal attention in small-scale living than in a regular psychogeriatric ward. Additionally, they appreciated the broadening of their tasks and the freedom to plan their day, thus promoting creativity among nursing staff.

The nursing staff also indicated that working in small-scale living is physically less intensive than the work in a regular psychogeriatric ward. Mentally and psychologically, however, small-scale living is demanding. It can be stressful to work and live with demented residents for 8 h a day. Nevertheless, nursing staff say that living together with the residents is also very satisfying. They feel a large commitment to their work, which is considered as very important. Residents can return a lot as well, for example, when residents react to positive attention.

Management indicated that nursing staff was specifically recruited. Their attitudes and visions of care giving were considered as very important. Treatment and direct contact with residents, for which communicative and social skills are essential, were paramount in small-scale living. Furthermore, staff members need to be able to work independently, be flexible, and have good organizational skills.

Te Boekhorst et al. (2008b) investigated differences in nursing staff's job characteristics in traditional nursing homes and small-scale living and the influence on well-being. Their results indicate that professional caregivers in small-scale living settings experienced a higher job satisfaction and less burn-out symptoms than those working at regular psychogeriatric wards. The nursing staff members were less emotionally exhausted, and experienced less depersonalization and an increased sense of personal accomplishment. These findings suggest that small-scale living facilities may have a positive effect on resilience for both nursing staff and residents.

Mediating job characteristics, including job autonomy, social support, and job demands may help explain these differences (te Boekhorst et al. 2008b). Nursing staff in small-scale living experienced more autonomy in their work; they had more control and decision authority. Furthermore, they experienced more social support from colleagues, although working alone more often. This is explained by a higher quality of contacts: the team shares responsibility for the residents' care and therefore interaction revolves around the residents, possibly increasing social support. Finally, staff in small-scale living experience less job demands, as measured in work and time pressure. Small-scale living is not guided by the routines of the organization, but by the needs and wishes of the residents.

Experiences from the United States

With the enactment of Medicare and Medicaid in 1965, nursing homes expanded rapidly and became the dominant modality for publicly funded long-term care in the United States. Nursing homes are licensed by the states in which they are located and certified to receive federal payments. They are expected to provide a broad range of services to a wide range of residents, including rehabilitation, end-of-life care, and ongoing long-term services for people with physical disabilities, cognitive impairment, or both. Considerable variation can be found across states, but the model nursing home has about 100 beds and is operated as a proprietary organization; most residents live in shared rooms. Although in the 1950s and early 1960s, elderly persons with Alzheimer's disease or other dementias often received custodial care in geriatric wards of state psychiatric hospitals, financial incentives operating since 1965 have led to the virtual elimination of long-stay care in psychiatric hospitals. Partly in response to quality problems, nursing homes have become strictly regulated; standards have been developed, nursing homes are inspected for compliance with those standards, penalties have been affixed, and comparative quality information has been made available to the public. Nursing homes have been criticized for the quality of their care, their regimentation, and the poor quality of life experienced by many residents (Shields 1988). Much of the critique can be summarized by the term "bed and body work," introduced by Gubrium (1975) to describe the task-oriented focus of the direct care workers. Three trends have influenced Alzheimer's care in nursing homes in the United States.

Dementia Special Care Units

Beginning in the 1970s, traditional nursing homes began to establish dementia special care units (SCUs). These units were ideally characterized as a defined section of the nursing home that is secure and locked and has a physical design suited to persons with dementia, staff specially trained in dementia care, specific programs designed for people with dementia, and defined admission and discharge criteria (Lawton 2001). In practice, by the mid-1990s, almost 25% of nursing homes had one or more dementia SCUs. These SCUs varied enormously, however, in their goals, target populations, and programs; they also differed in the extent to which the special training and programming occurred (see Maslow and Ory 2001). Most were not small, but rather home to approximately 40 people, comparable to other units. Some were designed to work with people who had few nursing needs, but exhibited so-called behavior problems with the plan that unit residents be discharged to a different unit for end-of-life care.

Residential Care and Assisted Living

A second trend in dementia care was that individuals with dementia began to utilize alternative residential programs rather than licensed nursing homes. Persons with dementia appeared to thrive in small group settings, such as family care homes or adult foster homes (Kane et al. 1991), perhaps because the settings were so similar to familiar living situations, were small, and easily negotiated because of the size.

Residential care settings, freed of the regulatory constraints associated with nursing homes, also developed dementia SCUs or dementia-specific settings organized into small living units in pods or small connected buildings. Apartment-style assisted living settings emerged in the late 1980s and expanded rapidly. Development were driven by an ideal of providing older people who needed the nursing-home level of care with normal living quarters and a program of services that emphasized individuality, choice, dignity, privacy, and normal life-style (Wilson 2007). Considerable work has been done to summarize accomplishments in assisted living, sometimes with special reference to dementia care (Kane et al. 2007; Zimmerman et al. 2001, 2005). In general, assisted living and other residential settings not licensed as nursing homes have become laboratories for new models of care.

Assisted living for old people has also been vigorously critiqued. First, depending on state regulations and the preferences operators, residents may be discharged to nursing homes when their acuity reaches some specified level (Mead et al. 2005). The smallest assisted living settings, including those licensed as adult foster homes in some states, are often literally in private home settings, and may be better able to retain residents when their health or cognitive conditions deteriorate, but, paradoxically, they may also have more rules governing the daily lives of residents (Eckert et al. 2009). Second, although assisted living settings have often managed to provide normal community living conditions, they rarely provide the organized health care services needed by so many older people (Kane and Mach 2007). Third, those assisted living settings for seniors that live up to the conceptual ideals of privacy, individualization, and function-enhancing amenities tend to exclude most low-income people and reject subsidization by the Medicaid program (Hernandez and Newcomer 2007).

In the last decade, most state governments have moved toward reducing their dependence on institutions for all populations needing long-term supportive services. There has been some critique, however, that residential care settings in the community can easily take on the qualities of institutions. A recent analysis suggested five criteria that could render a setting less institutional and more community oriented, namely: smaller scale; more residential physical features; more control, choice, and individualization for residents; more ability for residents to integrate with the larger community outside the setting, particularly on an individualized basis; and control over when and whether the person leaves the setting to go elsewhere, including to a more intensive care setting (Kane and Cutler 2009). Some analysts speculate that nursing home and residential care sectors will converge. If so, the hope is that the best elements of assisted living environments will be combined with the greater care capacity of nursing homes (Calkins and Keane 2008).

Culture Change Movement

A third influence on the development of small-scale nursing homes is broadly known as the culture change movement (Weiner and Ronch 2003). In general, the culture change movement is directed towards improving everyday life in nursing homes in such a way that residents experience more individualized care and have a better quality of life. This culture change is initiated through changes in architectural design to create more homelike normal environments and promote better functioning; changes in staff training and hierarchical roles based on the belief that frontline staff with greater power can offer improved flexibility to residents; and changes in programs and policies to minimize routines.

The environmental elements of culture change have often involved creating households of 8–10 people and structuring neighborhoods (i.e. clusters of households); residential kitchens and laundry areas may also be made available to residents. Private rooms are becoming more prevalent in nursing homes in general, partly because of the competition from other settings like residential care and partly because of the strong preferences that residents and family show for private rooms even for people with dementia (Kane et al. 1998). Some claim that people with dementia are calmer with private rooms. When residents have private rooms and private in suite bathrooms, some authorities argue that separation of people with dementia from those without dementia is less important.

The trend in nursing homes in the United States is towards more management at the unit level and replacement of large-scale dining with dining on specific units or choices of dining venues in a facility. A related trend is to permanently assign nursing staff, especially front-line nursing assistants, to particular units, and even to particular residents, for continuity of services.

Small-Scale Living in Nursing Homes in the United States

In the remainder of this section, we discuss just one type of small-scale nursing home emerging in the United States, the small-house nursing home, and its trademarked prototype, the Green House® setting. It is the most dramatic manifestation of small-scale nursing home because entirely separate buildings are used for each house, though several small houses can be linked administratively and hold a single nursing-home license. With a few exceptions, implementation to date has not been specific to dementia care, but many people with dementia have been served in the Green Houses and small-house nursing homes.

In 1991, William Thomas founded the *Eden Alternative* to combat what he called the scourges of nursing-home life – loneliness, boredom, and lack of meaning. The Eden Alternative envisaged a nursing home full of plants, animals, and children, but more importantly a setting with empowered frontline staff, flattened hierarchy, flexible routines, and room for spontaneity in residents' lives (Thomas 1994, 1996, 1999). Many care settings and state nursing-home trade associations became captivated by the ideals and values inherent in the approach.

Thomas came to believe that although the Eden Alternative correctly diagnosed a problem with nursing homes, its solution was insufficient, and that a complete transformation and de-institutionalization of the nursing home was required.

The articulation of the Green House idea began with that insight. The details of the model are highlighted in the next section, with more details available elsewhere (Rabig et al. 2006).

The Green House®Setting. The Green House, now a trademarked name, is a self-contained small house that is licensed as a nursing home or part of a nursing home and that serves no more than ten nursing-home residents. *Self-contained* means that the Green House should not be linked to any larger facility but be free standing with its own mechanical engineering systems, its own doors to the outside, and its own core staff. The physical environment includes a large family-style kitchen and dining area, and a living room with a fireplace (called the hearth). Meals are prepared in that kitchen, which is open to residents, and consumed in the dining area at a large family-style table. Each resident has a private room and en suite bathroom with a shower, an office/study for staff, a smaller sitting room (called a sunroom or a den), a patio, and an area with a whirlpool tub and hair dressing facilities complete the original plan. In an initial slogan, the physical setting was to be "warm, smart, and green." The latter referred to vegetation and growth, and "smart" referred to the plan that a variety of technologists would be employed to enhance care, functioning, and overall quality of life for the elders (the term for residents). The main manifestation of technology in the original prototypes was ceiling lifts that enabled one person to assist a transfer in and out of bed and from bed to toilet. Another mantra for the building was that nothing should be found in the Green House that would not be found in a private home. Institutional hallmarks such as medication carts were to be abolished. Most medications are, in fact, stored in a lockable wall cabinet in each elder's room.

The Green House transformed care arrangements as well as environmental plans. The core staff members of each Green House were the CNAs, who received additional training and had markedly expanded roles. Besides fulfilling all the ordinary responsibilities for personal care to meet ADL, IADL, and cognitive needs and assisting nurses with routine nursing care, they were charged to develop menus, prepare meals, serve meals, perform light housekeeping, and do the residents' personal laundry. They were also deemed resident *development specialists* who would know each elder well, implement plans to meet individual resident needs and fulfill personal preferences. In the Green House, this new type of personnel was called a Shahbaz (plural Shahbazim), a term suggested to remove all historical baggage associated with the designation "nurse's aide." In other models, they are sometimes called resident assistants or elder assistants. The Shahbazim were responsible for the life of the house. All professional staff required by law in nursing homes (e.g. nurses and director of nursing, medical director, activities director, social work director, dietician, therapists, etc.) were considered a clinical support team who visited the residents in the houses to provide direct care and support to Shahbazim. In clinical areas where they had legal responsibility (especially nursing), the clinical support team members provided direction and oversight to Shahbazim and otherwise acted as resource persons for the frontline staff. Adapted from work done by Yeatts et al. (2004) to establish functional work teams in traditional nursing homes, the frontline staff were constituted as self-directed work teams, and were responsible for their own scheduling and problem-solving (Rabig 2009). Rotating roles were assigned through the team, including house coordinator, coordinator for food, coordinator for housekeeping, scheduling coordinator, and later, quality of life coordinator. The Shahbazim did not report to nursing staff but to an administrator, known as a guide.

The final component of the model was an emphasis on quality of life, individualization of care, and integration with the community. The model envisaged a "sage," or wise community resource-person that would be an additional sounding board for Shabazim. Overall, the entire model emphasized quality of life outcomes. The Green House was not specifically an intervention designed to change the delivery of care, but to facilitate the Green House model some homes have streamlined medication regimens and improved communication about health-related changes.

Implementation of the Green House®Setting. The first implementation of the Green House was in a 140-bed traditional nursing home within a multilevel retirement community. The sponsor downsized its original setting and relocated 40 nursing-home residents to 4 Green Houses, which were constructed in a residential section of the campus. Two of these Green Houses were occupied by the former residents of a locked dementia SCU, and the other two were occupied by residents in the general campus, selected from volunteer applicants in order of their length of time in the retirement community.

This program was evaluated through a longitudinal study of quasi-experimental design that compared resident outcomes with those of two comparison groups – residents in the parent nursing home from which the Green House residents came and residents from a nursing home in another non-profit retirement campus about 90 miles away. The investigators hypothesized that Green House residents would have better quality of life, based on the 11 domains of quality of life measures developed specifically for nursing homes, than the two comparison groups and that Green House elders would be more satisfied with their care and would not suffer any deterioration of health and functional outcomes as measured by standardized quality indicators based on the minimum data set (Kane et al. 2003). All hypotheses were confirmed, and in fact some of the quality indicators were statistically significantly better for the Green House than the comparison groups, particularly the indicator on minimizing decline in physical functioning (Kane et al. 2007).

Family and staff members also benefit from involvement with the Green House. For example, family members maintained greater involvement with their relatives in the Green Houses and were more satisfied with their relatives' care than families with relatives in the other living facilities (Lum et al. 2008). Compared to the control groups, the CNA-level staff believed they knew their residents, had more sense that they could positively influence outcomes, and had great intrinsic and extrinsic job satisfaction.

Since the original implementation of the Green House model, the sponsoring nursing home in Tupelo has built additional Green Houses. The two Green Houses (Laney House and Page House) that were originally developed as dementia settings have retained their identity. Five years after implementation, most of the original residents in the houses were still living, though some had lost their ambulatory status or become less verbal. Staff turnover in those houses was also low. Newly admitted residents who might have qualified for the dementia SCU because of moderately advanced dementia with behavior issues tended to be admitted to those original dementia homes. But other Green Houses on the campus also served many elders with dementia, and no effort was made to relocate people who deteriorated.

In 2005, the Robert Wood Johnson Foundation funded a large 5-year project for rapid replication of Green Houses with the goal of implementing 50 new Green House programs and having widespread presence in most states. Counting the Mississippi programs, as of July 2009, at least 15 nursing-home Green House projects are operating in 11 states, and many more are in construction or under development. From review of the website, it appears that only one is planned to be a dementia-specific Green House.

In addition to the Green House projects, other firms are developing variations on the small-house theme that are similar but do not carry the Green House trademark. One such program has been developed by the Otterbein Retirement Homes of Ohio, a non-profit firm that operates a multi-level retirement campus. Two variations in this Otterbein initiative, called Avalon Neighborhoods by Otterbein, are noteworthy. First, the small-house nursing homes are situated away from the larger campuses in regular housing areas; and second, the projects designate 1–2 houses for post-acute care and short-stay rehabilitation. The long-stay houses tend to have a majority of residents with dementia, although they also serve residents without dementia. Four 5-house Avalon neighborhoods are already operating, and one of this chapter's authors (Kane) is leading a study particularly devoted to exploring lessons for Alzheimer's care emerging from the Avalon neighborhoods.

Conclusions and Implications

This chapter illustrated small-scale, homelike dementia care settings in the Netherlands and the United States, both examples from a cultural change movement in long-term care. The core values of various new models bear a strong resemblance to each other, emphasizing normalization of daily life, residents' autonomy and choices, individuality in service provision, and empowerment of front-line staff. Upholding these values provide opportunities to promote and enhance resilience.

Differences in implementation of small-scale living also exist between countries. This may be partially related to disparities in organization of health care services in general, and dementia care specifically. Additionally, some differences exist with respect to residents and staff. In the Netherlands, the development of small-scale living is mainly focused on people with dementia, although settings for other groups, such as people with traumatic brain injury or physical disabilities, have been created. Developments in the United States have created settings for frail people in general. Staffing levels may vary between both countries, although the core values of all-round nursing staff – providing personalized care – are similar. These developments result in certain challenges for clinical practice and future research.

Clinical Implications

There are several clinical implications for promoting positive growth and resilience in small-scale living. First, small-house models have shown "proof of concept"; they are operating successfully, they are liked by residents and their families, and tend to have waiting lists. Second, extraordinary skill development and empowerment has been observed among the CNAs and other nursing staff who work in these settings. Third, training of all personnel is essential to implement and sustain the model. Obviously the new elder assistant (referred to as the Shahbaz in the Green Houses) requires front-end training in a wide variety of topics, including culinary skills, managing kitchens laundries, housekeeping to conform to infection control standards, and team-building skills. Skills for effective communication with teammates, other nursing home personnel, families, and the general public are also crucial. Creativity, flexibility, and independence are important qualities for nursing staff in fulfilling these tasks.

Activities directors and occupational therapists are required to reinvent themselves and their programs because many of the large-group programs of conventional nursing-homes were no longer viable. Furthermore, although the small-house settings themselves permit a more normal rhythm of daily activity for each resident, activities personnel need to help frontline staff determine ways to take advantage of opportunities afforded by the physical settings, small community, and relaxed routines. New avenues for cooperation and negotiation of roles need to be sought in the future. Creative approaches to activities that build on the preferences and biographies of the residents, particularly those with dementia, are especially needed. Although the natural rhythms of the house, including cooking, provide a focus of interest, some residents with dementia seem not to have enough to do, and frontline care providers need suggestions for how they can trigger meaningful solo activities or interactions among residents who have more difficulty initiating activities because of cognitive impairment.

Future Research

The small-house and small-scale living models are now operational, and have proven their feasibility. Future research – both quantitative and qualitative – is necessary to refine the models. Based on our experiences, we recommend the following research areas:

1. Study of residents' characteristics and research into which residents reside best in small-scale, homelike settings. It is important to study how particular mixes of residents based on their physical and cognitive impairment influence the well-being of everyone in a small house. Additional studies of family members and staff, as well as the collective perspectives of all stakeholders also are warranted.
2. Examination of the appropriateness of small-scale living for late-stage dementia residents.

3. Post-occupancy evaluations to determine which aspects of the physical designs, fixtures, and furnishings and social and organizational environment work well and what could be improved. Additionally, greater detail and clarification of the concept of what constitutes small-scale, homelike settings is needed.
4. Investigation of the construction and operational costs of small-house nursing homes under differing assumptions of spaciousness, amenity level, and staffing.

References

Annerstedt, L. (1993) Development and consequences of group living in Sweden. A new mode of care for the demented elderly. *Social Science & Medicine 37*, 1529–1538

Calkins, M. P. (2001) *Creating successful dementia care settings.* Baltimore: Health Professions Press.

Calkins, M. P. & Keane, W. (2008) Tomorrow's assisted living and nursing homes: The converging worlds of residential long-term care. In S. M. Golant & J. Hyde (Eds.), *The Assisted living residence: a vision for the future* (pp. 86–118). Baltimore: Johns Hopkins Press.

Colvez, A., Joel, M. E., Ponton-Sanchez, A., & Royer, A. C. (2002) Health status and work burden of Alzheimer patients' informal caregivers: comparisons of five different care programs in the European Union. *Health Policy, 60*, 219–233.

Cutler, L. J., Kane, R. A., Degenholtz, H. B., Miller, M. J. & Grant L. (2007) Assessing and comparing physical environments for nursing home residents: using new tools for greater specificity. *The Gerontologist, 45*, 42–51.

de Rooij, I., Luijkx, K., Emmerink, P., Declercq, A., & Schols, J. M. (2009) Verhoogt kleinschalig wonen de kwaliteit van leven voor ouderen met dementie? (Does small-scale living increases quality of life for older people with dementia?). In H. Stoop & I. de Rooij (Eds.), *Grote kwaliteit op kleine schaal. Is kleinschalig wonen voor mensen met dementie een succesvolle parel in de ouderenzorg?* (pp. 43–52) Tilburg: Programmaraad Zorgvernieuwing Psychogeriatrie en De Kievitshorst/De Wever.

Declercq, A. (2009) Kleinschalig genormaliseerd wonen in Vlaanderen. (Small-scale normalized living in Flanders). In H. Stoop & I. de Rooij (Eds.), *Grote kwaliteit op kleine schaal. Is kleinschalig wonen voor mensen met dementie een succesvolle parel in de ouderenzorg?* (pp. 61–68) Tilburg: Programmaraad Zorgvernieuwing Psychogeriatrie en De Kievitshorst/De Wever.

Dettbarn-Reggentin, J. (2005) Studie zum Einfluss von Wohngruppenmilieus auf demenziell Erkrankte in stationären Einrichtungen. (Study on the influence of environmental residential groups on demented old people in nursing home residents). *Zeitschrift fur Gerontologie und Geriatrie, 38*, 95–100.

Eckert, J. K., Carder, P. C., Morgan, L. A., Frankowski, A. C., & Roth, E. G. (2009) *Inside assisted living: the Search for Home.* Baltimore: Johns Hopkins Press.

Foy-White-Chu, E., Graves, W. J., Godfrey, S. M., Bonner, A. & Sloane, P. (2009) Beyond the medical model: the culture change revolution in long-term care. *Journal of the American Medical Directors Association, 10*, 370–378.

Funaki, Y., Kaneko, F., & Okamura, H. (2005) Study on factors associated with changes in quality of life of demented elderly persons in group homes. *Scandinavian Journal of Occupational Therapy, 12*, 4–9.

Gubrium, J. F. (1975) *Living and dying at Murray Manor.* Charlottesville, VA: University of Virginia Press.

Hernandez, M & Newcomer, R (2007) Assisted living and special populations: what do we know about differences in use and potential access barriers? *The Gerontologist, 47 (Special Issue III)*, 110–117.

Kane, R. A., Baker, M. O., Salmon, J. & Veazie, W. (1998) *Consumer perspectives on private versus shared space in assisted living*. Washington, DC: AARP.

Kane, R. A., Chan, J., & Kane, R. L. (2007) Assisted living literature through May 2004: taking stock. *The Gerontolgist, 47 (Special Issue III),* 125–140.

Kane, R. A. & Cutler, L. C., (2009) Promoting home-like characteristics and eliminating institutional characteristics in community-based residential care settings: insights from an 8-state study. *Seniors Hoursing & Care Journal, 16,* 91–113.

Kane R. A., Kane R. L., Illston L. I., Nyman J., and Finch M. D. (1991) Adult foster care for the elderly in Oregon: a mainstream alternative to nursing homes? *American Journal of Public Health, 8,* 1113–1120.

Kane, R. A., Kling, K. C., Bershadsky, B., Kane, R. L., Giles, K., Degenholtz, H. B., Liu, J. & Cutler, L. J. (2003) Quality of life measures for nursing home residents. *Journal of Gerontology: Medical Sciences, 58A,* 240–248.

Kane, R. A., Lum, T., Cutler, L. J., Degenholtz, B., & Yu, A.-C. (2007) Resident outcomes in small-group-home nursing homes: a longitudinal evaluation of the initial Green House program. *Journal of the American Geriatrics Society, 55,* 832–839.

Kane, R. L. & Mach, Jr, J. R. (2007) Improving health care in assisted living. *The Gerontologist, 47 (Special Issue III),* 100–109.

Lawton, M. P. (2001) Quality of care and quality of life in dementia care units. In Noelker, L. S. & Harel, Z. (Eds). *Linking quality of care to quality of life* (pp. 136–161). New York: Springer.

Lawton, M. P. & Nahemow, L. (1973) Ecology and the aging process. In Eidorfer,C & Lawton, MP (Eds). *Psychology of adult development and aging* (pp. 619–674). Washington DC: American Psychological Association.

Lum, T. Y., Kane, R. A., Cutler, L. J., & Yu, T.-C. (2008) Effects of Green House® nursing homes on residents' families. *Health Care Financing Review, 30,* 37–51.

Maslow, K. & Ory, M. (2001) Review of a decade of special care unit research: Lessons learned. *Alzheimer's Care Today, 2,* 16–20.

Mead, L. C., Eckert, J.K., Zimmerman, S., & Schumacher, J. G. (2005) Sociocultural aspects of transitions from assisted living. *The Gerontologist, 45 (Special Issue 1),* 115–123.

Moise, P., Schwarzinger, M., & Um, M. (2004) *Dementia care in 9 OECD countries: a comparative analysis.* Paris: OECD.

Rabig, J.(2009) The effects of empowered work teams in the Greenhouse project. In Yeatts, D. E., McCready, C. M., & Noelker, LS (Eds.). *Empowered work teams in long-term care: strategies for improving outcomes for residents & staff.* Baltimore, MD: Health Professions Press.

Rabig, J., Thomas, W., Kane, R.A., Cutler, L.J., & McAlilly S. (2006) Radical redesign of nursing homes: applying the Green House concept in Tupleo, MS. *The Gerontologist, 46,* 533–39.

Schols, J. M. (2008) *Trends in Dutch nursing home care for demented patients.* Paper presented at the Dementia Fair Congress, Leipzig.

Schols, J. M., Crebolder, H. F., & van Weel, C. (2004) Nursing home and nursing home physician: the Dutch experience. *Journal of the American Medical Directors Association, 5,* 207–212.

Shields, R. R. (1988) *Uneasy endings: daily life in an American nursing home.* Ithaca, NY: Cornell University Press.

te Boekhorst, S., Depla, M. F., de Lange, J., Pot, A. M., & Eefsting, J. A. (2009) The effects of group living homes on older people with dementia: a comparison with traditional nursing home care. *International Journal of Geriatric Psychiatry, 24,* 970–978.

te Boekhorst, S., Depla, M. F. I. A., de Lange, J., Pot, A. M., & Eefsting, J. A. (2007) Kleinschalig wonen voor ouderen met dementie: een begripsverheldering (Small-scale group living for elderly with dementia: a clarification). *Tijdschrift voor Gerontologie en Geriatrie, 38,* 17–26.

te Boekhorst, S., Pot, A. M., Depla, M., Smit, D., de Lange, J., & Eefsting, J. (2008a) Group living homes for older people with dementia: the effects on psychological distress of informal caregivers. *Aging & Mental Health, 12,* 761–768

te Boekhorst, S., Willemse, B., Depla, M. F., Eefsting, J. A., & Pot, A. M. (2008b) Working in group living homes for older people with dementia: the effects on job satisfaction and burnout and the role of job characteristics. *International Psychogeriatrics, 20,* 927–940.

Thomas, W. H. (1999) *The Eden Alternative handbook: the art of building human habitats.* Sherburne, NY: Summer Hill Co.

Thomas, W. H. (1996) *Life worth living: how someone you love can still enjoy life in a nursing home: the Eden Alternative in action.* Acton, MA: VanderWyk Burnham.

Thomas, W. H. (1994) *The Eden alternative: nature, hope and nursing homes.* Sherburne, NY: Summer Hill Co.

Van Audenhove, C., Declercq, A., De Coster, I., Spruytte, N., Molenberghs, C., & Van den Heuvel, B. (2003) *Kleinschalig genormaliseerd wonen voor personen met dementie (Small scale normalized living for persons with dementia).* Antwerpen/Apeldoorn: Garant.

Verbeek, H., van Rossum, E., Zwakhalen, S. M., Kempen, G. I., & Hamers, J. P. (2009a) Small, homelike care environments for older people with dementia: a literature review. *International Psychogeriatrics, 21,* 252–264

Verbeek, H., van Rossum, E., Zwakhalen, S. M. G., Ambergen, T., Kempen, G. I. J. M., & Hamers, J. P. H. (2009b) The effects of small-scale, homelike facilities for older people with dementia on residents, family caregivers and staff: design of a longitudinal, quasi-experimental study. *BMC Geriatrics, 9(3).*

Verbeek, H., van Rossum, E., Zwakhalen, S. M. G., Kempen, G. I. J. M., & Hamers, J. P. H. (2008a) *Kleinschalig wonen voor ouderen met dementie. Een beschrijvend onderzoek naar de situatie in de provincie Limburg. (Small scale living for older people with dementia. A descriptive study to the situation in the province of Limburg).* Maastricht: University Press Maastricht.

Verbeek, H., Zwakhalen, S. M. G., van Rossum, E., Ambergen, T., Kempen, G. I. J. M. & Hamers, J. P. H. (2010). Small-scale, homelike facilities versus regular psychogeriatric nursing home wards: a cross-sectional study into residents' characteristics. *BMC Health Services Research* 10: 30

Weiner, A. S. & Ronch, J. L. (Eds) (2003) *Culture change in long-term care.* New York: Haworth Press.

Wilson, K. B. (2007) Historical evolution of assisted living in the United States, 1979 to the present. *The Gerontologist, 47 (Special Issue III)*: 8–22.

Yeatts, D. E., Ceady, C., Ray, B., DeWitt, A., & Queen, C. (2004) Self-managed work teams in nursing homes: implementing and empowering nurse aide teams. *The Gerontologist, 44,* 256–261.

Zeisel, J., Silverstein, N. M., Hyde, J., Levkoff, S., Lawton, M. P., & Homes, W. (2003) Environmental correlates to behavioral health outcomes in Alzheimer's Special Care Units. *The Gerontologist, 43,* 697–711.

Zimmerman, S. I., Sloane, P. D., & Ekert, J. K. (Eds) (2001) *Assisted living: needs, practices, and policies in residential care for the elderly.* Baltimore: Johns Hopkins Press.

Zimmerman, S., Sloan, P. D., Williams, C. S., Reed, P. S., Preisser, J. D., Eckert, J. L., Boustani, M., & Dobbs, D. (2005) Dementia care and quality of life in assisted living and nursing homes and assisted living. *The Gerontologist, 45 (Special Issue 1)*, 133–146.

Chapter 20
A Geriatric Mobile Crisis Response Team: A Resilience-Promoting Program to Meet the Mental Health Needs of Community-Residing Older People

Donna Cohen and B.L. King-Kallimanis

Mental health care for a rapidly aging population is now, and will continue to be, a significant public health challenge. By the middle of the century, 2050, it is estimated that there will be between 11 and 16 million persons aged 65 and older with Alzheimer's disease, a significant increase beyond the 5.1 million Americans in that age group with Alzheimer's disease in 2009 (Alzheimer's Association 2009). The number of persons aged 65 and older with other psychiatric disorders will more than double from about 7 million in 2000 to over 15 million in 2030, about 25% of the older population (Cohen and Eisdorfer 2011). Another 10–15% of older adults will experience significant emotional problems associated with the vicissitudes and stressful losses of later life.

Functional effectiveness and vitality are diminished when multiple illnesses, chronic conditions, injuries, and/or frailty interfere with physical and mental functioning. Prevalent chronic conditions in the population aged 65 and older include arthritis, hypertension, hearing and visual deficits, heart disease, diabetes, cancer, and stroke. Furthermore, emotional distress and psychiatric disorders occur in 25–50% of older persons with chronic illnesses (Hybels and Pieper 2009). Individually and collectively, these conditions negatively affect quality of life and contribute to functional decline, additional years spent in pain and misery, and increased dependency.

Unfortunately, mental health problems are usually not recognized, diagnosed accurately, or treated adequately in primary care settings, the de facto mental health system for older adults. Unrecognized and untreated, these illnesses decrease an individual's resiliency, diminishing his or her ability to recover and maintain well-being. Significant mental health problems interfere with cognitive, behavioral, emotional, and physical function which in turn may adversely affect an older adult's recognition that a problem exists, desire and/or ability to seek help, use of family and social supports, engagement in healthy behaviors, and successful coping with personal and life stressors.

A great deal can be done, however, to maximize resilience, functional effectiveness, and quality of life of older adults if they seek and find accessible services

D. Cohen (✉)
University of South Florida, Tampa, FL, USA
e-mail: cohen@fmhi.usf.edu

B. Resnick et al. (eds.), *Resilience in Aging: Concepts, Research, and Outcomes*,
DOI 10.1007/978-1-4419-0232-0_20, © Springer Science+Business Media, LLC 2011

where clinicians are trained to detect, diagnose, and treat psychiatric problems. Scholars estimate that one-third of older adults living in the community need mental health care but less than 3% are seen in outpatient mental health clinics, psychiatric hospitals, general hospitals with psychiatric units, and VA medical centers combined.

Clinical depression is one of the most common psychiatric disorders in older people, ranging in severity from mild to severe and life threatening (Heisel and Duberstein 2005). Twenty-five to thirty percent of older people living in the community report mild symptoms, and major depressive disorders occur in 1–9%, rates similar to those seen in younger populations (Blazer 2003). Untreated depression can be lethal, leading to suicide and homicide-suicide (Cohen and Kim 2007). Clinical depression is one of the most common risk factors for suicide, and the highest suicide rate occurs among men 65 years and older. Over 80% of suicides are men, and their suicide rates increase dramatically with advancing age. Older people also have homicide-suicide rates 2–3 times higher than younger persons, with over 90% of homicide-suicides perpetrated by men, 70% of whom have depression associated with caregiving strain (Cohen et al. 1998; Cohen 2002). Suicide rates do not increase with age in older women. Unfortunately, most older people do not seek or receive help for their depression, although as many as 70% have seen their primary care providers for medical consultation within 4 weeks of completing suicide or homicide-suicide.

The Need for Home and Community-Based Psychiatric Services

Traditional outpatient programs have not been responsive to the mental health needs of older people living in the community for several reasons, including the limited availability of mental health programs, the lack of staff knowledgeable about geriatric mental health care, the failure of older people and their family members to recognize the presence of mental health problems, the reluctance of older people to use services, and the many practical barriers to utilization of services, e.g. lack of transportation, impaired physical mobility.

Home and community based programs are needed to reach out to vulnerable older people in the community. Those among the old-old (ages 76–84) and oldest-old (ages 85 and older), especially, are often isolated from family, have limited mobility, and/or are homebound. Home-based crisis response teams with intensive care management appear to provide effective psychiatric management of mentally ill older persons who are homebound, leading to decreased frequency of psychiatric hospitalizations, reduced length of hospital stays, and stabilization at home (Dibben et al. 2008; Kohn et al. 2002). Unfortunately, few of these programs exist in the United States or the United Kingdom (Cooper et al. 2007; Richman et al. 2003).

The available literature describes four types of psychiatric home-based programs: crisis teams, mobile mental health teams without psychiatrists, mobile psychiatric teams without medical back-up, and multidisciplinary psychiatric mobile teams. However, most studies of these models have been descriptive and have not used uniform data collection to evaluate their effectiveness (Kohn et al. 2002).

The objective of this chapter is to provide a description and evaluation of a Geriatric Mobile Crisis Response Team (GMCRT) for older persons who were referred for mental health problems. Gulf Coast Jewish Family Services, a comprehensive mental health program in Florida, has successfully operated a GMCRT in two counties (Pinellas and Pasco counties) since 1994. An evaluation of the GMCRT in its first year of operation showed the effectiveness of the program in improving overall global functioning and reducing depression (Paveza 1996). Gulf Coast Jewish Family Services received a state contract to provide a similar program in South Broward county beginning in the summer 2005. Since characteristics of community populations, e.g. cultural diversity, health disparities, age distribution, may affect the operation of these types of programs, an evaluation was considered necessary for the first year to identify the effectiveness of the new program. These factors may be a barrier to knowledge about the treatability of mental disorders, willingness to seek help, and ability to participate in treatment. The findings from the evaluation will be integrated into an overall discussion of resilience maintenance among older adults with mental health diagnoses.

Geriatric Mobile Crisis Response Team Program

The GMCRT program, which is conducted in close coordination with Florida State Adult Protective Services, receives referrals from the Florida Department of Children and Families, social service agencies, home health agencies, law enforcement, aging network care managers, and others who deal with older adults. A very small number of clients self-refer. The GMCRT has a professional staff of three masters-level, licensed mental health professionals, and a consulting psychiatrist.

The GMCRT provides comprehensive in-home assessment, 24 h in-home crisis intervention, crisis intervention counseling, psychiatric evaluation, hospitalization when necessary, care planning, linkages with community services, as well as follow-up and intensive case management, with the overall goal of responding to the mental health needs of older persons and reducing the risk of suicide and self-injury. Clients who are seen after a referral are asked to sign a treatment consent form, and if they accept services, they are given a comprehensive mental status evaluation of behavioral and psychological functioning, then, if necessary, are seen by a psychiatrist in order to make triage decisions and create a care plan for intervention. Clients who are determined to be a danger to themselves and/or others and will not go to a psychiatric facility voluntarily are hospitalized under the state's civil involuntary commitment laws. Clients with Alzheimer's disease and related dementias are referred to local geriatric dementia services.

Evaluation of the Geriatric Mobile Crisis Response Team Program

The objectives of the evaluation were to determine whether the client population treated by the Broward County GMCRT would show a reduction in psychiatric symptoms and emotional distress and an improvement in functional effectiveness. Although the Florida Department of Children and Families provided funding for the clinical team, they did not allocate funds for the evaluation. Therefore, only two benchmark measures were included to measure outcome. The University of South Florida Institutional Review Board approved the evaluation study, which was based on secondary analysis of client admission and discharge data with all personal identifiers removed from client forms.

The client database included 42 persons enrolled, treated, and discharged between June 2005 and May 2006. No data were provided about the number of clients who refused services. The frequency of the diagnostic codes for those who accepted services were as follows: 43% with depressive disorders not otherwise specified; 43% with adjustment disorders with anxiety, depression, or both; 5% with major depressive disorder; and the remaining 9% with either dysthymia, alcohol abuse, panic disorder, or generalized anxiety disorder. A total of 10% described wanting to harm themselves, 5% wanted to harm themselves and others, and 2% wanted to harm another person.

The following client characteristics were included in the analysis: six sociode-mographic items (age, gender, race, marital status, educational attainment, and living arrangement); five health characteristics (presence of developmental disabilities, physical disabilities, and ADL impairments as well as whether a client was legally blind or legally deaf); two program variables (admission and discharge date); and two psychiatric outcome measures.

Client admission and discharge scores on two outcome measures were analyzed using a simple pre-test/post-test design to evaluate change in client status and the effectiveness of the team intervention: the Brief Psychiatric Rating Scale – BPRS (Overall and Gorham 1962) and the Global Assessment of Functioning Scale – GAF (APA 2000). Both are rating scales completed by the clinician.

The BPRS measures 24 psychiatric constructs, each rated on a 7-point scale of severity ranging from "not present" to "severe." The domains are somatic concern, anxiety, depression, suicidality, guilt, hostility, elevated mood, grandiosity, suspi-ciousness, hallucinations, unusual thought content, bizarre behavior, self-neglect, disorientation, conceptual disorganization blunted affect, emotional withdrawal, motor retardation, tension, uncooperativeness, excitement, distractibility, motor hyperactivity, and mannerisms and posturing. This instrument can be administered rapidly, has strong inter-rater and test–retest reliabilities, and is a validated measure of change. The GAF is a 100-point scale which allows clinicians to rate overall psy-chological and social impairment present in a person due to their psychiatric illness. It does not consider physical and environmental impairment. The GAF scores range from 1 to 100 and are divided into ten categories. Higher scores indicate a better level of overall psychosocial functioning. For example, a person with a score between 1 and 10 is seen as in persistent danger of hurting themselves or others, while a person scoring between 91 and 100 is functioning at a superior level. The GAF is included as Axis V in the Diagnostic and Statistical Manual of Mental Disorders of the American Psychiatric Association (APA 2000). Several additional measures were originally included in the evaluation: the Mini-Mental State Examination

(Folstein et al. 1975) and the Geriatric Depression Scale (Yesavage et al. 1983). However, staff did not administer them to a sufficient number of clients at admission and discharge to permit test–retest comparisons.

Table 20.1 provides demographic information on the 42 clients who were enrolled and discharged from the program. Women outnumbered men 4:1, and the men were significantly older than the women, an average age of 83 years vs. 76 years. The client population, both men and women, was largely non-Hispanic Caucasian (86%). A higher percentage of men were married compared to women, 50% vs. 6%, whereas more women were widowed, divorced, or separated than men, 91% vs. 50%. The majority of women lived alone (62%), whereas most men lived with a spouse or family member (75%). Table 20.2 shows that the sample did not include persons with developmental disabilities or those who were legally deaf; only one client was legally blind. Most of the clients, both men and women, were free of physical disabilities and ADL impairments.

The average duration of treatment for the population was 18 weeks (range 5–42 weeks), with 22 weeks for men and 18 weeks for women. A total of 70% of clients

Table 20.1 Socio-demographic characteristics of 42 clients treated by the Broward Geriatric Mobile Crisis Response Team

	Total	Men	Women
N	42	8 (19.0%)	34 (81.0%)
Age (Mean & SD)	77.7 ± 9.7	83.0 ± 9.8	76.5 ± 9.4
Race			
White	36 (85.7%)	7 (87.5%)	29 (85.3%)
Black	4 (9.5%)	0	4 (11.7%)
Hispanic	1 (2.4%)	1 (12.5%)	0
Other	1 (2.4%)	0	1 (2.9%)
Marital status			
Married	6 (14.3%)	4 (50.0%)	2 (5.9%)
Widowed	2 (50.0%)	3 (38.0%)	18 (52.9%)
Divorced/annulled	14 (33.3%)	1 (12.50%)	13 (38.2%)
Separated	1 (2.4%)	0	1 (2.9%)
Educational level			
Less than 12 years	9 (21.4%)	4 (50.0%)	5 (14.7%)
High school degree	15 (35.7%)	1 (12.5%)	14 (41.2%)
Some college	11 (26.2%)	1 (12.5%)	10 (29.4%)
College graduate	4 (9.5%)	1 (12.5%)	3 (8.8%)
Graduate school	3 (7.1%)	1 (12.5%)	2 (5.9%)
Living arrangement			
With spouse	4 (9.5%)	3 (37.5%)	1 (2.9%)
With child	8 (19.0%)	2 (25.0%)	6 (17.6%)
With other family	2 (4.7%)	1 (12.5%)	1 (2.9%)
Alone	22 (52.4%)	1 (12.5%)	21 (61.8%)
Supportive housing	6 (14.3%)	1 (12.5%)	3 (8.8%)
Other	1 (2.4%)	0	1 (2.9%)
Missing	1 (2.4%)		1 (2.9%)

Table 20.2 Health characteristics of 42 clients treated by the Broward Geriatric Mobile Crisis Response Team

	Total ($n = 42$)	Men ($n = 8$)	Women ($n = 34$)
Developmental disabilities			
Yes	0	0	0
No	42 (100%)	8 (100%)	34 (100%)
Legally deaf			
Yes	0	0	0
No	42 (100%)	8 (100%)	34 (100%)
Legally blind			
Yes	1 (2.4%)	0	1 (2.9%)
No	41 (97.6%)	8 (100%)	33 (97.1%)
Physical disabilities			
Yes	9 (21.4%)	2 (25.0%)	7 (20.6%)
No	33 (78.6%)	6 (75.0%)	27 (79.4%)
ADL impairments			
Yes	8 (19.0%)	0	8 (23.5%)
No	33 (78.6%)	8 (100%)	25(73.5%)
Missing	1 (2.4%)		1 (3.0%)

Table 20.3 Psychiatric status and functional performance of 42 clients treated by the Broward Geriatric Mobile Crisis Response Team

	Total ($n = 42$)	Men ($n = 8$)	Women ($n = 34$)
Duration of treatment (weeks)	18.6 ± 10.0	22.0 ± 13.6	17.8 ± 8.9
BPRS			
Admission	10.3 ± 5.1	6.5 ± 4.9	11.2 ± 4.8
Discharge	5.0 ± 3.9	3.5 ± 2.9	5.4 ± 4.1
	$t = 0.34$***		
GAF			
Admission	56.8 ± 6.0	57.2 ± 5.9	56.7 ± 5.9
Discharge	68.7 ± 6.9	69.5 ± 5.7	68.5 ± 7.2
	$t = -15.20$***		

***$p < 0.005$

achieved their goals and were discharged without a diagnostic code. With one exception, the remaining clients were discharged with the same diagnostic code assigned at admission. An individual diagnosed with depression not otherwise specified at admission was diagnosed with dementia not otherwise specified upon discharge. Only 5% were institutionalized over the course of treatment. As seen in Table 20.3, the client population showed a significant decrease in psychiatric symptoms on the BPRS, although the total scores for intake were in the very mild range of symptom presentation. There was a significant improvement on the GAF; the mean intake score of 56.8 indicated moderate difficulty in functioning whereas the mean discharge score of 68.5 indicated mild difficulty in functioning.

Case Summaries

AK. AK, a 76-year-old divorced woman, was referred by a community case manager because she was experiencing anxiety related to her medical conditions, lack of resources, and distress about family issues. When AK was evaluated by the team social worker, she reported that her biggest fears were of falling and not being able to continue to live in her apartment. She was also upset that her brother and sister were spreading untrue rumors about her. The social worker concurred that AK's anxiety was related to her physical limitations, not being able to live independently, and frustration with a long history of conflict with her siblings who lived in Ohio.

AK had an admitting BPRS score of 14 and a GAF of 50, and she was given a DSM-IV diagnosis of 300, Anxiety Not Otherwise Specified. The primary treatment objectives were to address AK's anxiety and concerns about her health, risk of falling, and sibling relationships in counseling and to link her with resources in the community to support her living safely at home. AK was given a weekly 1-h therapy session to deal with her issues as well as learn relaxation skills and assertive communication skills. She requested a female counselor who was provided for her therapy. AK was also referred to home health care to evaluate her needs for services, durable medical equipment, and physical therapy.

AK had excellent verbal and written skills and was highly motivated to meet her goals. She was discharged after 4 weeks with a BPRS of 4 and a GAF of 75. She was able to perform her personal care activities safely and independently with the use of assistive devices, including a walker and shower chair. AK was able to process the long term, chronic issues with her siblings and was able to use more effective coping styles to deal with the stress.

DG. DG, an 86-year-old divorced woman, was referred by Adult Protective Services (APS) because of a serious depression associated with multiple health conditions, relationship problems with her brother, and having been removed from her brother's home to an assisted living facility (ALF). When DG was evaluated by the team social worker, she reported that she was unhappy with the staff and the living conditions at the ALF, and she wanted a better relationship with her brother. DG also indicated that she wanted to hurt herself and had thought about suicide. The social worker observed that DG had little insight into her situation and the responsibility she had in making any improvements. DG was unwilling to discuss a treatment plan, blamed others for her problems, and would not acknowledge her role in bringing about the move or what she could do to change her situation.

DG had an admitting BPRS score of 26 and a GAF of 40, and she was given a DSM-IV diagnosis of 311, Depressive Disorder Not Otherwise Specified. The primary treatment objectives were to help DG understand how her behavior contributed to her interpersonal problems and to develop an understanding of how her depression was both a cause and a consequence of her conflicts with others. The team social worker provided short-term crisis counseling, case management, and tried to work on the relationship between DG and her brother. Although DG's brother agreed to joint sessions, he always cancelled claiming the issues were too stressful. The therapist tried to talk with DG to help her accept the impasse in this relationship, but she would not discuss the matter. DG remained unwilling to examine her own behavior and explore ways to improve her relationships with others, including the ALF staff. She had a MMSE score of 28, so the lack of insight was not due to cognitive impairment.

The therapist was able to work with DG to resolve some of the conflicts with the ALF administrator to make the transition easier as well as link DG to APS personnel to resolve frequent case management issues during treatment. DG became less depressed and more accepting of her living situation as well as the relationship with her brother. She was able to make some friends at the ALF, communicate her needs and preferences, and have a limited relationship with her brother. However, DG reported that her relationship with her brother was still stressful, and although she was resigned to living at the ALF, it too was stressful. DG used a walker and was able to dress, groom, and feed herself, but she required assistance with money and medication management. DG was discharged after 8 weeks with a BPRS of 19, a GAF of 50, and a discharge diagnosis which was the same as the admitting diagnosis. She had no thoughts of suicide or self-harm. APS was to follow up periodically after discharge.

MD. MD, a 75-year-old man, was referred by his daughter because he seemed to be having a recurrence of depression and increasing memory problems. MD had been successfully treated for depression in a psychiatric hospital 2 years prior, and he had been living independently in his home, with no physical limitations. However, his daughter had increasing concerns about his ability to continue to live alone and needing to be admitted to an ALF. When DM was evaluated by the team social worker, he was very alert, showed some memory loss, and talked about how he had enjoyed going to the gym, dancing, playing cards, and fishing. His wife had died 10 years prior, and DM had no history of psychiatric problems or substance abuse until the year after a heart attack when he developed a psychotic depression and admitted himself to the hospital.

DM had an admitting BPRS score of 32 and a GAF score of 65, and he was given a DSM-IV diagnosis of 311, Depressive Disorder Not Otherwise Specified. Although his score on the MMSE (23) suggested some mild memory impairment, he was not diagnosed with dementia at the time of screening. The social worker arranged for a psychiatric consultation, and DM was started on an antidepressant that had been beneficial during his previous treatment. He was also referred to a memory disorder clinic for an evaluation, where it was determined that DM had a vascular dementia The social worker conducted a functional evaluation, provided some short-term psychotherapy, and met several times with DM and his daughter. The social worker also provided a list of assisted living facilities for them to visit, and a month later DM moved into an ALF.

Value of Mobile Crisis Teams for Improving Mental Health and Functioning

The results of this descriptive evaluation study should be interpreted with care due to the small sample size. However, the results suggest that the mobile crisis response team intervention improved psychiatric symptoms and associated disability in this group of community-residing elderly with mental illness but with minimal if any cognitive impairment. The GAF score increased significantly, psychiatric conditions were resolved in 70% of enrolled clients, and 95% were able to stay in their homes. It cannot be determined whether this approach leads to better results compared to traditional outpatient psychiatric treatment because of the lack of a control group. However, it is likely that most of these clients would not have received services outside of the team outreach.

The percentage of clients who refused services is not known for this study, but 60% of clients referred to the GMCRT in Pinellas County refused services (Paveza 1996). The client sample in this study did not include persons with dementia, but other studies serving cognitively impaired clients as well as those with psychiatric problems showed that mobile crisis response teams were effective in decreasing psychiatric problems and increasing GAF scores (Kohn et al. 2002). This is an important finding because cognitively impaired individuals usually have more functional impairment.

Although the evaluation results suggest the effectiveness of the crisis team, they also highlight at least three other issues that need attention and resolution: (1) the need to reach out to persons who have more severe psychiatric problems; (2) the importance of finding ways to engage persons who otherwise would refuse service; and (3) the importance of finding ways to meet the needs of older persons of diverse racial and ethnic backgrounds. Other outreach models could be valuable to identify these groups and increase the likelihood that they would get needed treatment and remain in the community.

One such approach is the gatekeeper model developed by Raschko (1984) to identify older adults with psychiatric problems and at risk for suicide. The gatekeeper program trains community members employed in a number of service organizations, such as postal workers, meter readers, and bank tellers, teaching workers to be aware of changes in an older persons' functioning and alert appropriate professionals for needed services. The concept focuses on the fact that these employees are the people most likely to see the needs and vulnerabilities of older adults and be in the best position to take immediate steps to ensure their well-being. This program, which has been successfully replicated in all geographical regions, increases the likelihood of case detection over time, facilitates relationships with older persons in the community that may increase the likelihood of their engaging in services when needed, and provides a continuing check on people during and after services.

Home-based services and case management are critical to effectively respond to the mental health and functional needs of homebound older persons and maintain them in their homes. The lack of available and accessible home-based care is one of the best predictors of hospitalization and institutionalization of older persons with mental health problems and physical co-morbidities. However, the implementation of GMCRTs depends not only upon therapeutic effectiveness but also economic feasibility and the availability of home and community-based services in the community. Research with appropriate control groups is needed to determine whether these teams successfully treat psychiatric problems and improve functional effectiveness, decrease medical and psychiatric hospitalizations, postpone nursing home placement, and enhance quality of life in a cost-beneficial way. Even though mobile crisis response teams involve costs associated with the intensive case management and range of services offered, it is likely that the approach would be cost beneficial since untreated mental health problems in older adults are associated with overutilization of medical services and increased health care costs (Speer and Schneider 2003).

Mental Health and Resilience: Bouncing Back from Adversity

Resilience is defined as having good outcomes despite adversity and risk and can be described as maintaining the same level of the outcome or bouncing back after difficulties or hardships (Masten 2001; Netuveli et al. 2008). Using the latter definition, the preliminary evidence suggests that GMCRTs can be a resilience-promoting intervention. However, although the outcome measures indicated significant improvement from treatment, it is not possible too say whether indeed the population actually became more resilient as a result of their improved functioning.

Empirical studies of therapeutic interventions, such as mobile crisis outreach teams and the gatekeeper program, as well as longitudinal studies of older adults in the community should be research priorities. They should include measures of resilience and variables known to mediate resilience, including social supports and conditions, pre-morbid history of physical and mental functioning, cumulative life experiences with adversity, severity of exposure to adversity, self-perceptions, sense of control, optimism, coping styles, and limited resources, e.g. poverty (Hardy et al. 2004; Hildon et al. 2008, 2009).

The capacity to overcome the excess disability associated with mental health problems remains a challenge. Treating depression and other psychiatric problems may improve individual functioning but recovery does not necessarily mean that the individual has achieved mental health. We need to learn more about what the predictors of recovery from psychiatric problems are and to identify specific factors that promote mental health after recovery. It is also important to elucidate what aspects of resilience mediate an individual's ability to be compliant with long term treatment as well as endure the stress and strain of coping with chronic illnesses, including neurodegenerative processes that progressively incapacitate functional effectiveness and emotional well being.

References

Alzheimer's Association. (2009) *2009 Alzheimer's disease facts and figures*. Washington, DC: Alzheimer's Association.

American Psychiatric Association. (2000) *Diagnostic and statistical manual of mental disorders*, fourth edition, text revision. Washington, DC: American Psychiatric Association.

Blazer, D. (2003) Depression in late life: Review and commentary. *Journal of Gerontology Series A: Biological Sciences and Medical Sciences*, 58, 249–265.

Cohen, D. (2002) Estimating the incidence of homicide-suicide in the United States. *Journal of Mental Health and Aging*, 8, 179–182.

Cohen, D., & Eisdorfer, C. (2011) *An integrated textbook of geriatric mental health care.* Baltimore: Johns Hopkins University Press.

Cohen D., Eisdorfer, C., Llorente, M. (1998) Homicide-suicide in older persons. *American Journal of Psychiatry, 155,* 390–396.

Cohen, D., & Kim, H. (2007) Suicide in the older population. In K. Markides (Ed.), *The encyclopedia of health and aging* (pp. 545–548). New York: Sage Press.

Cooper, C., Regan, C, Tandy, A., Johnson, S., Livingston, G. (2007) Acute mental health care for older people by crisis resolution teams in England. *International Journal of Geriatric Psychiatry, 22,* 263–265.

Dibben, C., Saeed, H., Stagias, K., Khandaker, G., Rubinstein, J. (2008) Crisis resolution and home treatment teams for older people with mental illness. *Psychiatric Bulletin, 32,* 268–270.

Folstein, M., Folstein, S., McHugh, P. (1975) "Mini-mental state:" A practical method for grading the cognitive state of patients for the clinician. *Journal of Psychiatric Resesarch, 12,* 189–198.

Hardy, S., Concato, J., Gill, T. (2004) Resilience of community-dwelling older persons. *Journal of the American Geriatrics Society, 52,* 257–262.

Heisel, M., & Duberstein, P. (2005) Suicide prevention in older adults. *Clinical Psychology: Science and Practice, 12,* 242–259.

Hildon, Z., Montgomery, S., Blane, D., Wiggins, R., Netuveli, G. (2009) Examining resilience of quality of life in the face of health-related and psychosocial adversity at older ages: What is "right" about the way we age? *The Gerontologist,* doi: 10.1093/geront/gnp067.

Hildon, Z., Smith, G., Netuveli, G., Blane, D. (2008) Understanding adversity and resilience at older ages. *Society Health and Illness, 30,* 726–740.

Hybels, C., & Pieper, C. (2009) Epidemiology and geriatric psychiatry. *American Journal of Geriatric Psychiatry, 17,* 627–631.

Kohn, R., Goldsmith, E., Sedgewick, T. (2002) Treatment of homebound mentally ill elderly patients: The multidisciplinary psychiatric mobile team. *American Journal of Geriatric Psychiatry, 10,* 469–475.

Masten, A. (2001) Ordinary magic: Resilience processes in development. *American Psychologist, 56,* 227–238.

Netuveli, G., Wiggins, R., Montgomery, S., Hildon, Z., Blane, D. (2008) Mental health and resilience at older ages: Bouncing back after adversity in the British Household Panel Survey. *Journal of Epidemiology and Community Health Health, 62,* 987–991.

Overall, J. E., & Gorham, D. R. (1962) The Brief Psychiatric Rating Scale. *Psychological Reports, 10,* 799–812.

Paveza, G. (1996) *Technical report: Evaluation of the Geriatric Mobile Crisis Team.* Tampa, FL: Florida Mental Health Institute.

Raschko, R. (1984) Assertive at-home case management for impaired elderly persons – Elderly services program Spokane (Wash.) Community Mental Health Center. *Psychiatric Services, 39,* 1201–1202.

Richman, A., Wilson, K., Scally, L., Edwards, P., Wood, J. (2003) Service innovation: An outreach support team for older people with mental illness. *Psychiatric Bulletin, 27,* 348–351.

Speer, D., & Schneider, M. (2003) Mental health needs of older adults and primary care: Opportunity for interdisciplinary geriatric team practice. *Clinical Psychology: Science and Practice, 10,* 85–101.

Yesavage, J. A., Brink, T. L., Rose, T. L., Lum, O., Huang, V., Adey, M. B., Leirer, V. O. (1983) Development and validation of a geriatric depression screening scale: A preliminary report. *Journal of Psychiatric Research, 17,* 37–49.

Chapter 21
Optimizing Resilience in the 21st Century

Mary Hamil Parker

An individual's capacity to achieve, retain or regain a level of physical or emotional health after illness or loss may find support from new technologies for health care communication. Twenty-first century technologies also may fulfill additional components of resilience related to social functioning, morale, and bodily health – providing pleasurable activities and maintenance of contact with the world outside for those home or bed bound by illness or disability. Willingness to use technology may involve psychological factors such as receptivity, self-efficacy, and motivation, expressed in planning or acquisition of technologies for future needs or for future frailty.

Technologies related to health care are telehealth, electronic medical records, and telehome care. Technologies supporting independence and psychological resilience are safety monitoring and behavioral monitoring. Media applications, such as cell phones, the Wii, Facebook, and Twitter, have the potential to enhance and support social resilience. Most of these technology applications are based upon the same microprocessing chips and wireless, digital applications that have transformed worldwide communications – the way most people in the twenty-first century receive information, interact with others and carry out many tasks of daily life.

Compared to 1990, the array of technologies available for everyday activities has expanded exponentially; then, mass public access to Internet, cell phones, smart phones, Facebook, and Twitter were not contemplated. In the United States, access to broadband networks soon will be extended nationwide under Congressional mandates to the Federal Communications Commission (FCC) that every U.S. home have cost-free access to high-speed, broadband Internet service. In European countries, wide access already exists and there has been extensive governmental support for the development of technologies to assist older citizens.

M.H. Parker (✉)
Institute for Palliative & Hospice Training, Inc, Oak Park, VA, USA
e-mail: IPHT@comcast.net

B. Resnick et al. (eds.), *Resilience in Aging: Concepts, Research, and Outcomes*,
DOI 10.1007/978-1-4419-0232-0_21, © Springer Science+Business Media, LLC 2011

Age as a Predictor of Technology Use

Research and publications comparing computer and Internet usage of older and younger age groups have assessed elderly as resistant to technology (Charness and Boot 2009; Melenhorst et al. 2006). However, a 2007 Pew Research Center survey found 50% of Americans aged 65 and over had cell phones and that broadband use had tripled for these users between 2005 and 2008, the "biggest increase" was among those 70–75. The study suggested the aging-in of younger "Boomers" would create "access parity" . The 2009 Pew Survey showed that 38% of adults 65+ (Fox, Jones 2009; Fox, Jones 2009) use the Internet, 26% are home broadband users, and 16% access the Internet wirelessly, from computers or handheld devices (Raine 2010). The spread of wireless networks, digital phones and TV Internet access, should make Internet use "ageless."

Overcoming Accessibility Barriers

Universal accessibility principles and applications must be incorporated in cutting-edge technologies. Twenty-first century technology products should not place significant demands upon users with sensory, cognitive, and mobility/physical disabilities. Many consumers, regardless of age, have disabilities and require accommodating technologies. Stevie Wonder, a sight-impaired Motown musician, complained to the 2009 Consumer Electronics Show audience that touch screen technologies, using icons or keypads without auditory cues, disenfranchise sight-impaired users (Churchill 2009). Technologies that require voice commands and response to synthesized speech may disenfranchise the hearing impaired and those with speech difficulties or cognitive impairments. Recently, smart phone providers have recognized that mainstream consumers equally welcome large touch-screens, icons, and larger keyboards.

Privacy as a Barrier for Older Users

A recent study suggests elderly and younger people have the same concerns about privacy when accessing the Internet or using certain technologies (Beach et al. 2009). This study surveyed older, disabled, and nondisabled adults, age 65 and over, and "Baby Boomers," aged 45–64, to determine the conditions under which they would accept or reject the sharing of health information or the use of different types of technologies. Significant factors were the length of time required to learn use; the level of maintenance required, and whether the technology would improve quality of life and independent function in the community. Disabled persons were more willing to share personal health related information, if it would help them function in daily life, and more accepting of sharing and recording personal information than those who were not disabled. Most people were willing to share this information to family and health care providers and less willing to government agencies and insurance companies, particularly driving information. Respondents preferred systems that would support, rather than replace, the need for human inter-actions, particularly with family and other caregivers. The study suggests that care must be taken to design systems that are intuitive and user friendly.

A 2007 AARP survey of consumers 65 and over found 93% agreed computers, Internet and Personal Emergency Response Systems, are "a good thing," but most had "limited awareness" of technologies for social communication, personal safety, health and wellness (Barrett 2008).

Technologies to Assist Resilience with Health Issues

Electronic Personal Health Records

The twenty-first century technology affecting all Americans will be the implemen-tation of Electronic Medical Records (EMRs) by all health institutions receiving Federal funding. The 2009 American Recovery and Reinvestment Act (ARRA) required changes in regulations related to privacy and security breach notification of the Health Information Privacy and Accountability Act (HIPPA) that have impeded widespread U.S. public use of EMRs.

The 2009 Consumer Health and Informatics Conference, a collaboration of Federal agencies, explored the role of EMRs and Personal Health Records (PHRs) and how health information technologies could be used to implement preventive health behaviors to reduce disability and death due to cancer, heart disease, and diabetes (http://www.consumerhealthinformatics.org).

Project Health Design, Robert Wood Johnson Foundation (http://www.RWJF. org), produced examples of "next generation" personal health records that would promote resilience in users: (1) a computerized health record for breast cancer patients, which provides tools to integrate treatment scheduling, care planning, and evaluation of treatment options; (2) a hand held PDA, providing an electronic diary for pain and activity management to help patients and caregivers to manage medi-cations and control chronic pain; (3) a health record that helps people with diabetes track self-care, by recording and educating about daily behaviors; and (4) a com-puterized, voice activated "conversational assistant" to give congestive heart failure patients a daily "check-up," with reference to established treatment guidelines (http://www.projecthealthdesign.org).

Widespread use of electronic records will depend upon changes in Federal pro-grams, principally Medicare, to enable interstate transmission of health information and applications and reimburse for telehealth services in urban as well as rural areas. These changes will encourage acceptance by health insurers. *The New York Times* (Vance 2009) described the difficulties faced by a woman with amyotrophic lateral sclerosis (ALS), who wanted to use an iPhone, with added text-to-speech software so that she could carry her communications tool around with her as she went about daily activities. However, Medicare will only cover costs for a computer with a 2 lb. keyboard and a 6 in. screen with non-speech functions blocked. Since the iPhone could be used for non-medical, non-illness related uses: surf the Internet, view videos or play games; it could not be approved. A private insurer was quoted that if "enough people" requested common devices for medical purposes; the company would require "evidence-based data" to support payment for such use.

Telehealth

The U.S. Veterans Administration is in the forefront of developing telehealth and electronic medical records applications through its own systems. All veterans have EMRs. Internet technology is used for daily assessment and adjustment of care for frail community resident veterans. Pilot studies demonstrated that in-home therapy delivered by interactive video teleconferencing could successfully treat deficits in the performance of Activities of Daily Living tasks. Research has proved wireless video-conferencing to be a feasible way to provide individualized therapy in the home (Hoenig et al. 2006). The Miami University Medical Center T-Care Program blends care coordination with technology to reduce health care costs, by limiting or preventing hospitalizations and emergency room visits. An automated, telephone-based, in-home messaging device provides disease specific education for self-management and health care decision-making (http://www.umteleheath.com/projects/Miami-VA).

"Motiva," a commercial telehealth product of Royal Philips Electronics, uses the home television and a broadband Internet connection as an interactive health care platform that connects patients with chronic conditions – heart failure, diabetes, and pulmonary disease – to their health care providers to monitor vital signs. It provides daily feedback on measurements and personalized interactive health education content; surveys evaluate comprehension, motivation, and self-efficacy levels of patients (http://www.medical.philips.com).

The 2007 AARP survey reported "strong support" for telemedicine, with 75% of elderly responders willing to have a cardiologist diagnose or monitor a heart condition through electronic communications (Barrett 2008). The American Telemedicine Association (ATA) has been lobbying for changes in Medicare to cover telehealth medical services and remote disease management for the 34 million beneficiaries who live in metropolitan areas (http://www.americantelemedicine.org).

Monitoring to Promote Independence and Safety

Falls are a primary cause of injuries that challenge the physical, emotional, and psychological resilience of older people. Detection of falls and safety of individuals living alone is the goal of monitoring technologies. Little research has been done on the social, psychological, or self-efficacy effects of monitoring (Blaschke et al. 2009).

With active monitoring, the user may interact in some way with the technology, e.g., pressing a button, entering data, or information. Passive monitoring is present in the individual's living environment using wireless sensors to record activity of the individual on a relatively continuous basis and send data electronically to a central site where it is analyzed by computer to monitor safety and function. With Global Positioning Satellite (GPS) technology, wireless digital devices may be accessed almost anywhere, indoors, and out. Technologies specifically to assist people with dementia and their caregivers focus on safety, security, and social interaction. The ASTRID and ENABLE projects in Europe assessed the utility of various devices for people with dementia (Astell 2005). The use of tracking and surveillance equipment associated with law enforcement has been controversial.

Personal Emergency Response Systems

Andrew S. Dibner, PhD, and Susan Dibner, PhD developed the first monitoring technology to prevent premature institutionalization of elderly living alone because of family fears. The Personal Emergency Response System (PERS), marketed in 1974, required users to press a button on a landline telephone to dial the 24-h call center, which then contacted emergency services or a family member for assistance. Technology progressed to a portable device on a pendant or a bracelet with a tiny radio transmitter that sent the signal. With digital technology, alarms are sent wirelessly from a receiving box to the call center. Dibner found "positive psychological effects" resulting from PERS use, with subscribers reporting "an increased sense of security" and "strong anxiety-reducing effects for subscribers and their families" (Dibner 1985).

Lifeline (http://www.lifelinesys.com), now part of Phillips Medical Alert Systems, a U.S. subsidiary of Phillips Electronics, is used by an estimated 750,000 people in the US and Canada. New York State enacted legislation providing for Medicaid reimbursement for patients of certified home health agencies, whose PERS substituted for hours of safety monitoring by a personal care worker as part of the plan of care (Hyer and Rudnick 1994). At least 35 states now reimburse costs of PERS services under Medicaid. Compliance is a major issue, since PERS users must wear the device or have it within reach 24/7/365. After a fall, the PERS often would be found hanging from the refrigerator door or left on the bedside table. Some elders, who fell, would not send an alarm. People with memory impairment could not remember to push the button. In 2009, the Food and Drug Administration (FDA) issued an advisory safety alert in because people were being choked when PERS on neck chains were entangled in walkers, wheel chairs and bed guardrails (Lade 2009).

Lifeline's success fostered development of similar devices and services, many associated with security alarm services. An off-the-shelf PERS, available from electronics stores, can be programmed to send an alarm directly to a family member's cell phone; however, wireless "dead zones" limit effectiveness.

Most research on PERS has collected data on small numbers of users: characteristics, false alarms, falls, or alerts for other reasons and cost savings from reduction in hospital stays and postponed institutionalization (Edlich and Haines 2009).

A mail survey of PERS consumer satisfaction, with 618 clients of Victoria Lifeline in Manitoba, Canada and their designated responders, had a 53% response rate (Fallis et al. 2007). Most subscribers were satisfied, 79% were very satisfied. Men were more likely to use the PERS alarm than women. Sixty-seven percent of subscribers summoned emergency help at least once and these users were "significantly more satisfied" than those with no emergency use. Subscribers valued the "psychological comfort and reassurance of having the service." Both subscribers and responders said PERS provided "an all-important sense of security." In a study involving the home care experience of older widows, eight women, who had PERS experience and one of more falls, were asked about having a PERS (Porter 2003). Getting help after a fall and feeling safer with the ability contact help were main interview responses, also "shock" at hearing the "strange voices" of the PERS operators responding to accidental alerts or unexpected visits from responders to alerts from PERS operators. Porter concluded: "When the older person has a PERS, it might be more of a relief to family members and health care providers than it is to the older person." Dr. Porter is preparing to publish new research that includes data on PERS and fear of falling (PorterEJ@missouri.edu).

Twenty-First Century PERS Technologies

A twenty-first century PERS is a hands-free personal emergency response and fall prevention system, developed by the Intelligent Assistive Technology and Systems Lab (IATSL), University of Toronto (http://www.ot.utoronto.ca/iatsl), with funding from the Canadian National Science and Engineering Research Council (NSERC). The goal is to free users from the need to wear an alarm-sending device or press a button for help. The system links one or more ceiling mounted "vision sensor" units containing a non-recording video camera, a microphone, speakers, a voice processor, and a smoke detector. These send signals to a Central Control Unit that tracks a person moving about the home. Data, such as the dimensions of the tracked person's silhouette and shadows, rather than video photos, are analyzed to detect in real-time if there is an emergency such as a fall. The closest sensor unit uses speech recognition technology to have a dialogue with the person in distress to determine the type of assistance needed. Computer analysis of the dialogue has been developed to quickly assess the severity of the situation through a series of simple "yes" or "no" questions. The user can command a 911 call, speak with an operator or place a call to a neighbor or family member. If the user does not respond or the system does not understand the user's responses (e.g., severe injury, stroke, or unconsciousness), then the system automatically contacts an emergency response centre to summon aid. By responding to voice commands, rather than interpreting a fall using an accelerometer or vibration device, this system can respond to different types of incapacity (Alex.Mihailidis@utoronto.ca).

Another twenty-first century PERS application for falls, called "myPHD," incorporates passive and active monitoring, software-based data analysis, and web access.

AFrame Digital, Inc. (http://www.aframedigital.com) developed the myPHD with funds from Small Business Innovation Research (SBIR) contracts from the Defense Advanced Research Projects Agency (DARPA) and the National Institute on Aging, National Institutes of Health (NIH). The myPHD is worn 24-hours a day to monitor an individual's activity, location, and physiological status in real time, indoor and outside. The goal is to be able to continuously and non-intrusively monitor individuals to prevent falls and the medical complications that follow. The analog watch is lightweight, comfortable, and available in an array of colors – attributes based upon marketing research with 160 elderly. Caregivers or care managers have a mobile touch-screen device to receive alerts and check activity and health data.

AFrame Digital's research involves collaboration with the Virginia Institute of Technology, Locomotion Research Laboratory; the CREATE project at University of South Florida, and Florida State University. Studies remotely monitor elderly individuals and test external third-party devices that communicate with the AFrame system via a wireless Bluetooth gateway, a pulse-oximeter which provides both heart rate and blood-oxygen saturation level, a weight scale, a blood-pressure cuff, and a user-friendly device for responding to a daily health questionnaire.

Passive Monitoring

Over the past 10 years, research on passive monitoring of the functioning of older individuals within their living environments has evolved into products available in the marketplace. Some monitoring applications collect information unobtrusively, requiring little interaction from the user, summoning assistance on an as-needed basis or when data indicates a need for inquiry about the individual's health or wellbeing. "Behavioral monitoring" methods, based upon data recording trends in functional behavior, hold promise for moving beyond simple emergency response to helping elderly, disabled, and frail individuals to function better in their living environments by identifying changes needing preventive intervention to maintain independence.

QuietCare (http://www.GEhealthcare.com/AgingInPlace)

The basic concepts and methods used in behavioral monitoring systems were developed, researched, and patented, principally by David Kutzik, PhD and Anthony Glascock, PhD, both of Drexel University and Behavioral Informatics, Inc. (Glascock and Kutzik 2009). Their research resulted the QuietCare product that uses a simple array of wireless heat and motion sensors, strategically placed in the home, to monitor activity in the bedroom, bathroom, living area, use of the refrigerator, and access to medication. These sensors send signals periodically to a central data center, where data are interpreted by algorithms and related to behavioral norms established upon that individual's functional behavior over time. If the data indicate an emergency situation, such as unusual lack of activity, the possibility of a fall, environmental temperature above or below safe thresholds, a "red" alert is sent to a designated caregiver or responder. All the behavioral data are available on the Internet, through a secure access site, to care managers approved by the individual being monitored. The data array for a single time period is presented as green (normal activity), yellow (some departure from normal), or red (emergency alert) dots for each monitored activity.

For several years Charles G. Willems, Senior Staff, Zuyd University, Netherlands (c.g.m.h.willems@hszuyd.nl), has been conducting pilot research using QuietCare technology with clients of a care organization in supportive housing and living independently in the community.

The results of the pilots demonstrated that measurement of ADL activities provide a useful means to organize home care support but would require substantial changes in the way care is organized and delivered. A larger study is underway, funded by a Netherlands insurance company, to organize care in relation to data received from monitoring, particularly the intermediate, "yellow," alerts that indicate a change from usual patterns of behavior.

WellAWARE™ Systems (http://www.wellawaresystems.com)

The WellAWARE website shows how sensors are arrayed in a typical apartment to detect movement, temperature and humidity; a floor vibration sensor detects disabling falls, and bed sensors monitor sleep patterns and quality. Caregivers receive reports on behavior patterns and alerts. WellAWARE studied monitored residents in a Volunteers Of America (VOA) assisted living facility, assessing cost savings from reduction of hospitalizations, increased caregiver efficiency and reduced workload (Alwan et al. 2005; Alwan et al. 2006). The 21 residents monitored completed the Satisfaction with Quality of Life Scale (SWLS) pre and post installation of monitoring. The caregivers and facility management found the sensor data to be useful in care coordination and planning, data from residents of the memory care unit indicated nonverbal signs of pain and other behaviors.

Healthsense (http://www.healthsense.com)

The Healthsense, eNeighbor, uses tilt sensors on medicine boxes to monitor medication usage; motion detectors on walls to detect movement within rooms; contact sensors on kitchen cupboards and refrigerator doors to indicate that the resident is eating regularly; toilet sensors monitor toilet usage; pressure sensors on beds detect when a resident gets in or out of bed, and home-or-away sensors detect when the resident leaves or returns to the residence. Algorithms "predict" behavior based on a resident's habits and lifestyle; analysis of sensor data determines if the resident needs assistance and automatically issues alerts for help. A 2008 study surveyed 43 eNeighbor users in a senior residence, eight of whom had summoned emergency help, on perceived "level of independence" as a result of having the system (Meade 2008). Being able to get help quickly if they fall or become ill was "liked best," (rating of 3.9 on a four-point Likert scale) and next was the support to live independently (3.8). Caregiver staff positively assessed the effect of eNeighbor on residents and care delivery. On the negative side, some residents were annoyed by "false alarm" calls when no activity was sensed because they were reading or sleeping. Some said they disliked wearing the device around the neck and one person said monitoring was "like Big Brother."

Technologies Supporting Social Resilience

Smart Cell Phones

"Smart" cell phones able to access the Internet and mimic computers, provide platforms for resilience supportive applications, such as exercise, reminders, calls for help, contact with family and caregivers. Major providers now market phones with larger keypads, touch screens, icons, and other attributes more "friendly" to older users. The simple, low-cost "Jitterbug," (http://www.jitterbug.com), designed specifically to meet the needs of older consumers, offers 24-hour "live, registered nurses" to answer health questions. The twenty-first century smart phones will have biomedical/physical functioning supports, such as blood pressure monitoring, pulse, blood glucose and pulse-oxygen. Users of the "Seri Virtual Personal Assistant" (http://www.siri.com) will speak or write requests directly into the hand-held device.

Social Connectedness

The impact of technology on social relationships has primarily focused on young consumers and the dizzying speed with which new networking technologies have been introduced has not given time for research. However, media reports provide useful indicators that older consumers find social benefits from new technologies.

In a recent wedding announcement (Weddings/Celebrations Section, The New York Times, Sunday Styles, December 6, 2009, page 18), the bride, 71, and groom, 75, described how they carried on their "old-fashioned courtship" by e-mail.

Eric A.Taub, Personal Tech Editor for *The New York Times*, illustrated the social power of technology with a story about his 100-year-old Mother. In her last days of life, she expressed regret at not being able to see her family in California. Taub connected his computer with a web cam and used iChat to enable his Mother to see and speak with her great-grand children (Taub 2009).

The Nintendo Wii has become a staple for activities in U.S. senior programs, stimulating inter-center sports competitions via the Internet. In October 2009, the National Senior League, 182 teams in 102 senior living communities, launched an online Wii bowling section to track scores and determine division and national champions (http://www.nslgames.com). The Health Games Research project (http://www.healthgames.org), University of California, Santa Barbara (http://www.isber.ucsb.edu) funds research on interactive games to improve health, cognition, mobility/balance, and social networking of elderly. North Carolina State University (gainsthroughgaming.org) and Georgia Institute of Technology (http://www.gatech.edu), are studying the cognitive effects of the Wii and video games.

The "Eons" Internet site (http://www.eons.com) targets Boomers and seniors, offering brain fitness and other games, special interest communities and updates via Twitter. Nielsen, December 10, 2009, reported a survey of on-line destinations of users over 65. In the previous 30 days, Google Search was the No. 1 online destination, with 10.3 million unique visitors, second was Windows Media Player, 8.2 million, and Facebook was third, 7.9 million visitors (http://blog.nielsen.com/nielsenwire). In 2008, a *Nielsen* survey of the same age group ranked, Facebook, No. 45. In 2009, VibrantNation.com, an online site for mature women received on-line responses from 20,000 women, aged 50 and over, 63% owned an iPod or other MP3 player, and 30% used Skype (Reily 2009).

Social Networking and Activities

It'sNever2Late (IN2L) (http://www.in2l.com), a touch-screen computer and Internet technology, enables older adults to communicate with family members and participate in stimulating activities. Mather LifeWays Institute on Aging is conducting a case-control study evaluating the use of IN2L. "Resilience" is defined as a personality resource, evidenced by self-confidence, self-efficacy, and intellectual capabilities. Preliminary statistics show 43% of participants engaged in learning at least once a week, 41% in mind exercises, 41% in communication, 36% in communication with families and others, 34% in hobbies, but less than 10% in physical exercise. Over 21% participated in TV games, the most popular activity. Staff reported that IN2L activities increased interactions and relationships among residents, staff, and resident families; 70% reported staff learned more about residents and 50% said elders were interacting more with staff and had improved relationships. Significant differences were found between residents classified as "low resilience" compared to those with "high resilience." Among high resilience residents, 31% reported "very good or excellent" health and 58% were rated as "more active"; compared to the low resilience residents, 65% of whom reported "fair or poor" health and 75% were rated as less active (Hollinger-Smith 2009).

Technology Use in Resilience Supportive Communities

To provide examples of how twenty-first century technologies can be used to create "resilience supportive" communities, Mary H. Parker, PhD, interviewed staff and residents of Selfhelp Community Services, Inc., New York, NY (http://www.selfhelp.net) and Lutheran Life Communities, Arlington Heights, IL, http://www.lutheranlifecommunities.org (Parker 2009).

Selfhelp Community Services

Established in 1936 to assist holocaust survivors, Selfhelp has taken an active approach to the integration of technologies into its services. Leo M. Asen, Vice President, Senior Communities, said that the Selfhelp Board and executive management made a conscious decision to incorporate technology in the "way it does business" providing services and programs for residents in senior housing and other community programs. Selfhelp annually serves over 20,000 aging, frail, and at-risk New York City residents. Selfhelp operates 6 senior facilities housing over 1,000 older people of many nationalities. It has four programs in housing facilities that have become Naturally Occurring Retirement Communities (NORCs), six senior activity centers, an adult daycare program for people with Alzheimer's disease, several homecare programs and three case management programs.

Since 1996, Selfhelp has placed over 80 QuietCare passive monitoring units; at present over 30 clients have monitoring. New monitoring clients are also issued a personal emergency response (PERS) to enable them to send their own alerts for help. Two women in their 90's, who have received passive monitoring and case management for several years, said monitoring was their choice and enabled them to live alone, feel confident and safe alone. One woman said that she had lived alone for many years, but felt "more secure" with the monitoring, which also gave her sons "peace of mind." By telephone, her son, who was vacationing over 100 miles distant, said he had checked his computer that morning and noted his Mother was up, breakfasted, and moving around her apartment. The other woman, who had a history of falls, said she felt "confident" in her ability to live alone with monitoring. Her son said prior to monitoring he made frequent daily phone calls to his Mother and, if she did not answer the phone, he would drive to her apartment to see if she was OK. Both women said that with monitoring, family members are less concerned about them living alone. One woman said: "Now, I ask about their health."

Under a grant from the New York State Department of Health, Selfhelp's Medicare-certified home health agency offers telehealth-monitoring of blood pressure, weight, and glucose to elderly with chronic disease. A 30-day, 1–3 daily dosage medication dispenser provides reminders and notification to caregivers of missed doses.

Selfhelp is extremely supportive of computer use by residents and other program participants; training is provided by a professional instructor. A wireless hotspot is at one senior center and residents use computers located in some of the residential facility lobbies. Touch-screen computer terminals are in several locations, so seniors can drop by either daily or several times a week to exercise memory skills with "brain fitness" programs. The Nintendo Wii provides exercise and socialization within the senior centers; bowling and similar sports are most popular.

A "virtual" senior center is being developed using the ItsNever2Late platform to enable residents and community clients, who can no longer easily leave their homes, to participate by Internet in senior center programming. Selfhelp is constructing a residential "smart" building, equipped to handle current and future technology applications.

Lutheran Life Communities

The Arlington Heights, IL, campus has over 1,300 clients in independent and assisted living and the three levels within its memory support program, with 24-hour nursing, Medicare-certified skilled nursing and rehabilitation therapy. Residents in assisted living and independent living have PERS services.

Using ItsNever2Late, residents engage in activities, such as a simulated bicycle ride led by one resident, with a controller and "pedals," followed by residents, "pedaling" themselves on a "virtual ride" down a country road. Staff training fostered greater use of IN2L in programming for residents and as a rehabilitation and therapeutic tool. A work group of therapists, trained by IN2L, developed a manual identifying specific therapeutic uses, such as individuals needing cognitive stimulation may use a computer game to stimulate memory or a word game as part of speech therapy. The height of the computer can be adjusted for standing balance and functional reach therapy, using simulated driving, tic-tac-toe, or another game for restorative therapy.

Activities Directors use both IN2L and Wii activities. Several residents have used the IN2L touch screen to teach staff how to play games like bridge and poker. A new resident, became more involved when a nurse aide brought up the real estate listing of her former home on the computer and showed her how it was being marketed. The staff has started to develop resident life stories; all residents will have their own page, identified by an icon, showing their selected photos and information about their life experiences. The WII is used primarily for programs such as golf and bowling, something that residents enjoy from earlier life activities, providing exercise even in winter.

Organizations Funding Research on Technology

Only when beneficial technologies leave the laboratory, are tested with real users and enter the market can Americans benefit. The lack of evidence-based research is a major impediment to widespread adoption or adaptation of generally available technologies for resilience-related needs of elderly. U.S investors require proof of marketability and return on investment, rather than evidence of efficacy to finance new market entries. Research is needed to create the evidence base for ways technologies support the resilient abilities of users, improving well-being and quality of life.

The Robert Wood Johnson Foundation (rwjf.org) Pioneer research projects have explored resilience-related benefits from Personal Health Records and digital games. The INTEL Corporation employs social science researchers to understand the ways elderly would use technology to deal with daily needs and activities and also provides grants to university research (http://www.intel.com/healthcare/research). The Alzheimer's Association and INTEL collaborate in the Everyday Technologies for Alzheimer Care (ETAC) grants to develop new technologies to assist people with dementia (Dishman and Carrillo 2007). The Center for Technology and Aging, Oakland, CA (http://www.techandaging.org) provides grants to support the diffusion of technologies that assist in the care of chronic conditions and improve the independence of older adults. Many Federal agencies fund Small Business Innovation Research (SBIR) and Small Business Technology Transfer Research (STTR) grants and contracts for new technologies and products directed to meeting needs of older and disabled people.

References

Alwan, M., Dalal, S., Mack, D., Kell, S., Turner, B., Leachtenauer, J., Felder, R. (2006), Impact of monitoring technology in assisted living: Outcome Pilot, IEEE Transactions on Information Technology in Biomedicine, 10(1), 192–198.

Astell, A. (2005) Developing technology for people with dementia, Psychiatric Times, XXII, 13. Available at http://www.psychiatrictimes.com.

Barrett, L.L. (2008) 'Healthy @ Home', AARP Knowledge Management. Available at http://assets.aarp.org/rgcenter/il/healthy_home.pdf (Retrieved January 15, 2010).

Beach, S., Schultz, R., Downs, J., Matthews, J., Barron, B., Seelman, K. (2009). Disability, age, and informational privacy attitudes in quality of life technology applications: results from a national Web survey, ACM Transactions on Accessible Computing (TACCESS), 2, 1.

Blaschke, C.M., Freddolino, P., Mullen, E. (2009) Ageing and technology: a review of the research literature, British Journal of Social Work, 39(4), 641–656.

Charness, N., Boot, W.R. (2009) Aging and information technology use: potential and barriers, Current Directions in Psychological Science, 18(5), 253–258.

Churchill, R. (2009) Stevie wonder speaks at the annual consumer electronics show in Las Vegas, MSNBC News, 1/9/09.

Dibner, A.S. (1985). Effect of personal emergency response system on hospital use. Watertown, MA: Lifeline Systems, Inc.

Dishman, E., Carrillo, M.C. (2007) Perspective on everyday technologies for Alzheimer's care: research findings, directions, and challenges. Alzheimer's & Dementia, 3, 227–234.

Edlich, R., Haines, M. (2009) Scientific Basis for Selection of Personal Emergency Response Systems. Available at http://www.liveabled.com/manual/EmergResponseSyst.htm (Retrieved January 27, 2010).

Fallis, W., Silverthorne, D., Franklin, J., McClement, S. (2007) Client and responder perceptions of a personalized emergency response system: lifeline, Home Health Care Services Quarterly, 26(3), 1–21.

Glascock, A.P., Kutzik, D.M. (2009) The impact of behavioral monitoring technology on the provision of health care in the home, Journal of Universal Computer Science, 12(1), 59–79.

Hoenig, H., Sanford, J., et al. (2006) Development of a tele-technology protocol for in-home rehabilitation, Journal of Rehabilitation Research & Development, 43(2), 287–298.

Hollinger-Smith, L. (2009) It's Never 2 Late Program Evaluation for The Green House® Project Available at lhollinger-smith@MatherLifeWays.com.

Hyer, K., Rudnick, L. (1994) The effectiveness of personal emergency response systems in meeting the safety monitoring needs of home care clients, Journal of Nursing Administration, 24(6), 39–44.

Internet User Profiles Reloaded: Updated Demographics for Internet, Broadband and Wireless Users, January 5, 2010, Pew Research Center Publications. Available at http://pewresearch. org/pubs/1454/demographic-profiles-internet-broadband-cell-phone-wireless-users (Retrieved January 15, 2010).

Lade, D. (2009) Officials issue alert on personal emergency response systems, AARP Bulletin Today. October 30, 2009, bulletin.aarp.org/.../2009 (Retrieved January 28, 2010).

Meade, C. (2008) eNeighbor technology and its effect on Senior Living – a primary research study, 11th Annual Zieglar Senior Living Finance + Strategy Conference. Available at http:// www.ziegler.com

Melenhorst, A., Rogers, W.A., Bouwhuis, D.G. (2006). Older adults' motivated choice for technological innovation: Evidence for benefit-driven selectivity. Psychology and Aging, 21, 190–195.

Neilsen Six Million More Seniors Using the Web than Five Years Ago December 10, 2009. Available at http://blog.nielsen.com/nielsenwire/ (Retrieved January 28, 2010).

Parker, M. (2009) Interviews with Leo M. Asen and Selfhelp Services Staff and Residents, July 27, 2009. Telephone interview with Amy Iacch, RN, LNHA, Corporate Clinical Specialist, Lutheran Life Communities, August 4, 2009.

Porter, E.J. (2003) Moments of apprehension in the midst of a certainty: Some frail older widow's lives with a personal emergency response system, Qual Health Res, 13, 1311–1323.

Raine, L. "Internet,Broadband, and Cell Phone Statistics," Jan. 5, 2010, Pew Internet and American Life Project. (Retrieved January 28, 2010).

Reily, S. (2009) VibrantNation.com tech Survey: Boomer Women Are Early Adopters of New Consumer Electronics, Posted on Wednesday, February 25, 2009 (Retrieved January 25, 2010).

Taub, E. (2009) Helping Grandpa Get His Tech On, The New York Times, October 29, 2009, B8. Available at http://www.NYTimes.com (Retrieved January 28, 2010).

Vance, A. (2009) Insurers Fight Speech-Impairment Remedy, The New York Times, September 15, 2009, 1-A. Available at http://www.NYTimes.com (Retrieved January 28, 2010).

Chapter 22
Resilience in the Workplace: Job Conditions that Buffer Negative Attitudes Toward Older Workers

Jacquelyn B. James, Elyssa Besen, and Marcie Pitt-Catsouphes

In the United States and abroad, older people are vulnerable to negative perceptions and stereotyping, and in some instances outright discrimination (Hedge et al. 2006). These vulnerabilities are especially problematic today due to the increasing demands for employment opportunities among older workers. Are there protective factors that render older workers resilient to these vulnerabilities? Are there things that employers of older workers can do to buffer these vulnerabilities?

Forty years of research documents the negative stereotypes about the capabilities of older workers (Hedge et al. 2006). Most of these stereotypes have been challenged, even refuted, by the bulk of empirical research (see, e.g., McEvoy and Cascio 1989; Ng and Feldman 2008), yet they remain. Recent research reveals their intransigence, especially among younger co-workers (James et al. 2007). It may be the case that negative attitudes and misperceptions about the capabilities of older workers accumulate over time and lead to a slow erosion of older employees' well-being, in a way that may be similar to the way "microaggressions," as described by Sue et al. (2007b), erode the self-esteem of racial minorities. Seldom, however, are these forms of adversity examined for their effects on older workers themselves. In addition, there has been limited attention focused on protective factors that might minimize the typical negative outcomes of negative attitudes toward older workers.

The purpose of this chapter is to examine the impact of negative attitudes toward older individuals in today's workplace and explore factors mitigating against them. We propose that there are both internal and external factors that contribute to individuals' sensitivity to the stress associated with negative attitudes. Drawing from conceptions of diversity among other underrepresented groups (Mor Barak 2005), we will explore the extent to which experiences on the job are protective factors against the harmful effects of negative attitudes. In the context of work, job conditions such as supervisor support and work team inclusion may serve as external protective factors, while employees' dispositions or sources of psychological hardiness, such as one's core sense of self, may act as internal protective factors against the harmful effects of daily microaggressions expressed as negative attitudes

J.B. James (✉)
Boston College, Boston, MA, USA
e-mail: Jamesjc@bc.edu

B. Resnick et al. (eds.), *Resilience in Aging: Concepts, Research, and Outcomes,*
DOI 10.1007/978-1-4419-0232-0_22, © Springer Science+Business Media, LLC 2011

J.B. James et al.

toward late-career workers. We also examine the extent to which job conditions and core sense of self modify the relationships between positive attitudes and the two outcome variables, mental health and employee engagement.

Age: The Twenty-First Century Workforce Diversity Challenge

In recent decades, the U.S. workforce has become progressively more diverse in terms of age. During the 1950s, the 65 and older workforce was relatively small in comparison to other age groups (Toossi 2002). Recent pressure to continue work into later life, however, has meant that today's older workers represent a substantial portion of the U.S. workforce, a trend that is expected to continue in the coming decades. There are now increasing numbers of workplaces where individuals who range widely in age work side by side (Toossi 2006). In fact, in 2007, 14.8% of the labor force was between ages 16 and 24, 68.4% was between ages 25 and 54, and 16.8% were ages 55 or older (Toossi 2006). It is said that "age is the new diversity" (Capowski 1994).

In the current swirl of economic turmoil, dramatic investment/pension losses, and doubts about the sustainability of social security in the United States, many workers who thought they were nearing retirement age are being forced to rethink their plans, which will further increase this trend of extended labor force participation among older adults. The *Boston Globe* recently published a story bemoaning the lack of jobs available to younger workers due to current older workers' reluctance to retire (Gavin 2009, February 28). The point was to bring out the old saw that older workers should make room for younger workers who need to get started on their careers. The story is but one example of the kind of age and generation polemics that have been circulating in the popular press and that have been perpetuated by some organizational consultants, suggesting that people of such wide age ranges and career stages have trouble working together (Lancaster and Stillman 2005). While this literature includes negative (and some positive) stereotypes of both older and younger workers, older workers are a special case due to the fact that, as the *Globe* story indicates, they are expected to vacate their positions.

Negative Stereotypes of Older Workers

One of the more persistent and hard to dispel notions about older workers is that they are hard to train (i.e., slow to learn) or disinterested in learning. In addition, they are often thought to be less productive, less physically able, less ambitious, and less adaptable compared to younger workers (Hassell and Perrewe 1995; Ng and Feldman 2008; Rosen and Jerdee 1976). In a recent study, 44% of the employers surveyed felt that their late-career workers are reluctant to try new technologies, 38% felt their late-career workers are burnt out, and 28% felt they are reluctant to travel (Pitt-Catsouphes et al. 2007). These negative stereotypes associated with older workers may be one form of ageism in the workforce (McCann and Giles 2002). Indeed, age discrimination claims have been on the rise for some time, with a recent spike (approximately a 30%

increase over last year, from 2007 to 2008) that has made news in the *Washington Post* (U.S. Equal Employment Opportunity Commission 2010; Vogel 2009).

Studies have shown that ageism is experienced by many older workers. In a recent AARP survey, 60% of respondents between ages 45 and 74 reported that they believe that age discrimination is present in the workplace, and of those, 45% think it is very common (Groeneman 2008). In that same study, 13% of respondents between ages 45 and 74 felt that they were treated worse by their employer in comparison to other workers as a result of their age (Groeneman 2008). Whether or not discrimination is involved, negative attitudes in the workplace constitute a serious problem for older workers. They are "detrimental to both individual and organizational productivity, and although legislation can mandate particular organizational policies, it cannot dictate attitudes or behaviors" (Hedge et al. 2006, 46).

How Do Negative Attitudes Affect Older Workers?

Sue, et al. (2007a) have described a phenomenon whereby racial minorities experience "brief and commonplace daily verbal, behavioral, and environmental indignities, whether intentional or unintentional, that communicate hostile, derogatory, or negative racial slights and insults to the target person or group..." (p.72), referred to as "microaggressions." These slights and insults are often experienced as challenges to the self esteem and/or well-being of their targets. Microaggressions are often out of the awareness of the perpetrator and sometimes take the form of "subtle snubs or dismissive looks, gestures, and tones" (Sue, et al. 2007b, p. 273).

We assert that microaggressions are not limited to insults having to do with race; insults having to do with age also have pernicious effects. Any type of slight, from an inappropriate tease ("old man," "gramps") to an outright slur ("greedy geezer," "old bag") is an instance of negative attitudes and assumptions that are degrading to older people. In our view, when these incidents happen repeatedly, day after day, they may be considered age-related microaggressions. As such, they are likely to have a negative impact on the well-being and the work-related outcomes of older workers. It is interesting to note that James et al. (2008) found that perceptions of unfairness toward older workers predicted lower well-being and employee engagement for all but the youngest workers (under age 30). Thus, negative attitudes and perceptions affect the organizational climate whether one is a member of the targeted group or not.

As was previously mentioned, there are many negative and mostly erroneous attitudes about the capabilities of older workers. In fact, prejudice about age is the most socially acceptable prejudice there is in America (Hedge et al. 2006). Older people themselves, who have internalized the negative attitudes so prevalent in our society, are just as likely to hold such attitudes as are younger people (Levy and Banaji 2002). Older workers constitute a very heterogeneous group; however, and older workers respond in different ways to the challenges associated with negative attitudes that may be present at their places of work. To the extent that there may be protective factors that foster resilience in older workers against the damaging effects of such negative attitudes, it would be beneficial to both employers as well as to employees to discover them.

Resilience and the Workplace

Throughout the life course, individuals are faced with many hardships that range from single traumatic events to pervasive adversity over many years. Some individuals are able to thrive despite such experiences, while others seem to falter. We are learning that it is not simply luck that puts people in one category or the other. Those who seem to effectively cope in stressful situations, or who do not manifest the negative outcomes typical of those who have similar experiences, are said to be resilient. Resilience has been defined in many different ways by different people. Summarizing broadly, the definitions primarily conceptualize resilience either as an outcome of some event/situation or as a process leading to an outcome (Kaplan 1999).

Definitions in which resilience is viewed as an outcome focus on the idea that resilience occurs as an unusual response to a stressor. For example, resilience was defined by Masten (1989) as "the positive side of adaptation after extenuating circumstances" [as cited in Ryff et al. (1998, 70)]. In this sense, a person is thought to be resilient when showing a positive outcome despite a significant adversity which has typically resulted in a negative outcome.

In contrast, definitions of resilience as a cause or influence focus on the idea that individuals may possess certain personal characteristics that protect them from negative outcomes typical of others. One of these characteristics is "hardiness." Psychological hardiness is a quality of an individual defined as having high "commitment (belief in the importance and value of oneself and one's experiences or activities), control (the belief that life events and experiences are predictable and consequences of one's actions), and challenge (the belief that change is normal and represents a positive rather than threatening circumstance)" (Kaplan 1999, 20–21). It is thought that hardy individuals may be better able to withstand significant stressors in their environments due to their atypical cognitive and behavioral responses to events (Crowley et al. 2003). In addition, research has shown a link between other instantiations of psychological hardiness such as high self-efficacy, high self-esteem, and internal locus of control, with positive outcomes despite significant risk factors (Cappella and Weinstein 2001; Kaplan 1999; Kumpfer 1999; Wanberg and Banas 2000). According to this conceptualization, resilience is similar to a stable personality trait.

The study of resilience has traditionally focused on people who are either (a) growing up under adverse conditions, such as poverty, extreme violence, parental mental illness, or tragic life events (Luthar et al. 2000) or (b) coming to terms with extremely traumatic events, life-threatening situations such as rape or some other form of sexual abuse (Bonanno 2004; James et al. 1997; Liem et al. 1997). More pertinent to the research presented here, some studies have examined resilience in the face of the indignities of aging. Staudinger et al. (1999), for example, found that certain aspects of personality and emotional response sets are related to satisfaction with aging, which they conceptualized as resilience. In addition, Ryff et al. (1998) suggested that psychological resources such as positive self-perceptions and social comparisons are protective factors for psychological well-being among older adults. In recent years, the study of resilience has been broadened to include everyday stressors.

Martin and Marsh (2008) proposed a new construct, "buoyancy," to describe everyday resilience which is defined as "an individual's capacity to successfully overcome setbacks and challenges that are typical of the ordinary course of everyday life" (p. 169). From this perspective, individuals may show resilience to chronic stress in their everyday environments, or as mentioned above, older workers may be resilient in the face of perceived negative assumptions and stereotypes held about them by their younger coworkers.

Regardless of the definition, the study of resilience involves the recognition of risk factors and the search for protective factors. Risk factors heighten the chances of negative outcomes and may be internal or external (Keyes 2004). Protective factors work to buffer against the negative effects of the risk factors and like risk factors, they may also be internal or external (Kaplan 1999). Simply put, protective factors serve to increase the likelihood of a person's resilience in the face of risk factors. For example, a risk factor for many children is growing up in an impoverished environment, but a protective factor in that situation may be strong social support from parents and peers. If a child in such an environment shows positive developmental outcomes, the child may be thought of as resilient and the protective factor of social support the buffer. Similarly, work overload is a risk factor for lower job satisfaction, but supervisor support may be a protective factor against the negative effects of work overload.

Facilitators of Resilience in the Workplace

There are both internal and external factors that can contribute to individuals' sensitivity to and hardiness in response to the stresses associated with negative attitudes. While employees' dispositions or sources of psychological hardiness (such as one's core sense of self) may act as internal protective factors against the harmful effects of daily microaggressions expressed as negative attitudes toward late-career workers, job conditions such as supervisor support and work team inclusion may serve as external protective factors.

Numerous studies have found that high levels of social support help buffer against the negative outcomes seen with many risk factors (Bonanno et al. 2007; McCalister et al. 2006; Wilks and Croom 2008). Accordingly, social support at work may serve as a protective factor for older workers against the negative attitudes that they are exposed to in many places of work. Supervisor support is defined as "the degree to which employees form impressions that their superiors care about their well-being, value their contributions, and are generally supportive" (Dawley et al. 2008, 238). It is thought to affect work-related outcomes such as job satisfaction and turnover intentions (Ng and Sorensen 2008). It is possible that a highly supportive supervisor relationship could serve as a buffer for the deleterious effects of negative attitudes toward older workers.

The extent to which one is made to feel that he or she is a crucial part of the work team may also buffer negative attitudes that could be present at the workplace. Often referred to as "inclusion," it refers to "the degree to which individuals feel part of critical organizational processes such as access to information and resources, involvement in work groups, and the ability to influence the decision making process" (Mor Barak and Cherin 1998, 48). Work team inclusion has a substantial impact on employees' experiences and has been linked to many work-related outcomes, as well as outcomes of well-being (Mor Barak et al. 1998). High levels of work team inclusion may foster feelings of being part of a supportive work environment which may in turn protect older workers from the negative attitudes of others.

Age & Generations Study

To explore outcomes associated with negative attitudes toward late-career workers we used data from the larger *Age & Generations Study* (Pitt-Catsouphes et al. 2009). The *Age & Generations Study* gathered information about employee well-being in today's multigenerational workforce. Employees completed a survey between November 2007 and March 2008, asking a series of questions about the following topics: employees' perceptions of their work, organization/department as a whole, work group, supervisor/team leader, work style, and outlook on life. In total, 2,210 employees from 12 departments in nine organizations participated in this study. The data were weighted so that each organization was equally represented in the sample.

For the purposes of this investigation, our sample focused on older workers. Older workers are often defined based on chronological age (Greller and Simpson 1999; Riach 2007), but the term "older worker" has been applied to a large range of ages from 40 to over 75 (Hedge et al. 2006; Kooij et al. 2008). Acknowledging the large range of ages that has been used to describe older workers (Kooij et al. 2008; Pitt-Catsouphes and Smyer 2007), we adopted a definition congruent with American Discrimination in Employment Act which protects anyone 40 and over from age discrimination. Consequently, our sample of older workers includes workers aged 40 or older.

The participating organizations in the *Age & Generations Study* are affiliated with a range of industry sectors: two of the organizations are in the educational services industry; two are in health care and social assistance; one is in retail trade; two are in finance and insurance; one is in professional, scientific, and technical

Table 22.1 Characteristics of the sample

	Employees aged 40 years or older
Approximate number of participants	1,000
Percentage of women	65.7
Percentage of men	34.3
Percentage of full-time employees	87.8
Percentage of part-time employees	12.2
Percentage of hourly employees	44.8
Percentage of salaried employees	55.2
Median wage for hourly employees	$29/h
Median salary for salaried employees	$84,244.54/year
Average age of employees	51 years
Percentage age 40–49	43.1
Percentage age 50–59	42.8
Percentage age 60–65	10.1
Percentage age 65 or older	4.0
Percentage with supervisory responsibilities	49.0
Percentage reporting that they have an additional job with a second employer	7.7
Percentage of temporary employees	4.8
Percentage of consultants	2.4
Percentage reporting that they were "working in retirement," i.e., they had officially retired from a previous job	5.7

services; and one is in the pharmaceutical industry. Five of the participating organizations have a worksite located outside of the United States and four do not. All of the organizations in our sample were considered large businesses, each having over 1,000 employees: four of the organizations had between 1,000 and 10,000 employees; four had between 10,000 and 50,000 employees; and one had over 50,000 employees. While four of the participating organizations were for-profit, five were nonprofit.

Table 22.1 summarizes some of the employee characteristics in the sample for employees aged 40 or older.

Attitudes at Work

As part of the *Age & Generations Study*, employees were asked about their perceptions of workers at different career stages. In this study, we used measures of attitudes toward late-career workers as a proxy for attitudes toward older workers. Respondents were asked how true it was that late-career workers (1) are productive; (2) take initiative; (3) add creativity to projects; (4) have high levels of skills

Table 22.2 Means and standard deviations for the attitudes toward late-career team members ($N = 910$)

In general, how true do you think the following statements are for the members of your team who are late career?	Mean	Standard deviation	Range
Late-career employees are productive	3.18	0.69	1–4
Late-career employees take initiative	2.88	0.82	1–4
Late-career employees add creativity to projects	2.76	0.79	1–4
Late-career employees have high levels of skills compared to what is needed for their jobs	3.00	0.77	1–4
Late-career employees are often our best employees	2.92	0.75	1–4

compared to what is needed for their jobs; and (5) are often our best employees (see Table 22.2). A composite score was then created by taking the mean of these five items. Lower scores indicate less positive attitudes toward late-career team members and higher scores indicate more positive attitudes. These results suggest that workers aged 40 or older are more positive about older workers (in general) being productive and having high levels of skills compared to their assessment of older workers having what is needed for their jobs. By contrast, workers 40 and older were less positive about their ability to add creativity to projects. When the responses to the individual items regarding attitudes toward late-career team members were aggregated, we found that the attitudes are significantly less positive among workers under age 40 ($M = 2.81$, SD = 0.58) than among those age 40 or older ($M = 2.95$, SD = 0.56), $t(1,745) = 5.01$, $p = 0.001$.

Relationships Between Negative Attitudes and Important Outcomes: Mental Health and Engagement

Building on previous work suggesting that negative attitudes are very stressful for those experiencing them (Sue et al. 2008), we examined the extent to which attitudes toward late-career team members predict outcomes of well-being for employees aged 40 or older. To measure personal and organizational outcomes, we used a measure of mental health (personal well-being) and employee engagement (active involvement with and commitment to the organization). Mental health was measured using the eight-item SF-8 (Ware et al. 2001). Sample items include, "During the past 4 weeks, how much have you been bothered by emotional problems (such as feeling anxious, depressed, or irritable)?" and "During the past 4 weeks, how much energy did you have?" Employee engagement was measured using a nine-item adapted version of the Utrecht Work Engagement Scale (Schaufeli and

Table 22.3 Standardized regression estimates of measures of well-being on attitudes toward late-career workers ($N = 737$)

Predictor	Mental health B	Employee engagement B
Gender[a]	0.105**	0.108**
Marital status[b]	0.012	–0.021
Parental status[c]	–0.028	–0.118**
Ethnicity[d]	–0.083*	–0.111**
Education[e]	0.039	–0.007
Income	0.074*	0.089*
Age	0.199***	0.171***
Attitudes toward late-career team members	0.136***	0.265***
R^2	0.077***	0.124***

Note: Gender, marital status, parental status, ethnicity, education, income, and age are controls
*$p<0.05$, **$p<0.01$, ***$p<0.001$
[a]Reference = female
Reference = married or cohabitating
[c]Reference = has no children
[d]Reference = white
[e]Reference = bachelors degree or higher

Bakker 2004). Sample items include "At my work, I feel bursting with energy" and "I am immersed in my work."[1]

As can be seen in Table 22.3,[2] after controlling for key demographic characteristics and dependent care responsibilities, an increase in positive attitudes toward late-career team members is associated with an increase in well-being and employee engagement. Of course, the reverse is also true; negative attitudes toward late-career team members are associated with lower well-being and lower employee engagement. These findings suggest that negative attitudes toward late-career team members can contribute to the erosion of older workers' well-being and depress their employee engagement scores in a way similar to the way the microaggressions erode the self-esteem and well-being of racial minorities. As such, they are a significant risk factor for poor mental health outcomes among older workers.

---

[1]According to Kahn (1990), employee engagement is the "harnessing of organizational members' selves to their work roles; in engagement, people employ and express themselves physically, cognitively, and emotionally during role performances" (p. 694). Generally, engaged employees are those who have a "sense of energetic and effective connection with their work activities and they see themselves as able to deal completely with the demands of their job" (Schaufeli et al. 2002, 73; see also Pitt-Catsouphes and Matz-Costa 2009). Angle and Perry (1983) suggest that this type of "harnessing" of the self is a function of the way that employees have been treated by the organization.

[2]It is interesting to note that this finding is consistent for workers under the age of 40. For these workers, negative attitudes towards late-career team members are also related to lower levels of mental health and employee engagement.

Protective Factors

Having found that attitudes toward late-career team members are related to well-being and employee engagement, we wanted to explore the extent to which some older workers are more susceptible to the stress associated with them than other older workers, as Kang and Chasteen (2009) have suggested. Using a model of resilience proposed by Luthar (1991) as a framework, who examined personal attributes that moderated the relationship between the risk factors of life stress and low socioeconomic status and the outcomes of social competence, we assessed what factors moderate the relationship between the risk factor (negative attitudes) and the outcomes (mental health and employee engagement). Specifically, we looked at the extent to which certain job conditions and the personal disposition of core self-evaluations (CSE) moderate the relationship between negative attitudes toward late-career team members and mental health and employee engagement for workers aged 40 or older. We used the measures listed in Table 22.3 and examined the moderating effects of potential internal (CSE as dispositional "hardiness") and external protective factors (supervisor support and work team inclusion as job conditions) on the relationship between attitudes toward late-career team members and the well-being outcomes.

Supervisor support was measured using an eight-item adapted scale (Bond et al. 2002; Greenhaus et al. 1990; Mor Barak and Cherin 1998). Sample items include "My team leader/supervisor gives me helpful feedback about my performance" and "My team leader/supervisor cares about whether or not I achieve my career goals." Inclusion was measured using a ten-item adapted scale (Bond et al. 2002; Mor Barak and Cherin 1998). Sample items include "I have a say in the way my work group performs its tasks" and "I am able to influence decisions that affect my work group." The CSE is a higher order construct comprised of neuroticism (reverse scored), locus of control, self-esteem, and self-efficacy. It was measured using the 12-item CSE Scale (Judge et al. 2003). Sample items include "When I try, I generally succeed" and "I determine what will happen in my life."

Protective Factors for Older Workers

As can be seen in Table 22.4,[3] direct effects were found between CSE (but not supervisor support or team inclusion) and mental health. Supervisor support, team inclusion, and CSE also contributed to the explanation of the variation in the measure of employee engagement.

---

[3]When looking at workers under the age of 40, CSE does not significantly moderate the relationship between attitudes towards late-career team members and mental health. In addition, for workers under the age of 40, supervisor support, work team inclusion, and CSE all do not significantly moderate the relationship between attitudes toward late-career team members and employee engagement. This suggests that these moderators may be unique to older workers.

Table 22.4 Standardized regression estimates of measures of well-being on attitudes toward late-career workers and supervisor support, inclusion, and CSE ($N = 737$)

Predictor	Mental health B	Employee engagement B
Gender[a]	0.029	0.074*
Marital status[b]	−0.018	−0.052
Parental status[c]	0.034	−0.073*
Ethnicity[d]	−0.065*	−0.086**
Education[e]	−0.008	−0.050
Income	0.030	0.023
Age	0.138***	0.142***
Attitudes toward late-career team members	0.016	0.122***
Supervisor support	0.061	0.119**
Attitudes by supervisor support	0.022	0.098*
Inclusion	−0.048	0.121**
Attitudes by inclusion	−0.016	−0.151***
CSE	0.559***	0.380***
Attitudes by CSE	−0.071*	−0.106***
R^2	0.360***	0.358***

Note: Gender, marital status, parental status, ethnicity, education, income, and age are controls

*$p<0.05$, **$p<0.01$, ***$p<0.001$

[a]Reference = female

[b]Reference = married or cohabitating

[c]Reference = has no children

[d]Reference = white

[e]Reference = bachelors degree or higher

Core self-evaluations moderated the relationship between attitudes toward late-career team members and mental health for older workers. Supervisor support, work team inclusion, and CSE all moderated the relationships between attitudes toward late-career team members and employee engagement among older workers. The significant interactions between attitudes and CSE in predicting mental health, and the interactions between attitudes and CSE, supervisor support, and inclusion in predicting employee engagement suggest that CSE, supervisor support, and inclusion serve as protective factors against attitudes toward late-career team members (cf. Luthar 1991).

To further examine the moderating effects of supervisor support, work team inclusion, and CSE as either protective or vulnerability processes, we plotted the relationships between the significant moderators and attitudes toward late-career team members for mental health and employee engagement for older workers (see Figs. 22.1–22.4). If the outcomes of mental health and employee engagement are high when the moderators are at higher levels despite high levels of negative attitudes toward late-career team members, then the moderators are protective factors in our conception of resilience; however, if the reverse is true and the outcomes of

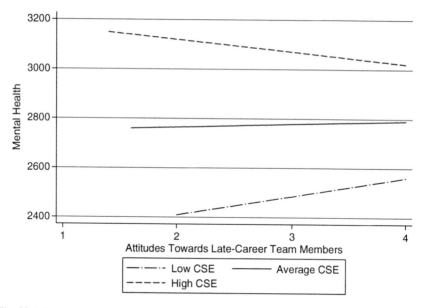

Fig. 22.1 Moderating effect of core self-evaluations (CSE) on the relationship between attitudes toward late-career team members and mental health

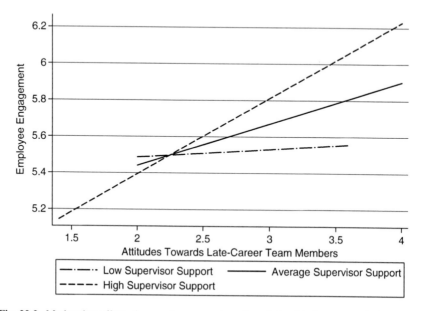

Fig. 22.2 Moderating effect of supervisor support on the relationship between attitudes toward late-career team members and employee engagement

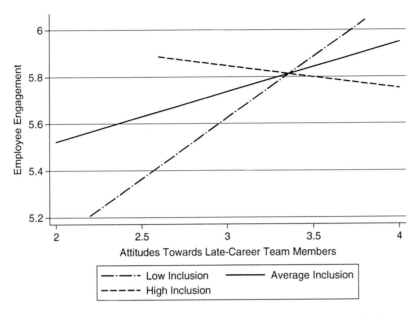

Fig. 22.3 Moderating effect of work team inclusion on the relationship between attitudes toward late-career team members and employee engagement

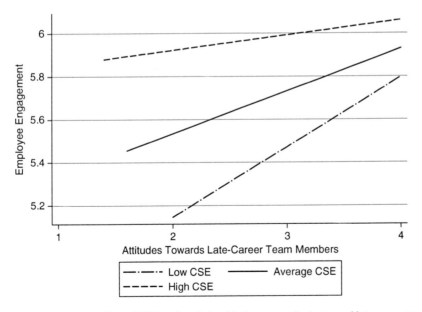

Fig. 22.4 Moderating effect of CSE on the relationship between attitudes toward late-career team members and employee engagement

mental health and engagement are lower, then the moderators are considered to be vulnerability factors. Thus, when protective factors against negative attitudes toward late-career team members are present, a person is thought to be resilient.

As can be seen in Fig. 22.1, when the risk factor of negative attitudes toward late-career team members is present, workers with low CSE have lower mental health than workers with average or high CSE. As attitudes toward late-career team members become more positive and are no longer a risk factor, the effect of the attitudes on mental health decreases. This suggests that CSE serve as a protective factor against the effects of the negative attitudes on mental health in a way that is similar to the way that "hardiness" has functioned in previous studies (Crowley et al. 2003; Kaplan 1999).

As can be seen in Fig. 22.2, contrary to our expectations, employee engagement was not higher for workers with high supervisor support when the risk factor of negative attitudes toward late-career team members was present. This suggests that supervisor support is not a protective factor against negative attitudes. However, as the attitudes toward late-career team members become more positive, employee engagement is greater for workers with high supervisor support than for those with average or low supervisor support.

Another important potential external protective factor is work team inclusion. As can be seen in Fig. 22.3, when attitudes toward late-career workers are very negative and the risk factor is present, workers with high levels of work team inclusion have higher employee engagement than workers with average or low work team inclusion. However, as attitudes become more positive and they are no longer a risk factor, the effect of work team inclusion on levels of engagement diminishes. This finding suggests that work team inclusion is a protective factor against the effects of negative attitudes on work-related well-being.

The moderating effect of CSE on the relationship between attitudes toward late-career team members and employee engagement is similar to the effect for mental health. As can be seen in Fig. 22.4, when attitudes toward late-career team members are the most negative, workers with high CSE have the greatest employee engagement compared to workers with average or low CSE, but CSE have little effect on employee engagement when attitudes are more positive and are no longer a risk factor. This suggests that CSE or hardiness is a protective factor against the effects of the negative attitudes on employee engagement.

Conclusions

While resilience remains a complex and multifaceted variable, our findings show that it is a useful construct for understanding the on-the-job experiences of today's older workers. It would be easy (but a mistake) to assume from preliminary analyses that job conditions have little to do with mental health in the workplace. Indeed, our findings suggest that job conditions have no direct effect on the relationship between attitudes toward late-career team members and mental health. When conceptualizing vulnerabilities among older workers or late-career team members such as negative attitudes, and examining the data for buffers against these vulnerabilities, our focus shifts not only from direct, negative effects but also to a more positive frame. Instead of what's wrong in the workplace, it is helpful to expand on what is working well.

Findings indicate that there are both internal and external buffers against the age-related microaggressions older workers are subjected to. Specifically, high CSE served as a significant protective factor against the risk factor of negative attitudes on both mental health and employee engagement. Work team inclusion was an important moderator of the relationship between attitudes toward late-career team members and employee engagement but not mental health. These findings suggest that CSE and work team inclusion are particularly important for older workers' employee engagement when attitudes toward late-career team members are negative. In addition, having more positive attitudes toward late-career team members in general is related to greater employee engagement and mental health in older workers regardless of job conditions and personal dispositions.

Contrary to our expectations, the job condition operationalized as supervisor support was not a protective factor. Even so, the significant interaction between attitudes toward late-career team members and supervisor support revealed that for more positive attitudes, employee engagement is greater for workers with high levels of supervisor support when compared to workers with average or low supervisor support. Although not necessarily a protective factor, supervisor support is an important factor in the life of older workers, especially when the organizational climate is favorable toward late-career workers.

As we conclude this chapter, we must grapple with an important question: why should employers care about protecting older workers from daily slights and degradations? First, as employers come to see the value of older workers for their good work ethic, their ease with customers, and their reliability (James et al. 2008; Munnell et al. 2006; Pitt-Catsouphes et al. 2007), they also want them to be happy and satisfied; there is concern with their well-being. Second, as employers work with intergenerational teams and struggle with a reeling economy, employers want to know what will engage these employees and ensure their commitment to the organization. Workers who are "engaged," for example, tend to be less stressed and more satisfied with their lives; they also tend to use less health care, take fewer sick days, be more productive, and stay longer with their organizations than their less engaged counterparts (Gallup Organization 2003, 2006). Given the relationship we have found between protective factors against negative attitudes and engagement, it would seem to be in employers enlightened self-interest to take an interest enhancing the resilience of their older workers.

Employers can take a number of steps to promote the development of work environments that protect older workers against the microaggressions associated with ageism. As a first line of defense, employers should gather information (either formally or informally) to assess the extent to which (and in what types of situations) employees perceive ageism at the workplace. Following this type of culture audit, employers can take steps, such as supervisor training and team building experiences that promote supervisor support and a climate of inclusion.

Some employers might also find that job redesign (i.e., adjusting some aspects of jobs so that they better fit with the needs and preferences of older workers) is an effective approach as one study found that job redesign that results in skill variety, increased task significance and autonomy can enhance resilience (Badran and Kafafy 2008).

Decades of research suggest that negative stereotypes against older workers are entrenched and it may take time to replace assumptions about the limitations of older workers with new perspectives about the assets that older workers can bring to the workplace. In the mean time, it is the responsibility of employers to create work environments that help foster resilience that can help older workers maintain their engagement in and enjoyment of meaningful jobs.

Acknowledgments This study was supported by a grant from the Alfred P. Sloan Foundation to the Sloan Center on Aging & Work. We also want to acknowledge the contributions made by the organizations that participated in the *Age & Generations Study* and the work of other members of the research team, including Michael Smyer, Ph.D., co-principal investigator.

References

Angle, H. L., & Perry, J. L. (1983). Organizational commitment: Individual and organization influences. *Work and Occupations, 10*, 123–146.

Badran, M., & Kafafy, J. (2008). The effect of job redesign on job satisfaction, resilience, commitment and flexibility: The case of an Egyptian public sector bank. *International Journal of Business Research, 8*(3), 27–41.

Bonanno, G. A. (2004). Loss, trauma, and human resilience: Have we underestimated the human capacity to thrive after extremely aversive events? *American Psychologist, 59*(1), 20–28.

Bonanno, G. A., Galea, S., Bucciarelli, A., & Vlahov, D. (2007). What predicts psychological resilience after disaster? The role of demographics, resources, and life stress. *Journal of Consulting and Clinical Psychology, 75*(5), 671–682.

Bond, J. T., Thompson, C., Galinsky, E., & Prottas, D. (2002). *Highlights of the national study of the changing workforce: Executive summary*. New York, NY: Families and Work Institute.

Capowski, G. (1994). Ageism: The new diversity issue. *Management Review, 83*(10), 10.

Cappella, E., & Weinstein, R. S. (2001). Turning around reading achievement: Predictors of high school students' academic resilience. *Journal of Educational Psychology, 93*(4), 758–771.

Crowley, B. J., Hayslip, B., Jr., & Hobdy, J. (2003). Psychological hardiness and adjustment to life events in adulthood. *Journal of Adult Development, 10*(4), 237–248.

Dawley, D. D., Andrews, M. C., & Bucklew, N. S. (2008). Mentoring, supervisor support, and perceived organizational support: What matters most? *Leadership & Organization Development Journal, 29*(3), 235–247.

Gallup Organization. (2003). Bringing work problems home. *Gallup Management Journal*. Retrieved from http://gmj.gallup.com.

Gallup Organization. (2006). Gallup study: Engaged employees inspire company innovation. *Gallup Management Journal*. Retrieved from http://gmj.gallup.com.

Gavin, R. (February 28, 2009). Feeling jobbed work for teens scarcer as elders defer retirement. *The Boston Globe*, pp. A1.

Greenhaus, J. H., Parasuraman, S., & Wormley, W. M. (1990). Effects of race on organizational experiences, job performance evaluations, and career outcomes. *Academy of Management Journal, 33*(1), 64–86.

Greller, M. M., & Simpson, P. (1999). In search of late career: A review of contemporary social science research applicable to the understanding of late career. *Human Resource Management Review, 9*(3), 309–347.

Groeneman, S. (2008). *Staying ahead of the curve 2007: The AARP work and career study*. Washington, DC: AARP. Retrieved from http://assets.aarp.org/rgcenter/econ/work_career_08.pdf.

Hassell, B. L., & Perrewe, P. L. (1995). An examination of beliefs about older workers: Do stereotypes still exist? *Journal of Organizational Behavior, 16*(5), 457–468.

Hedge, J. W., Borman, W. C., & Lammlein, S. E. (2006). *The aging workforce: Realities, myths, and implications for organizations*. Washington, DC: American Psychological Association.

James, J. B., Liem, J. H., & O'Toole, J. G. (1997). In search of resilience in adult survivors of childhood sexual abuse: Linking outlets for power motivation to psychological health. In A. Lieblich, & R. Josselson (Eds.), *American psychological association conference, psychosocial and behavioral factors in women's health: Creating an agenda for the 21st century, May 1994, Washington, DC* (pp. 207–233). Thousand Oaks, CA: Sage Publications, Inc.

James, J. B., Swanberg, J. E., & McKechnie, S. P. (2007). *Generational differences in perceptions of older workers' capabilities* (Issue Brief No. 12). Chestnut Hill, MA: Boston College Center on Aging & Work/Workplace Flexibility. Retrieved from http://agingandwork.bc.edu/documents/IB12_OlderWorkers%20Capability.pdf.

James, J. B., Swanberg, J. E., & McKechnie, S. P. (2008). *The citisales study of older workers: Employee engagement, job quality, health, and well-being* (Research Highlight No. 5). Chestnut Hill, MA: Sloan Center on Aging and Work at Boston College. Retrieved from http://agingandwork.bc.edu/documents/RH05_Citisales_2008-11-13b.pdf.

Judge, T. A., Erez, A., Bono, J. E., & Thoresen, C. J. (2003). The core self-evaluations scale: Development of a measure. *Personnel Psychology, 56*(2), 303–331.

Kahn, W. A. (1990). Psychological conditions of personal engagement and disengagement at work. *Academy of Management Journal, 33*(4), 692–724.

Kang, S. K., & Chasteen, A. L. (2009). The development and validation of the age-based rejection sensitivity questionnaire. *The Gerontologist, 49*(3), 303–316.

Kaplan, H. B. (1999). Toward an understanding of resilience: A critical review of definitions and models. In M. D. Glantz, & J. L. Johnson (Eds.), *Resilience and development: Positive life adaptations* (pp. 17–83). Dordrecht, Netherlands: Kluwer Academic Publishers.

Keyes, C. L. M. (2004). Risk and resilience in human development: An introduction. *Research in Human Development, 1*(4), 223–227.

Kooij, D., de Lange, A., Jansen, P., & Dikkers, J. (2008). Older workers' motivation to continue to work: Five meanings of age: A conceptual review. *Journal of Managerial Psychology, 23*(4), 364–394.

Kumpfer, K. L. (1999). Factors and processes contributing to resilience: The resilience framework. In M. D. Glantz, & J. L. Johnson (Eds.), *Resilience and development: Positive life adaptations*. (pp. 179–224). Dordrecht, Netherlands: Kluwer Academic Publishers.

Lancaster, L., & Stillman, D. (2005). *When generations collide: Who they are, why they clash, how to solve the generational puzzle at work* (1st Collins Business ed.). New York: Collins Business.

Levy, B. R., & Banaji, M. R. (2002). Implicit ageism. In T. D. Nelson (Ed.), *Ageism: Stereotyping and prejudice against older persons* (pp. 49–75). Cambridge, MA: The MIT Press.

Liem, J. H., James, J. B., O'Toole, J. G., & Boudewyn, A. C. (1997). Assessing resilience in adults with histories of childhood sexual abuse. *American Journal of Orthopsychiatry, 67*(4), 594–606.

Luthar, S. S. (1991). Vulnerability and resilience: A study of high-risk adolescents. *Child Development, 62*(3), 600–616.

Luthar, S. S., Cicchetti, D., & Becker, B. (2000). The construct of resilience: A critical evaluation and guidelines for future work. *Child Development, 71*(3), 543–562.

Martin, A. J., & Marsh, H. W. (2008). Workplace and academic buoyancy: Psychometric assessment and construct validity amongst school personnel and students. *Journal of Psychoeducational Assessment, 26*(2), 168–184.

Masten, A. S. (1989). Resilience in development: Implications of the study of successful adaptation for developmental psychopathology. In D. Cicchetti (Ed.), (pp. 261–294). Hillsdale, NJ, England: Lawrence Erlbaum Associates, Inc.

McCalister, K. T., Dolbier, C. L., Webster, J. A., Mallon, M. W., & Steinhardt, M. A. (2006). Hardiness and support at work as predictors of work stress and job satisfaction. *American Journal of Health Promotion, 20*(3), 183–191.

McCann, R., & Giles, H. (2002). Ageism in the workplace: A communication perspective. In T. D. Nelson (Ed.), *Ageism: Stereotyping and prejudice against older persons* (pp. 163–199). Cambridge, MA: The MIT Press.

McEvoy, G. M., & Cascio, W. F. (1989). Cumulative evidence of the relationship between employee age and job performance. *Journal of Applied Psychology, 74*(1), 11–17.

Mor Barak, M. E. (2005). *Managing diversity: Toward a globally inclusive workplace.* Thousand Oaks, CA: Sage Publications.

Mor Barak, M. E., & Cherin, D. A. (1998). A tool to expand organizational understanding of workforce diversity: Exploring a measure of inclusion-exclusion. *Administration in Social Work, 22*(1), 47–64.

Mor Barak, M. E., Cherin, D. A., & Berkman, S. (1998). Organizational and personal dimensions in diversity climate: Ethnic and gender differences in employee perceptions. *Journal of Applied Behavioral Science, 34*(1), 82–104.

Munnell, A. H., Sass, S. A., & Soto, M. (2006). *Employer attitudes towards older workers: Survey results.* Chestnut Hill, MA: Center for Retirement Research at Boston College. Retrieved from http://crr.bc.edu/images/stories/Briefs/wob_3.pdf.

Ng, T. W. H., & Feldman, D. C. (2008). The relationship of age to ten dimensions of job performance. *Journal of Applied Psychology, 93*(2), 392–423.

Ng, T. W. H., & Sorensen, K. L. (2008). Toward a further understanding of the relationships between perceptions of support and work attitudes: A meta-analysis. *Group & Organization Management, 33*(3), 243–268.

Pitt-Catsouphes, M., & Matz-Costa, C. (2009). *Engaging the 21st century multi-generational workforce: Findings from the age & generations study* (Issue Brief No. 20). Chestnut Hill, MA: Sloan Center on Aging & Work at Boston College. Retrieved from http://agingandwork. bc.edu/documents/IB20_Engagement_2009–02–10.pdf.

Pitt-Catsouphes, M., & Smyer, M. A. (2007). *The 21st century multi-generational workplace* (Issue Brief No. 09). Chestnut Hill, MA: Boston College Center on Aging & Work/Workplace Flexibility. Retrieved from http://agingandwork.bc.edu/documents/IB09_MultiGenWorkplace_001.pdf.

Pitt-Catsouphes, M., Smyer, M. A., Matz-Costa, C., & Kane, K. (2007). *The national study report: Phase II of the national study of business strategy and workforce development* (Research Highlight No. 04). Chestnut Hill, MA: The Center on Aging & Work/Workplace Flexibility. Retrieved from http://agingandwork.bc.edu/documents/RH04_NationalStudy_03–07_004.pdf.

Pitt-Catsouphes, M., Matz-Costa, C., & Besen, E. (2009). *Age and generations: Understanding experiences at the workplace* (Research Highlight No. 6). Chestnut Hill, MA: Sloan Center on Aging and Work at Boston College. Retrieved from http://agingandwork.bc.edu/documents/ RH06_Age&Generations_2009–03–20.pdf.

Riach, K. (2007). 'Othering' older worker identity in recruitment. *Human Relations. Special Issue: Human Relations, 60*(11), 1701–1726.

Rosen, B., & Jerdee, T. H. (1976). The nature of job-related age stereotypes. *Journal of Applied Psychology, 61*(2), 180–183.

Ryff, C. D., Singer, B., Love, G. D., & Essex, M. J. (1998). Resilience in adulthood and later life: Defining features and dynamic processes. In J. Lomranz (Ed.), *Handbook of aging and mental health: An integrative approach* (pp. 69–96). New York, NY: Plenum Press.

Schaufeli, W. B., Salanova, M., González-Romá, V., & Bakker, A. B. (2002). The measurement of engagement and burnout: A two sample confirmatory factor analytic approach. *Journal of Happiness Studies, 3*(1), 71–92. doi:10.1023/A:1015630930326

Schaufeli, W. B., & Bakker, A. B. (2004). Job demands, job resources, and their relationship with burnout and engagement: A multi-sample study. *Journal of Organizational Behavior, 25*(3), 293–315.

Staudinger, U. M., Freund, A. M., Linden, M., & Maas, I. (1999). Self, personality, and life regulation: Facets of psychological resilience in old age. In P. B. Baltes, & K. U. Mayer (Eds.), *The Berlin aging study: Aging from 70 to 100* (pp. 302–328). New York, NY: Cambridge University Press.

Sue, D. W., Bucceri, J., Lin, A. I., Nadal, K. L., & Torino, G. C. (2007a). Racial microaggressions and the Asian American experience. *Cultural Diversity and Ethnic Minority Psychology, 13*(1), 72–81.

Sue, D. W., Capodilupo, C. M., Torino, G. C., Bucceri, J. M., Holder, A. M. B., Nadal, K. L., et al. (2007b). Racial microaggressions in everyday life: Implications for clinical practice. *American Psychologist, 62*(4), 271–286.

Sue, D. W., Capodilupo, C. M., & Holder, A. M. B. (2008). Racial microaggressions in the life experience of black Americans. *Professional Psychology: Research and Practice, 39*(3), 329–336.

Toossi, M. (2002). A century of change: The U.S. labor force, 1950–2050. *Monthly Labor Review, 125*(5), 15.

Toossi, M. (2006). Labor force projections to 2016: More workers in their golden years. *Monthly Labor Review, 130*(11), 33–52.

U.S. Equal Employment Opportunity Commission. (2010). Change statistics FY 1997 through FY 2009. Washington, DC: Equal Employment Opportunity Commission. Retrieved from http://www.eeoc.gov/eeoc/statistics/enforcement/charges.cfm

Vogel, S. (July 16, 2009). Age discrimination claims jump, worrying EEOC, worker advocates. *The Washington Post*, pp. A21.

Wanberg, C. R., & Banas, J. T. (2000). Predictors and outcomes of openness to changes in a reorganizing workplace. *Journal of Applied Psychology, 85*(1), 132–142.

Ware, J. E., Kosinski, M., Dewey, J. E., & Gandek, B. (2001). *How to score and interpret single-item health status measures: A manual for users of the SF-8 health survey*. Lincoln, RI: Quality Metric Inc.

Wilks, S. E., & Croom, B. (2008). Perceived stress and resilience in Alzheimer's disease caregivers: Testing moderation and mediation models of social support. *Aging & Mental Health, 12*(3), 357–365.

Chapter 23
Conclusion

Barbara Resnick

This book provides a comprehensive look at the many aspects of resilience and the ways in which older adults can build resilience and overcome challenges experienced throughout the aging process. The chapter authors provide several different definitions of resilience. For example, Allen et al. (Chap. 1) describes resilience as a dynamic process of maintaining positive adaptation and effective coping strategies in the face of adversity, or simply stated resilience is a dynamic process of adaptation to adversity. Hochholter et al. (Chap. 2) refer to resilience as an extraordinary and positive response to a challenge or stressor, and Rosowsky in Chap. 3 notes that resilient older adults are able to tolerate the vicissitudes of aging and defray the overhead of growing old. Across the many definitions and descriptions of resilience provided, resilience is conceptualized to reflect an effective response to some type of adversity or challenge, whether it is physical, psychological, economic, political, environmental, or social.

Resilience is thus central to aging because adversity is inevitable at points throughout the lifespan and certainly as we age. Some adults will be fortunate enough to survive till old age, with "old" varying from 50 to 75 years of age (World Health Organization 2010) without multimorbidity. Even for these individuals, there will be some physical and sensory changes and psychosocial challenges common to older adults such as role loss, loss of friends and family, or a beloved pet. Responses to these challenges are as varied as the challenges themselves. Some individuals become depressed or disengaged when faced with age-associated changes such as graying of hair or wrinkling of skin. Others respond by seeking cosmetic intervention, using appropriate behavioral interventions (facial exercises), humor, or simply take pride in the changes as a badge of honor associated with growing old (e.g. I earned these gray hairs!).

B. Resnick (✉)
University of Maryland, Baltimore, MD, USA
e-mail: barbresnick@gmail.com

B. Resnick et al. (eds.), *Resilience in Aging: Concepts, Research, and Outcomes*,
DOI 10.1007/978-1-4419-0232-0_23, © Springer Science+Business Media, LLC 2011

Resilience and Aging Well

Even in the face of normal aging, resilience is relevant and being resilient is likely central to aging well. Successful aging is generally conceptualized as the older adult who has, by virtue of good luck, family history, and adherence to healthy lifestyle behaviors, avoided physical, cognitive, or functional changes that influence quality of life or active engagement. The image of a successful older adult tends to be the 95-year-old runner who wins his or her age group in the Boston marathon, or the individual featured on greeting cards who can display flexibility that most of us never could achieve as children. The truly successful older individual, however, is someone who has demonstrated resilience and at age 95, with multiple morbidities optimizes function, volunteers or continues to be actively aged in meaningful activities, or is simply happy reviewing his or her prior life activities. It is the individual who has a hip fracture and engages fully in rehabilitation activities and remains determined to return home, or the individual who recognizes cognitive changes with a decline in short-term memory and buys a bigger calendar to write more reminders or cues.

Resilience and Exercise

Exercise, and adherence to exercise throughout life, has been described as one of the best interventions to optimize the likelihood of aging successfully (Depp and Jeste 2006). There is no question that there are numerous, well-supported benefits to exercise throughout the lifespan. For example, exercise can decrease progression of degenerative joint disease (Netz et al. 2005), prevent osteoporosis of the lumbar spine (Palombaro 2005), decrease incidence of falls and fear of falling (Oliver et al. 2008), increase gait speed (Smith et al. 2006), increase muscle strength and overall fitness and function (Ada et al. 2006; Liu and Latham 2009), improve cognitive function (Angevaren et al. 2008), and improve quality of life and overall well-being (Netz et al. 2005). It is those who are resilient, however, who have the motivation, determination, and impetus to engage in regular exercise activities, regardless of underlying physical challenges, pain, or fear. Thus, it may not simply be exercise that is the secret to successful aging. Rather, it may be the individual's resilience and ability to adapt to physical challenges or overcome other barriers to engaging in exercise such as time, competing activities, and responsibilities.

Moving Forward and Preparing the Baby Boomers

Throughout this book we embrace the conceptualization of resilience as a process or behavioral response that can be strengthened, improved, and called upon to establish, maintain, or regain a state of physical, psychological, or emotional equilibrium over time. Building resilience should be a lifelong process and can be facilitated through numerous pathways and approaches. Interventions can focus on such things as developing positive interpersonal relationships, incorporating social connectedness with a willingness to extend oneself to others, developing and recognizing strong internal resources, having an optimistic or positive affect, keeping things in perspective, setting goals and taking steps to achieve those goals, developing and maintaining high self-esteem and high self-efficacy, building one's determination, and developing or expanding one's sense of spirituality, which involves a sense of purpose, belonging, or a belief in a higher power and a sense of curiosity, awe, or wonder.

Interventions to stimulate and build resilience can be organized around three areas: (1) developing disposition attributes of the individual such as vigor, optimism, and physical robustness; (2) improving socialization practices; and (3) strengthening self-efficacy, self-esteem, and motivation through interpersonal interactions as well as experiences. The chapters in this book provide wonderful examples of how to recognize, develop, and strengthen resilience in older adults across all the three areas. There are examples and discussions of using civic engagement and volunteer or paid employment to achieve physical, emotional, and psychosocial benefits. Preparing current work environments to assure the safety and optimal job satisfaction of older employees is critical. Likewise environmental interventions to assure that older adults can travel to and safely access sites of employment (volunteer or paid employment) as well as community resources and activities are critical. The Age-Friendly New York City Project provides a wonderful model for how to comprehensively evaluate and implement interventions to optimize the physical environment in cities for older individuals to build resilience and facilitate successful aging.

There are also numerous examples throughout the chapters to address the special challenges of optimizing resilience and successful aging among older adults with cognitive impairment. Using narratives is one way in which older adults with cognitive impairment can share life stories with families and have such stories become enduring heirlooms for future generations. Social remembering and talking with others about shared experiences is another way in which to engage an individual with cognitive impairment in an enjoyable successful experience that builds self-esteem. I do this often in my own clinical practice as I have patients and had the opportunity to work with them for over 25 years. Together we share much history and I stimulate their memories of prior successful recoveries and engage them in drawing on those experiences. In the wonderful project, Meet Me at the MoMA, there is evidence of how enlivening creativity and drawing on past and current creative abilities and interests can have an important impact on older adults with cognitive impairment. Similar use of creative endeavors can be implemented in care facilities or home settings.

The Baby Boomers may be a generation that is more comfortable with self-help and support group activities compared to the current cohort of older adults. Self-help, self-care, or support activities may be tremendously important for older adults with chronic illnesses to strengthen resilience and live out their remaining years with multiple chronic conditions. Another special group of old adults anticipated to grow exponentially in the future are those with lifelong mental health disabilities (e.g. depression, bipolar, anxiety, schizophrenia, or personality disorders). These individuals may benefit from self-help activities such as exercise. Alternatively, as seen in the description of the Geriatric Mobile Crisis Response Team, such individuals may need one-on-one intervention to strengthen resilience through counseling, appropriate medication management, or connections to community resources.

Spirituality, whether this be the traditional involvement of older adults with religious groups or organizations or a sense of spirituality through one's beliefs, is another way in which older adults help themselves obtain and maintain a sense of resilience. Spirituality can be thought of as a relationship with a Transcendent Being and a desire to expand that relationship and find meaning and purpose in all, but particularly challenging life experiences. Thus, many older adults draw on their spirituality to build resilience. As seen in Chap. 17, older adults that are caregivers gain a sense of resilience through spiritual activities and beliefs as they live with the challenges of providing care for an older spouse, partner, relative, or friend. Cultural sensitivity and understanding are crucial to support of spiritual beliefs and building resilience across different communities and religious affiliations. Although spirituality may help build resilience, it is important to be certain that an individual is not deferring to a Transcendent Being to help with recovery following an acute event, rather than engaging in the necessary behaviors to optimize recovery.

As stated in the Institute of Medicine Report, Retooling for an Aging America: Building the Health Care Workforce (Institute of Medicine Report 2008), the number of older adults in the United States will almost double between 2005 and 2030, and the nation is not prepared to meet their social and health care needs. We therefore have a tremendous opportunity and responsibility to work together to help all Americans develop, strengthen, and maintain optimal resilience to face the challenges and appreciate the positive aspects of aging. We all have within us the capacity to age well with resilience. Some individuals have innate resilience and/or a well-practiced resilience and they will age with grace on their own. Others will need the guidance of professionals, use of social resources, services, or organized religious groups and the environmental support to strengthen or sustain resilience and overcome challenges. As you face your own aging and as you work with others, be creative, be optimistic, draw on your past successes and reach out to seek and accept help from others to be resilient, maintain resilience, and age well as you help those for whom you provide care to do likewise.

References

Ada L, Dorsch S, & Canning CG. (2006) Strengthening interventions increase strength and improve activity after stroke: a systematic review. Aust J Physiother, 52(4), 241–248.

Angevaren M, Aufdemkampe G, Verhaar HJ, Aleman A, Vanhees L. (2008) Physical activity and enhanced fitness to improve cognitive function in older people without known cognitive impairment. Cochrane Database Syst Rev, 16(2):CD005381.

Depp CA, & Jeste DV. (2006) Definitions and predictors of successful aging: a comprehensive review of larger quantitative studies. Am J Geriatr Psychiatry, 14(1), 6–20.

Institute of Medicine Report. (2008) Retooling for an Aging America: Building the Health Care Workforce.   http://www.iom.edu/Reports/2008/Retooling-for-an-Aging-America-Building-the-Health-Care-Workforce.aspx.

Liu CJ, & Latham NK. (2009) Progressive resistance strength training for improving physical function in older adults. Cochrane Database Syst Rev, 8(3), CD002759.

Netz Y, Wu MJ, Becker BJ, & Tennenbaum G. (2005) Physical activity and psychological well being in advanced age: A meta-analysis of intervention studies. Psychol Aging, 20(2), 272–284.

Oliver D, Connelly JB, Victor CR et al. (2008) Strategies to prevent falls and fractures in hospitals and care homes and effect of cognitive impairment: systematic review and meta-analyses. Age Ageing, 37(6), 621–627.

Palombaro KM. (2005) Effects of walking-only interventions on bone mineral density at various skeletal sites: a meta-analysis. J Geriatr Phys Therapy, 28(3), 102–107.

Smith TP, Kennedy SL, Smith M, Orent S, & Fleshner M. (2006) Physiological improvements and health benefits during an exercise-based comprehensive rehabilitation program in medically complex patients. Exerc Immunol Rev 12, 86–96.

World Health Organization. (2010) Definition of Aging. Available at http://www.who.int/healthinfo/survey/ageingdefnolder/en/index.html.

Index

Breinigsville, PA USA
01 November 2010
248298BV00004B/38/P

9 781441 902313